Barbara O'Neill
Natural Remedies Secret Collection

35 Books in 1

The Definitive Guide to Barbara O'Neill's Studies and Teachings to Uncover What the Pharmaceutical Industru Doesn't Want You to Know

Melissa Hudson

© **Copyright 2024 - All rights reserved.**

The content contained within this book may not be reproduced, duplicated or transmitted without direct written permission from the author or the publisher. Under no circumstances will any blame or legal responsibility be held against the publisher, or author, for any damages, reparation, or monetary loss due to the information contained within this book. Either directly or indirectly.

Legal Notice:

This book is copyright protected. This book is only for personal use. You cannot amend, distribute, sell, use, quote or paraphrase any part, or the content within this book, without the consent of the author or publisher.

Disclaimer Notice:

All effort has been executed to present accurate, up to date, and reliable, complete information. No warranties of any kind are declared or implied. Readers acknowledge that the author is not engaging in the rendering of legal, financial, medical or professional advice. The content within this book has been derived from various sources. Please consult a licensed professional before attempting any techniques outlined in this book.

By reading this document, the reader agrees that under no circumstances is the author responsible for any losses, direct or indirect, which are incurred as a result of the use of information contained within this document, including, but not limited to, errors, omissions, or inaccuracies.

Table of Contents

Introduction 11

Book 1: Introduction to Barbara O'Neill's Philosophy 12

    The Origins of Natural Healing 12

    Barbara's Journey: From Nurse to Natural Health Expert 12

    The Importance of Holistic Health 13

    The Power of Prevention 13

    Barbara's Fight Against the Pharmaceutical Industry 13

    Building a Non-Toxic Lifestyle 14

Book 2: Nutrition and Its Role in Healing 15

    Understanding the Power of Nutrition 15

    Key Nutrients for Optimal Health 15

    How Diet Impacts the Immune System 16

    Nutritional Deficiencies and Their Consequences 16

    Whole Foods vs. Processed Foods 17

    Therapeutic Diets for Specific Conditions 17

    Superfoods for Healing and Vitality 18

Book 3: Detoxification and Cleansing 19

    The Body's Natural Detox Mechanisms 19

    Identifying Toxins in Everyday Life 19

    The Role of the Liver in Detoxification 20

    Detoxifying with Herbs and Natural Remedies 21

    Colon Cleansing for Optimal Health 22

    Fasting as a Detox Strategy 23

    Detoxification Protocols for Chronic Conditions 24

    Post-Detoxification: Maintaining a Clean System 25

Book 4: The Power of Herbs in Healing 26

    History and Uses of Medicinal Herbs 26

    How Herbs Work with the Body 27

    Common Herbs for Everyday Ailments 28

    Anti-Inflammatory Herbs and Their Benefits 29

    Herbal Treatments for the Digestive System 30

    Immune-Boosting Herbs for Preventative Care 31

    How to Grow and Harvest Medicinal Herbs 32

    Making Herbal Preparations at Home 33

Safety and Precautions with Herbal Use 34

Book 5: Natural Remedies for Women's Health 36

Hormonal Balance and Natural Approaches 36

Herbs and Supplements for Menstrual Health 37

Natural Solutions for Menopause Symptoms 39

Fertility and Pregnancy: Safe Natural Remedies 40

Breast Health and Cancer Prevention 41

Managing Stress and Emotional Health in Women 43

Detoxification for Women's Hormonal Health 44

Supporting Thyroid Function Naturally 46

Osteoporosis Prevention and Natural Remedies 47

Building Long-Term Health and Wellness 49

Book 6: The Immune System and Natural Defense 51

Understanding the Immune System 51

Strengthening the Immune System with Nutrition 52

The Role of Probiotics in Immune Health 53

Herbal Immune Boosters and Adaptogens 55

Natural Remedies for Autoimmune Disorders 56

Managing Allergies Naturally 57

How to Fight Infections with Natural Treatments 59

Seasonal Illnesses: Cold, Flu, and Immunity 60

Daily Habits for Immune System Maintenance 61

Book 7: Natural Remedies for Men's Health 64

Supporting Prostate Health Naturally 64

Natural Solutions for Erectile Dysfunction 65

Boosting Testosterone Levels Naturally 67

Detoxification for Men's Hormonal Balance 69

Cardiovascular Health: Natural Approaches 71

Maintaining Vitality and Longevity 73

Book 8: Gut Health and Digestion 75

The Gut-Brain Connection and Its Importance 75

Healing Leaky Gut Syndrome Naturally 75

Probiotics and Digestive Health 76

Herbal Remedies for Digestive Disorders 77

Managing Food Intolerances and Sensitivities 78

Natural Approaches for IBS and Colitis 79

Supporting the Liver for Better Digestion 80

Balancing the Microbiome for Optimal Health 82

Book 9: Stress Relief and Emotional Well-Being 83
Understanding the Impact of Stress on the Body 83
Herbal Adaptogens for Stress Management 84
Nutrition for Mental Clarity and Stress Reduction 85
Managing Anxiety and Depression Naturally 87
Sleep Hygiene for Stress Relief 88
Emotional Detoxification Practices 89
Building Emotional Resilience 90

Book 10: Cancer Prevention and Natural Healing 92
Understanding the Body's Natural Defenses Against Cancer 92
Nutrition and Lifestyle Changes for Cancer Prevention 93
Detoxification Protocols for Cancer Patients 94
Herbal Support for Cancer Treatment 95
Immune System Boosters for Cancer Recovery 96
Managing Side Effects of Conventional Cancer Treatments 97
Mental and Emotional Support for Cancer Patients 99

Book 11: Cardiovascular Health and Longevity 101
Understanding Heart Health from a Holistic Perspective 101
Nutrition and Herbs for Healthy Blood Pressure 102
Reducing Cholesterol Levels Naturally 104
The Role of Stress in Cardiovascular Health 105
Exercise and Its Role in Heart Health 107
Supporting Circulation with Natural Remedies 108

Book 12: Natural Skin and Hair Care Remedies 110
Detoxifying Your Skin Naturally 110
Essential Oils for Skincare 111
Herbal Hair Treatments 112
Nutrition for Radiant Skin and Hair 114
Avoiding Toxins in Beauty Products 116

Book 13: Hormonal Health and Balance 118
Understanding the Endocrine System 118
Managing Hormonal Imbalances Naturally 119
Herbs for Adrenal and Thyroid Support 121
Supporting Women's Hormonal Health 122
Natural Approaches to PMS and Menopause 124
Boosting Fertility Naturally 126
Nutrition and Lifestyle for Hormonal Balance 128
Preventing Hormonal Disruptions from Environmental Toxins 129

Book 14: Respiratory Health and Natural Remedies ... 131
Understanding the Respiratory System ... 131
Herbal Remedies for Respiratory Infections ... 132
Managing Asthma and Allergies Naturally ... 133
Detoxifying the Lungs ... 135
Breathing Techniques for Lung Health ... 136
Herbs and Essential Oils for Sinus Health ... 139

Book 15: Managing Diabetes and Blood Sugar Naturally ... 141
Understanding Diabetes and Blood Sugar Imbalance ... 141
Nutritional Strategies for Managing Blood Sugar ... 142
Herbs That Support Blood Sugar Regulation ... 143
Preventing Diabetes with a Natural Lifestyle ... 144
Supplements for Blood Sugar Control ... 145
Daily Habits to Maintain Healthy Glucose Levels ... 147

Book 16: Eye Health and Vision Restoration ... 149
The Importance of Nutrients for Eye Health ... 149
Herbal Remedies for Eye Strain and Fatigue ... 150
Protecting Your Eyes from Environmental Damage ... 151
Natural Approaches to Improving Vision ... 152
Preventing Eye Diseases with Nutrition and Herbs ... 153
Exercises for Eye Strength and Focus ... 154

Book 17: Detoxification and Heavy Metal Cleansing ... 156
Understanding the Impact of Heavy Metals on Health ... 156
Chelation Therapy and Natural Detoxification ... 157
Herbal and Nutritional Support for Heavy Metal Detox ... 158
How to Avoid Heavy Metal Exposure ... 160
Daily Detox Habits for a Clean Body ... 161
Rebuilding Health After Heavy Metal Exposure ... 163
Liver Support for Efficient Detoxification ... 164

Book 18: Healing Inflammation Naturally ... 167
The Root Causes of Inflammation ... 167
Anti-Inflammatory Foods for Everyday Health ... 168
Herbal Remedies for Reducing Inflammation ... 169
The Role of the Gut in Inflammation ... 169
Managing Chronic Inflammatory Conditions ... 170
Exercise and Lifestyle Changes for Inflammation ... 172
Understanding the Link Between Inflammation and Disease ... 173

Book 19: Bone and Joint Health with Natural Remedies ... 175

    Understanding Bone Health and Aging 175

    Natural Remedies for Arthritis and Joint Pain 176

    Nutritional Support for Strong Bones 177

    Herbal Approaches to Bone Healing 178

    Preventing Osteoporosis Naturally 180

    Maintaining Joint Mobility and Flexibility 181

    Exercises and Habits for Long-Term Bone Health 184

Book 20: Gut-Brain Connection and Mental Health 186

    Understanding the Gut-Brain Axis 186

    Healing the Gut to Improve Mental Clarity 187

    Probiotics for Mental Health 188

    How Nutrition Affects Mood and Emotions 189

    Herbal Remedies for Anxiety and Depression 190

    The Role of Detoxification in Mental Wellness 191

    Mindfulness and Mental Well-Being 192

Book 21: Natural Remedies for Children's Health 193

    Strengthening Children's Immune System Naturally 193

    Herbal Remedies for Common Childhood Illnesses 194

    Natural Approaches to Managing ADHD 195

    Nutrition for Healthy Growth and Development 196

    Remedies for Skin Conditions in Children 197

    Managing Allergies and Asthma in Children 198

    Building Emotional Resilience in Kids 200

Book 22: Healing the Liver and Gallbladder Naturally 202

    The Role of the Liver and Gallbladder in Detoxification 202

    Signs of Liver Overload and How to Address Them 202

    Herbal Remedies for Liver Support 203

    The Gallbladder Cleanse and Its Benefits 204

    Nutrition for Liver Health 205

    Managing Gallstones Naturally 206

    Daily Practices for Liver and Gallbladder Maintenance 207

Book 23: Weight Loss and Metabolic Health with Natural Approaches 208

    Understanding the Metabolism and Weight Management 208

    Natural Appetite Suppressants and Fat Burners 209

    Herbs for Supporting Metabolic Function 211

    Balancing Blood Sugar for Weight Control 212

    The Role of Detoxification in Weight Loss 214

    Managing Emotional Eating with Natural Remedies 216

  Nutritional Strategies for Sustainable Weight Loss 217

Book 24: Skin Healing and Beauty from Within 220

  The Importance of Nutrition for Skin Health 220

  Herbal Remedies for Acne and Blemishes 221

  Essential Oils for Skin Radiance 222

  Healing Eczema and Psoriasis Naturally 223

  Detoxifying the Skin Through Natural Methods 224

  Preventing Premature Aging with Natural Products 225

  DIY Natural Beauty Recipes for Radiant Skin 227

Book 25: Natural Remedies for Allergies and Asthma 229

  Understanding the Root Causes of Allergies 229

  Herbal Remedies for Respiratory Health 230

  Managing Seasonal Allergies Naturally 231

  Preventing Asthma Attacks with Natural Approaches 232

  Foods and Supplements for Allergy Relief 233

  Detoxifying the Body to Reduce Allergic Reactions 234

  Detoxifying the Body to Reduce Allergic Reactions 235

Book 26: Digestive Health and Natural Solutions for IBS 236

  Identifying the Causes of Irritable Bowel Syndrome (IBS) 236

  Herbal Remedies for IBS Relief 237

  The Role of Probiotics in Digestive Health 238

  Nutritional Strategies for Soothing the Digestive System 239

  Managing Stress to Improve IBS Symptoms 240

  Daily Practices for Long-Term Digestive Wellness 241

Book 27: Strengthening the Immune System with Natural Approaches 243

  Understanding the Immune System's Role in Health 243

  Herbal Immune Boosters 244

  Nutritional Support for Immune Strength 245

  The Role of Probiotics in Immune Function 246

  Managing Autoimmune Disorders Naturally 247

  Daily Habits to Maintain a Strong Immune System 248

  Preventing Infections with Natural Remedies 249

Book 28: Detoxing the Body for Optimal Health 251

  The Importance of Regular Detoxification 251

  Liver and Kidney Cleansing Protocols 252

  Herbal Detox Remedies for the Body 253

  The Role of Water in Detoxification 254

  Detoxing Heavy Metals and Environmental Toxins 255

    Supporting the Lymphatic System in Detox 256

    Colon Cleansing and Gut Health 257

Book 29: Dr. Barbara Cookbook 259

    Breakfast 20 recipes 259

    Lunch 20 recipes 268

    Dinner 20 recipes 276

    Snacks 20 recipes 283

    Desserts 20 recipes 287

Book 30: Natural Remedies for Chronic Fatigue 292

    Understanding Chronic Fatigue and Its Causes 292

    Herbal Remedies for Energy Boosting 292

    Nutritional Support for Fighting Fatigue 293

    Managing Adrenal Fatigue Naturally 294

    The Role of Detoxification in Fatigue Recovery 295

    Restoring Sleep and Energy Levels Naturally 295

Book 31: Healing Infections with Natural Remedies 297

    The Body's Natural Defense Against Infections 297

    Herbal Antibiotics and Antivirals 298

    Supporting the Immune System During Infections 299

    Managing Bacterial and Fungal Infections Naturally 300

    Detoxifying After Infections 301

    Probiotics and Gut Health During Infections 302

    Preventing Future Infections with Lifestyle Changes 304

Book 32: Encyclopedia of Healing Herbs 306

    Introduction to Herbal Medicine 306

    100 Healing Herbs 307

Book 33: Natural Pain Management Strategies 312

    Understanding Chronic Pain and Its Causes 312

    Herbal Pain Relievers for Common Conditions 313

    Managing Joint and Muscle Pain Naturally 314

    Detoxifying the Body to Alleviate Pain 316

    Mind-Body Techniques for Pain Management 317

    Long-Term Strategies for Pain-Free Living 318

Book 34: Enhancing Longevity with Natural Approaches 320

    The Science of Longevity and Aging 320

    Anti-Aging Nutritional Strategies 321

    Herbs and Supplements for Healthy Aging 322

    Detoxing for Longevity and Vitality 323

Managing Stress for a Longer Life 325

The Role of Physical Activity in Aging Gracefully 326

Preventing Age-Related Diseases Naturally 327

Book 35: Natural Remedies for Cardiovascular Health **329**

The Role of Nutrition in Heart Health 329

Herbal Remedies for Lowering Blood Pressure 330

Managing Cholesterol Naturally 331

Strengthening Blood Vessels with Natural Solutions 332

Detoxing for Heart Health 333

Preventing Heart Disease with a Holistic Lifestyle 334

Conclusion **336**

Introduction

Welcome to a journey of natural healing and wellness inspired by the profound insights of Barbara O'Neill. Known for her holistic approach to health, Barbara O'Neill believes in the body's remarkable ability to heal itself when provided with the right tools. Her philosophy centers around using nature's resources—nutritious food, herbs, detoxification, and simple remedies—to achieve optimal health and prevent disease.

In this book, we'll explore the key elements of her philosophy, which focuses on understanding how our bodies work and how we can support them naturally. Barbara emphasizes the importance of balancing all aspects of life—nutrition, exercise, emotional well-being, and proper rest. She teaches that true healing goes beyond treating symptoms; it involves addressing the root causes of illness, nurturing the body, mind, and spirit.

As you delve into the chapters, you'll find practical advice and natural solutions for various health issues, from boosting your immune system to managing stress and improving gut health. Each chapter is designed to provide you with easy-to-follow guidance on how to integrate these natural practices into your daily life.

Whether you're new to natural healing or looking to deepen your understanding, this book offers a comprehensive guide to living a healthier, more balanced life. Barbara O'Neill's compassionate and empowering approach will inspire you to take control of your health, making informed choices that lead to lasting well-being.

Book 1: Introduction to Barbara O'Neill's Philosophy

The Origins of Natural Healing

Natural healing is rooted in the belief that the body has an innate ability to heal itself when given the right tools and environment. Barbara O'Neill has always been drawn to this philosophy, inspired by traditional practices that have been passed down for generations. Long before modern medicine, people relied on natural remedies like herbs, clean water, sunlight, and fresh air to maintain their health.

Barbara's approach to natural healing stems from the idea that the human body is designed to be self-sustaining. She believes that instead of masking symptoms, we should focus on supporting the body's healing processes. By understanding the simple, natural ways the body works, we can help prevent disease and support overall wellness.

At the heart of Barbara's teachings is the idea that healing doesn't need to be complicated. It's about reconnecting with nature, using wholesome foods, and making lifestyle choices that enhance our body's natural defenses. Whether it's through detoxification, proper nutrition, or even the importance of rest, Barbara encourages people to embrace natural, sustainable approaches to health.

Barbara's Journey: From Nurse to Natural Health Expert

Barbara O'Neill's path to becoming a leading voice in natural health began in a very conventional way—as a nurse. Her early years in healthcare were spent working in traditional medical settings, where she witnessed the immense value of modern medicine. However, she also saw its limitations. While the treatments she administered were often effective in addressing symptoms, they didn't always promote long-term wellness or get to the root cause of health issues.

This experience sparked something in Barbara—a desire to explore other ways of healing that could complement, or even surpass, conventional methods. She became increasingly curious about how lifestyle, diet, and the natural environment could support the body's natural ability to heal. Over time, this curiosity evolved into a deep passion for natural health.

Barbara's shift from nursing to natural health wasn't immediate. It was a gradual journey filled with study, personal research, and a strong conviction that true health is about more than just managing disease—it's about nurturing the body's inherent wisdom. She learned from various experts, traveled, and gathered knowledge from both traditional practices and modern science.

As she embraced natural health, Barbara began to teach others about these holistic methods, helping people take charge of their own well-being. Her background in nursing gave her a unique perspective, allowing her to combine the best of both worlds—bridging the gap between medical science and natural healing.

Today, Barbara is a well-respected natural health expert, and her journey continues to inspire countless individuals to explore the benefits of natural healing. This subchapter will take you through Barbara's transformation and the key moments that led her to where she is today.

The Importance of Holistic Health

Holistic health is at the core of Barbara O'Neill's philosophy, emphasizing that true wellness goes beyond simply treating symptoms. Instead, it's about looking at the whole person—mind, body, and spirit—and understanding how these elements work together to create balance and health.

Barbara believes that health cannot be compartmentalized. It's not just about what you eat or how much you exercise, but also about emotional well-being, stress management, and the environment you live in. For example, a nutrient-rich diet might support physical health, but if stress and anxiety are overwhelming, it can still take a toll on overall wellness. Holistic health encourages us to address all aspects of life to promote healing and vitality.

Barbara's approach encourages people to be proactive about their health, making thoughtful choices that support balance in every area. Whether it's through proper nutrition, regular movement, sufficient rest, or nurturing positive relationships, she teaches that each piece of the puzzle plays a vital role in our overall well-being.

The Power of Prevention

Barbara O'Neill is a firm believer in the power of prevention as a cornerstone of good health. Rather than waiting for illness to strike, her philosophy encourages people to take proactive steps to maintain wellness and avoid common health issues. Prevention, she teaches, is not just about avoiding disease but about creating a lifestyle that supports long-term vitality and balance.

At the heart of Barbara's approach is the understanding that many health problems, especially chronic diseases, are largely preventable. Conditions like heart disease, diabetes, and obesity are often the result of poor lifestyle choices—such as an unhealthy diet, lack of exercise, and unmanaged stress. By making small but consistent changes, like eating nourishing foods, moving regularly, and managing stress, we can significantly reduce the risk of developing these conditions.

Barbara also emphasizes that prevention is empowering. When we actively choose to take care of ourselves—whether through nutrition, exercise, or mindfulness—we regain control over our health. Prevention becomes a way of life, not something we think about only when a problem arises.

Barbara's Fight Against the Pharmaceutical Industry

Barbara O'Neill has long been a vocal advocate for natural healing, and her stance has often put her at odds with the pharmaceutical industry. Her concerns stem from what she sees as an over-reliance on medications to treat symptoms rather than addressing the root causes of health problems. While she acknowledges that pharmaceuticals have their place in emergency medicine,

Barbara believes that they are often prescribed unnecessarily, leading to a cycle where people depend on drugs instead of exploring natural, preventive solutions.

Barbara's fight against the pharmaceutical industry isn't just about challenging the system; it's about educating individuals to take charge of their health. She encourages people to ask critical questions, to understand what's being prescribed, and to consider natural alternatives wherever possible. She emphasizes that many conditions, especially chronic illnesses, can be managed through lifestyle changes, proper nutrition, and natural remedies.

One of her key arguments is that pharmaceutical companies often prioritize profits over people's health. She highlights how heavily the industry influences modern healthcare, from the medications prescribed to the information made available to patients. This, she believes, has led to a system where natural treatments and preventive care are often overlooked.

Building a Non-Toxic Lifestyle

Barbara O'Neill emphasizes the importance of living a non-toxic lifestyle as a key component of maintaining good health. She believes that the modern world exposes us to a variety of harmful chemicals and toxins, from the foods we eat to the products we use in our homes. Over time, these toxins can accumulate in the body, weakening the immune system and leading to chronic illnesses. To counteract this, Barbara advocates for a lifestyle that minimizes exposure to these harmful substances.

Building a non-toxic lifestyle begins with awareness. Barbara encourages individuals to take a closer look at their everyday choices, from the cleaning products under the sink to the foods in the pantry. Many conventional household items contain chemicals that can be harmful over time, while processed foods often carry artificial additives, preservatives, and pesticides. By switching to natural alternatives, such as organic foods and eco-friendly products, we can greatly reduce our toxic load.

Barbara also emphasizes the importance of the environment in which we live. Simple changes, like using natural cleaning products, choosing non-toxic skincare, and filtering the water we drink, can have a profound impact on our well-being. Reducing exposure to harmful chemicals creates a cleaner, healthier living space for both the body and the mind.

Book 2: Nutrition and Its Role in Healing

Understanding the Power of Nutrition

Nutrition is at the heart of Barbara O'Neill's approach to healing. She believes that food is not just fuel; it is medicine. The power of nutrition lies in its ability to nourish the body at a cellular level, providing the essential vitamins, minerals, and nutrients that our bodies need to function optimally and heal naturally.

Barbara teaches that a well-balanced, nutrient-rich diet can be the key to preventing and even reversing many chronic health conditions. She emphasizes the importance of eating whole, unprocessed foods—like fresh fruits, vegetables, nuts, seeds, and whole grains—that are full of life-giving nutrients. These foods provide the body with the building blocks it needs to repair, regenerate, and thrive.

One of the most powerful aspects of nutrition, according to Barbara, is its role in reducing inflammation, boosting the immune system, and supporting the body's detoxification processes. For example, antioxidant-rich foods, such as berries and leafy greens, help protect cells from damage, while fiber-rich foods aid digestion and help eliminate toxins. The right foods can also balance hormones, stabilize blood sugar, and enhance mental clarity, all of which contribute to overall well-being.

In this subchapter, we'll explore how making mindful, intentional choices about what we eat can transform our health. Barbara encourages us to think of food not just as a necessity, but as a vital tool in the journey toward healing and vitality. By understanding the power of nutrition, we can take control of our health and unlock the body's true potential for self-healing.

Key Nutrients for Optimal Health

When it comes to achieving optimal health, Barbara O'Neill emphasizes the importance of focusing on key nutrients that support the body's vital functions. These essential nutrients, when consumed through a wholesome and balanced diet, act as the foundation for healing and maintaining long-term wellness.

Barbara highlights the role of vitamins and minerals as crucial elements in this process. For instance, vitamin C is a powerful antioxidant that helps boost the immune system and promotes skin health. Similarly, vitamin D, often known as the "sunshine vitamin," is essential for bone health and plays a role in mood regulation. Many people, however, are deficient in this vitamin, which is why Barbara encourages outdoor activities and vitamin D-rich foods like fish and fortified products.

Minerals such as magnesium are equally important, as they support muscle function, reduce inflammation, and help manage stress. Foods like leafy greens, nuts, and seeds are excellent sources of magnesium and can easily be included in daily meals.

Omega-3 fatty acids, found in fatty fish like salmon and in flaxseeds, are another key nutrient Barbara often talks about. These healthy fats are vital for brain health, reducing inflammation, and supporting heart health. Incorporating these healthy fats into the diet can lead to improved mental clarity and cardiovascular function.

Additionally, fiber plays a key role in digestion and detoxification. Whole grains, fruits, and vegetables are rich in fiber, which helps cleanse the digestive system and promote gut health—an area that Barbara views as central to overall well-being.

How Diet Impacts the Immune System

Barbara O'Neill places great emphasis on the connection between diet and the immune system. According to her teachings, the foods we eat have a direct impact on how well our bodies can defend against illness and maintain overall health. A strong immune system starts with proper nutrition, as it provides the essential building blocks that the body needs to stay resilient and fight off infections.

Barbara believes that certain foods can either boost or weaken the immune system. For instance, a diet rich in processed foods, refined sugars, and unhealthy fats can contribute to chronic inflammation, which compromises immune function. On the other hand, a diet full of whole, nutrient-dense foods like fresh fruits, vegetables, and healthy fats strengthens the body's natural defenses.

Antioxidant-rich foods such as berries, citrus fruits, and leafy greens are particularly important because they help neutralize harmful free radicals, protecting cells from damage. Foods high in vitamin C, like oranges and red peppers, are well-known immune boosters, helping the body produce more white blood cells, which are essential in fighting infections.

Barbara also highlights the importance of probiotics in maintaining a healthy gut, which is where a large part of the immune system resides. Fermented foods like yogurt, sauerkraut, and kefir introduce beneficial bacteria that support gut health, promoting a balanced and efficient immune response.

Nutritional Deficiencies and Their Consequences

Barbara O'Neill underscores the critical role that proper nutrition plays in maintaining health, and she's particularly concerned about the consequences of nutritional deficiencies. When our diets lack essential nutrients, it can lead to a range of health issues, affecting everything from our energy levels to our immune function.

For instance, a deficiency in vitamin D can result in weakened bones, increased risk of fractures, and even mood disorders like depression. Since vitamin D is crucial for calcium absorption, its lack can lead to conditions like osteoporosis, particularly in those who don't get enough sunlight or consume fortified foods.

Iron deficiency is another common issue, particularly among women. Iron is vital for producing hemoglobin, the protein in red blood cells that carries oxygen throughout the body. A lack of iron can lead to anemia, causing fatigue, weakness, and pale skin. Barbara recommends incorporating iron-rich foods like leafy greens, legumes, and lean meats to combat this deficiency.

Vitamin B12 deficiency can lead to neurological issues, including numbness and tingling, as well as cognitive problems like memory loss. This vitamin is primarily found in animal products, so those following a plant-based diet need to be especially mindful of their intake and consider fortified foods or supplements.

Omega-3 fatty acids are essential for heart and brain health, and a deficiency can contribute to inflammation and cognitive decline. Including sources like fatty fish, flaxseeds, and walnuts in your diet can help maintain optimal levels of these crucial fats.

Whole Foods vs. Processed Foods

Barbara O'Neill is a strong advocate for choosing whole foods over processed foods, believing that this choice can significantly impact overall health and healing. Understanding the differences between these two types of foods is key to making better dietary decisions that support well-being.

Whole foods are foods that are as close to their natural state as possible. They are minimally processed and free from artificial additives, preservatives, and excessive sugars. Examples include fresh fruits, vegetables, whole grains, nuts, seeds, and lean proteins. Barbara highlights that whole foods are rich in essential nutrients like vitamins, minerals, fiber, and antioxidants. These nutrients are crucial for maintaining a healthy immune system, supporting digestion, and reducing inflammation.

On the other hand, processed foods often undergo extensive manufacturing processes that strip away much of their nutritional value. They can be loaded with unhealthy fats, refined sugars, sodium, and artificial additives. Common examples include sugary snacks, fast food, and pre-packaged meals. Barbara points out that these foods can contribute to chronic health problems such as obesity, heart disease, and diabetes, as they often provide empty calories without the essential nutrients needed for optimal health.

Barbara encourages a shift towards whole foods by focusing on meals made from fresh, unprocessed ingredients. This approach not only supports better health but also fosters a more mindful and satisfying eating experience. By choosing whole foods, individuals can provide their bodies with the nutrients they need to function at their best and promote long-term healing.

Therapeutic Diets for Specific Conditions

Barbara O'Neill advocates for therapeutic diets as a powerful way to manage and even alleviate various health conditions. By tailoring nutrition to address specific issues, individuals can support their bodies in healing and restoring balance. Here's a look at how certain diets can be used therapeutically for different conditions:

Anti-Inflammatory Diet: This diet is designed to reduce inflammation throughout the body, which is beneficial for conditions like arthritis, autoimmune diseases, and chronic inflammatory conditions. It focuses on consuming foods high in antioxidants and omega-3 fatty acids, such as berries, leafy greens, nuts, seeds, and fatty fish. Barbara emphasizes the importance of avoiding inflammatory triggers like refined sugars, trans fats, and processed foods.

Low-FODMAP Diet: For individuals suffering from irritable bowel syndrome (IBS) or other digestive issues, the Low-FODMAP diet can be highly effective. It involves reducing intake of foods that are high in fermentable oligosaccharides, disaccharides, monosaccharides, and polyols. These include certain fruits, vegetables, and dairy products. By eliminating these triggers, many people experience relief from bloating, gas, and abdominal pain.

Mediterranean Diet: Known for its heart-health benefits, the Mediterranean diet emphasizes whole grains, healthy fats (such as olive oil), lean proteins (like fish and poultry), and plenty of fruits and vegetables. Barbara recommends this diet for its potential to lower the risk of cardiovascular diseases and support overall wellness.

Gluten-Free Diet: For those with celiac disease or gluten sensitivity, a strict gluten-free diet is essential. This means avoiding all foods that contain gluten, a protein found in wheat, barley, and rye. Barbara advises focusing on naturally gluten-free foods such as fruits, vegetables, meat, and gluten-free grains like quinoa and rice.

Ketogenic Diet: The ketogenic diet, which is high in fats and low in carbohydrates, can be beneficial for certain neurological conditions and for managing weight. It shifts the body into a state of ketosis, where it burns fat for fuel instead of carbohydrates. Barbara notes that while this diet can be effective for some, it's important to consult with a healthcare provider to ensure it's appropriate for individual health needs.

Superfoods for Healing and Vitality

When it comes to boosting health and vitality, Barbara O'Neill champions the inclusion of superfoods in our diets. These nutrient-dense foods are packed with vitamins, minerals, and antioxidants that can significantly enhance the body's healing processes and overall well-being. Here's a closer look at some of Barbara's favorite superfoods and how they contribute to health:

Blueberries: Often hailed as a top superfood, blueberries are rich in antioxidants known as flavonoids, which help protect the body's cells from damage. They also offer anti-inflammatory benefits and support brain health. Barbara recommends adding them to smoothies or yogurt for a delicious, health-boosting snack.

Spinach: This leafy green is a powerhouse of vitamins A, C, and K, as well as minerals like iron and magnesium. Spinach supports immune function, promotes healthy skin, and helps with energy production. Barbara suggests incorporating spinach into salads, soups, or as a side dish.

Chia Seeds: These tiny seeds are packed with omega-3 fatty acids, fiber, and protein. They support heart health, aid in digestion, and help keep you feeling full longer. Barbara often includes chia seeds in her morning oatmeal or smoothies for an extra nutritional boost.

Turmeric: Known for its bright yellow color and strong anti-inflammatory properties, turmeric contains curcumin, a compound that helps reduce inflammation and supports joint health. Barbara recommends using turmeric in cooking, such as in curries or soups, or as a supplement for its health benefits.

Walnuts: Rich in omega-3 fatty acids and antioxidants, walnuts are great for heart health and cognitive function. They also provide essential nutrients like vitamin E and magnesium. Barbara advises eating a handful of walnuts as a snack or adding them to salads and baked goods.

Ginger: With its anti-inflammatory and digestive benefits, ginger is a versatile superfood. It can help with nausea, improve digestion, and reduce inflammation. Barbara incorporates fresh ginger into teas, smoothies, and stir-fries for its healing properties.

Quinoa: This whole grain is a complete protein, meaning it contains all nine essential amino acids. It's also high in fiber, vitamins, and minerals. Barbara suggests using quinoa as a base for salads, side dishes, or as a substitute for rice.

Book 3: Detoxification and Cleansing

The Body's Natural Detox Mechanisms

Barbara O'Neill emphasizes the incredible efficiency of the body's natural detoxification systems. Our bodies are equipped with sophisticated mechanisms that work tirelessly to eliminate toxins and maintain balance. Understanding how these processes work can help us support and enhance our body's own detox efforts.

Liver: The liver is a key player in detoxification. It processes and breaks down toxins, drugs, and other harmful substances. Barbara highlights the liver's role in converting these toxins into less harmful substances that can be excreted. Supporting liver health with a balanced diet rich in antioxidants and avoiding excessive alcohol can help it function optimally.

Kidneys: The kidneys filter blood, removing waste products and excess fluids, which are then excreted as urine. Barbara points out that staying hydrated is crucial for kidney health, as water helps the kidneys flush out toxins effectively. Drinking plenty of water and consuming foods that support kidney function, like cranberries and beets, can aid this process.

Lungs: Our lungs play a vital role in removing gaseous wastes, such as carbon dioxide, from the body. Barbara recommends practices that support lung health, such as deep breathing exercises and avoiding exposure to pollutants, to ensure the lungs can efficiently expel waste gases.

Skin: The skin is not just a protective barrier; it also aids in detoxification through sweating. Barbara encourages regular physical activity and saunas, which can help promote sweating and thus support the elimination of toxins through the skin.

Digestive System: The digestive system helps remove waste through bowel movements. Barbara emphasizes the importance of a fiber-rich diet, which supports healthy digestion and regular bowel movements, aiding in the removal of toxins and waste products from the body.

Lymphatic System: The lymphatic system helps remove toxins and waste products from the cells. It also plays a role in immune function. Barbara suggests incorporating activities that stimulate lymphatic flow, such as exercise and dry brushing, to support this crucial system.

Identifying Toxins in Everyday Life

Barbara O'Neill believes that being aware of the toxins we encounter in our daily lives is crucial for maintaining health and supporting our body's natural detoxification processes. Many everyday products and environmental factors can introduce harmful substances into our bodies, but with a bit of knowledge, we can make more informed choices to minimize our exposure.

Household Cleaning Products: Many common cleaning products contain chemicals that can be harsh on both the environment and our health. Barbara points out that ingredients like ammonia, bleach, and synthetic fragrances can release toxins into the air and affect indoor air quality.

Opting for natural cleaning solutions or DIY alternatives, such as vinegar and baking soda, can help reduce exposure to these harmful substances.

Personal Care Products: From shampoos to lotions, many personal care products include chemicals like parabens, phthalates, and sulfates. These ingredients can potentially disrupt hormonal balance and cause other health issues. Barbara recommends choosing products with natural ingredients or those labeled as free from harmful additives.

Processed Foods: Packaged and processed foods often contain artificial additives, preservatives, and high levels of refined sugars and unhealthy fats. Barbara emphasizes the importance of reading labels and opting for whole, unprocessed foods whenever possible to avoid these hidden toxins.

Plastic Containers: Certain plastics can leach harmful chemicals, such as BPA (bisphenol A), into food and beverages. Barbara suggests using glass or stainless steel containers instead of plastic, particularly for food storage and water bottles.

Air Pollution: Outdoor air pollution from vehicle emissions, industrial activities, and other sources can introduce toxins into the environment. Barbara recommends spending time in green spaces and using air purifiers at home to help reduce exposure to airborne pollutants.

Water Quality: Contaminants such as heavy metals, chlorine, and pesticides can affect water quality. Barbara advises using a water filter that removes these impurities or choosing bottled water from trusted sources to ensure clean drinking water.

Pesticides and Herbicides: Residues from pesticides and herbicides on fruits and vegetables can contribute to toxin intake. Barbara recommends washing produce thoroughly and choosing organic options when possible to minimize exposure.

The Role of the Liver in Detoxification

Barbara O'Neill often highlights the liver's pivotal role in the body's detoxification process. As one of our most vital organs, the liver works tirelessly to filter and process the substances that enter our system. Understanding how it functions can help us appreciate its importance and take steps to support its health.

Filtering Toxins: The liver acts as the body's primary filter, processing blood coming from the digestive tract. It identifies and breaks down toxins, including drugs, alcohol, and environmental pollutants, turning them into less harmful substances. Barbara emphasizes that a well-functioning liver is essential for removing these toxins efficiently and keeping our system balanced.

Metabolism of Nutrients: Beyond detoxification, the liver also plays a crucial role in metabolizing nutrients from the foods we eat. It converts proteins, fats, and carbohydrates into energy and stores essential vitamins and minerals. Barbara notes that a healthy liver helps ensure that our bodies get the most out of the nutrients we consume.

Detoxification Pathways: The liver uses two main phases to detoxify substances:

- Phase 1: In this phase, the liver transforms toxins into intermediate compounds through various enzymes. These intermediate compounds are often more reactive and need further processing.
- Phase 2: Here, the liver conjugates these intermediate compounds with molecules like glucuronide, sulfate, or glutathione, making them easier to excrete. Barbara explains that both phases are essential for effectively neutralizing and eliminating toxins from the body.

Supporting Liver Health: To keep the liver functioning optimally, Barbara recommends maintaining a healthy lifestyle. This includes eating a balanced diet rich in antioxidants, staying hydrated, and avoiding excessive alcohol consumption. Foods like garlic, beets, and leafy greens can support liver function and promote detoxification.

Recognizing Liver Stress: Signs of liver stress or dysfunction can include fatigue, jaundice (yellowing of the skin), and digestive issues. Barbara advises seeking medical advice if you experience these symptoms, as they may indicate a need for additional support or treatment.

Detoxifying with Herbs and Natural Remedies

Barbara O'Neill champions the use of herbs and natural remedies as effective tools for supporting the body's detoxification processes. These natural solutions can gently enhance the body's ability to cleanse itself, providing a complementary approach to more conventional detox methods. Here's a closer look at some of Barbara's favorite herbs and remedies for detoxification:

Milk Thistle: Renowned for its liver-supporting properties, milk thistle contains silymarin, a compound that helps protect liver cells from damage and supports their regeneration. Barbara often recommends milk thistle as a natural remedy to bolster liver function and enhance detoxification.

Dandelion Root: Dandelion root is a potent herb that supports both liver and kidney function. It acts as a diuretic, helping to flush out excess fluids and toxins from the body. Barbara suggests drinking dandelion root tea or incorporating it into your diet to support overall detoxification.

Cilantro: Cilantro is known for its ability to help remove heavy metals from the body. Barbara highlights its role in chelation, which binds to toxins and aids in their elimination. Adding fresh cilantro to salads, soups, or smoothies can be a tasty way to incorporate this herb into your diet.

Turmeric: This bright yellow spice contains curcumin, which has powerful anti-inflammatory and antioxidant properties. Barbara uses turmeric to support liver health and enhance its detoxification abilities. It can be added to curries, smoothies, or taken as a supplement.

Ginger: Ginger is a versatile root that helps improve digestion and reduce inflammation. Barbara often recommends ginger tea or incorporating fresh ginger into meals to aid in detoxification and support overall digestive health.

Green Tea: Rich in antioxidants, particularly catechins, green tea supports liver function and helps neutralize free radicals in the body. Barbara advises drinking green tea regularly to boost your antioxidant intake and support detoxification.

Activated Charcoal: Known for its ability to adsorb toxins, activated charcoal can be used to help remove harmful substances from the digestive tract. Barbara suggests using it under guidance, as it can bind to both toxins and essential nutrients, so timing and dosage are important.

Lemon Water: Starting your day with a glass of lemon water can help stimulate digestion and support liver function. The vitamin C in lemons helps boost the body's natural detoxification processes, according to Barbara's recommendations.

Colon Cleansing for Optimal Health

Barbara O'Neill underscores the importance of colon health in the broader context of detoxification and overall well-being. The colon, or large intestine, plays a crucial role in eliminating waste and maintaining a healthy digestive system. A well-functioning colon supports effective detoxification and can contribute to overall vitality. Here's how Barbara approaches colon cleansing for optimal health:

Understanding Colon Cleansing: Colon cleansing involves techniques designed to remove accumulated waste and toxins from the colon. Barbara explains that while the body's natural processes usually handle waste removal effectively, occasional cleansing can help maintain colon health and enhance overall detoxification.

Dietary Fiber: One of the simplest and most effective ways to support colon health is by increasing dietary fiber. Barbara recommends consuming a diet rich in fruits, vegetables, whole grains, and legumes. Fiber adds bulk to stool, promotes regular bowel movements, and helps prevent constipation, ensuring that waste is efficiently expelled from the body.

Hydration: Staying well-hydrated is essential for a healthy colon. Barbara highlights that water helps keep stool soft and supports the overall digestive process. Drinking plenty of water throughout the day can aid in maintaining regular bowel movements and preventing dehydration.

Probiotics: Probiotics are beneficial bacteria that support gut health and can aid in digestion. Barbara suggests incorporating probiotic-rich foods, such as yogurt, kefir, and fermented vegetables, into your diet to promote a healthy balance of gut flora and enhance colon function.

Herbal Teas: Certain herbal teas can support colon cleansing and digestion. Barbara recommends teas made from ingredients like peppermint, ginger, and senna. These herbs can help soothe the digestive system and promote regular bowel movements.

Colon Hydrotherapy: For those interested in a more intensive approach, Barbara discusses colon hydrotherapy, also known as colonic irrigation. This process involves flushing the colon with water to remove waste. While it can be beneficial, Barbara advises consulting with a healthcare professional before undergoing this treatment.

Avoiding Processed Foods: Reducing or eliminating processed foods and those high in sugars and unhealthy fats can help support colon health. Barbara emphasizes choosing whole, unprocessed foods to reduce the burden on the colon and support overall digestive function.

Regular Exercise: Physical activity promotes healthy digestion and regular bowel movements. Barbara encourages incorporating regular exercise into your routine, as it can help stimulate the digestive system and support colon health.

Fasting as a Detox Strategy

Fasting is a powerful tool in the realm of detoxification, and Barbara O'Neill recognizes its potential for enhancing health and well-being. When done thoughtfully, fasting can give the body a chance to reset, repair, and rejuvenate. Here's how Barbara explains fasting as a detox strategy:

What is Fasting? Fasting involves abstaining from all or certain types of food and drink for a specific period. Barbara explains that there are various forms of fasting, including intermittent fasting, extended fasting, and periodic fasting. Each type offers unique benefits and can be tailored to individual needs.

Intermittent Fasting: This popular fasting method involves cycling between eating and fasting periods within a 24-hour day. Barbara highlights how intermittent fasting can help regulate blood sugar levels, improve metabolism, and support weight management. It's a flexible approach that can easily be integrated into daily routines.

Extended Fasting: Extended fasting typically lasts for more than 24 hours and can be done for a few days or longer. Barbara notes that while extended fasting can provide deeper detoxification benefits, it requires careful planning and should be done under medical supervision to ensure safety and effectiveness.

Periodic Fasting: This involves fasting for a set period, such as one day a week or a few days each month. Barbara suggests that periodic fasting can help give the digestive system a break and promote overall health without the need for daily restriction.

Detoxification Benefits: During fasting, the body can focus on detoxification and repair. Barbara explains that fasting triggers autophagy, a process where cells clean out damaged components and regenerate. This can help improve cellular health and support the body's natural detoxification processes.

Supporting the Fast: To get the most out of a fasting regimen, Barbara advises staying hydrated by drinking plenty of water and herbal teas. It's also important to consume nutrient-dense foods during eating periods to ensure that the body gets essential vitamins and minerals.

Listening to Your Body: Barbara emphasizes the importance of listening to your body during fasting. If you experience symptoms like dizziness, fatigue, or extreme hunger, it may be a sign that the fasting approach needs adjustment. Fasting should feel supportive, not overwhelming.

Combining with Other Practices: For enhanced detoxification, Barbara suggests combining fasting with other supportive practices, such as gentle exercise, adequate sleep, and stress management. These holistic approaches can amplify the benefits of fasting and support overall well-being.

Detoxification Protocols for Chronic Conditions

Barbara O'Neill emphasizes that detoxification can play a significant role in managing and alleviating chronic conditions. While detoxifying the body can support overall health, addressing chronic health issues often requires a more tailored approach. Here's a look at how Barbara recommends using detoxification protocols to support those with chronic conditions:

Understanding Chronic Conditions: Chronic conditions, such as diabetes, autoimmune diseases, and chronic fatigue syndrome, often involve long-term inflammation and toxin buildup in the body. Barbara highlights that detoxification can help reduce the toxic load and support the body's natural healing processes.

Customized Detox Protocols: Barbara believes that a one-size-fits-all approach doesn't work for chronic conditions. Instead, she recommends customizing detox protocols based on the specific condition and individual needs. Consulting with a healthcare professional can help create a personalized plan that addresses unique health concerns.

Anti-Inflammatory Diet: For many chronic conditions, inflammation is a key issue. Barbara suggests following an anti-inflammatory diet, which includes foods rich in antioxidants and omega-3 fatty acids. This diet can help reduce inflammation and support overall detoxification. Foods like berries, leafy greens, fatty fish, and turmeric are beneficial.

Gentle Detox Practices: When dealing with chronic conditions, Barbara recommends starting with gentle detox practices. This can include methods such as drinking herbal teas, increasing fiber intake, and staying hydrated. These approaches help support the body's natural detoxification processes without overwhelming it.

Supportive Supplements: Certain supplements can aid in detoxification and support chronic condition management. Barbara suggests considering supplements such as milk thistle for liver health, probiotics for gut balance, and omega-3 fatty acids for reducing inflammation. Always consult with a healthcare provider before starting new supplements.

Managing Stress: Chronic stress can exacerbate many health conditions and impede detoxification. Barbara emphasizes the importance of incorporating stress management techniques, such as meditation, deep breathing exercises, and gentle physical activity, into your routine to support overall health.

Regular Monitoring: For individuals with chronic conditions, it's important to monitor progress and adjust detox protocols as needed. Barbara advises keeping track of symptoms and working closely with a healthcare professional to make any necessary changes to the detox plan.

Holistic Approach: Detoxification for chronic conditions is most effective when combined with a holistic approach. This includes not only dietary changes but also addressing lifestyle factors such as sleep, exercise, and mental health. Barbara encourages a comprehensive strategy to support overall well-being.

Post-Detoxification: Maintaining a Clean System

After completing a detoxification program, maintaining a clean system is key to sustaining the benefits and supporting long-term health. Barbara O'Neill emphasizes that the post-detox phase is just as important as the detox itself. Here's how Barbara suggests keeping your body in optimal condition after a detox:

Transition Gradually: After a detox, it's important to transition back to regular eating slowly and mindfully. Barbara recommends reintroducing foods gradually to monitor how your body responds. Start with easily digestible foods and slowly add in more complex items to avoid overwhelming your system.

Focus on Whole Foods: To maintain a clean system, Barbara advises continuing to eat a diet rich in whole foods. Prioritize fresh fruits, vegetables, whole grains, and lean proteins. These nutrient-dense foods support overall health and help keep the body's detoxification systems functioning well.

Stay Hydrated: Hydration is crucial for ongoing detoxification. Barbara suggests drinking plenty of water throughout the day to help flush out toxins and support kidney function. Herbal teas and infused water with lemon or cucumber can also be refreshing options.

Maintain Regular Exercise: Physical activity helps to stimulate circulation and support the body's natural detox processes. Barbara encourages incorporating regular exercise into your routine, such as walking, yoga, or strength training, to promote overall wellness and maintain a clean system.

Practice Stress Management: Chronic stress can hinder the body's ability to detoxify effectively. Barbara highlights the importance of managing stress through relaxation techniques such as meditation, deep breathing exercises, and engaging in activities that bring you joy and relaxation.

Monitor Your Health: Keeping track of how you feel post-detox can help identify any changes or issues that arise. Barbara suggests paying attention to your energy levels, digestion, and overall well-being. If you notice any concerns, consult with a healthcare professional for guidance.

Support Gut Health: A healthy gut is essential for ongoing detoxification. Barbara recommends consuming probiotic-rich foods, such as yogurt and fermented vegetables, and eating a diet high in fiber to support a balanced gut microbiome and optimal digestive function.

Avoid Toxins: To maintain the benefits of detoxification, it's helpful to minimize exposure to toxins. Barbara advises reducing intake of processed foods, artificial additives, and environmental pollutants. Choosing organic foods and natural cleaning products can also contribute to a cleaner lifestyle.

Incorporate Detox-Friendly Habits: Continue to adopt detox-friendly habits, such as having a daily green smoothie, enjoying a cup of detoxifying herbal tea, or incorporating lemon water into your morning routine. These practices can support ongoing detoxification and overall health.

Book 4: The Power of Herbs in Healing

History and Uses of Medicinal Herbs

Medicinal herbs have been an integral part of human healing practices for centuries, offering a natural and holistic approach to health. Barbara O'Neill explores the rich history and diverse uses of these remarkable plants, highlighting their enduring significance in wellness.

A Storied History: The use of medicinal herbs dates back to ancient civilizations, where they were revered for their healing properties. Barbara delves into how early cultures, including the Egyptians, Greeks, and Chinese, relied on herbs to treat ailments and maintain health. These ancient practices laid the foundation for modern herbal medicine.

Traditional Wisdom: Many traditional healing systems, such as Ayurveda and Traditional Chinese Medicine (TCM), have deep roots in the use of medicinal herbs. Barbara explains how these traditions used herbs not just for treating illness but also for promoting balance and harmony within the body. Ayurvedic texts and TCM herbal formularies are filled with insights into the healing potential of various herbs.

Herbal Knowledge Across Cultures: From Native American tribes to Indigenous peoples of the Amazon, different cultures have contributed to the global understanding of medicinal herbs. Barbara highlights how these diverse traditions have shared knowledge about herbs, leading to a rich tapestry of herbal remedies and practices.

Common Medicinal Herbs and Their Uses: Barbara introduces several well-known medicinal herbs and their uses. For example, Echinacea is celebrated for its immune-boosting properties, Ginger is known for aiding digestion and reducing nausea, and Turmeric is prized for its anti-inflammatory effects. Each herb has a unique set of benefits that can support various aspects of health.

Modern Applications: Today, medicinal herbs are used in a variety of forms, including teas, tinctures, capsules, and topical applications. Barbara discusses how modern herbalists and healthcare practitioners integrate these traditional remedies into contemporary wellness practices. Many herbs are now recognized and supported by scientific research for their therapeutic benefits.

Growing and Harvesting Herbs: Barbara emphasizes the importance of knowing how to grow and harvest medicinal herbs. Whether you have a garden or prefer to purchase herbs, understanding how to properly cultivate and prepare these plants ensures that you get the most benefit from them.

Safety and Efficacy: While medicinal herbs offer many benefits, Barbara stresses the importance of using them safely and effectively. It's crucial to consult with a knowledgeable herbalist or healthcare provider to ensure that the herbs you choose are appropriate for your specific health needs and to avoid potential interactions with other medications.

Integrating Herbs into Daily Life: Barbara encourages incorporating medicinal herbs into your daily routine. This could mean sipping a soothing herbal tea, using herbal remedies for common ailments, or incorporating herbs into your cooking for added flavor and health benefits.

How Herbs Work with the Body

Herbs have an incredible ability to support and enhance our health, but how exactly do they work within our bodies? Barbara O'Neill provides insight into the fascinating ways herbs interact with our systems, helping us to understand their powerful effects.

Natural Compounds in Herbs: Herbs contain a variety of natural compounds, such as alkaloids, flavonoids, and essential oils. Barbara explains that these compounds have specific properties that can influence the body's functions. For example, alkaloids can have stimulating effects, while flavonoids often provide antioxidant benefits.

Synergy with Body Systems: Herbs work in harmony with the body's various systems, including the digestive, immune, and circulatory systems. Barbara highlights how different herbs can target specific areas. For instance, Peppermint can soothe the digestive tract, Echinacea can support the immune system, and Ginkgo Biloba can enhance circulation.

Supporting Detoxification: Many herbs assist the body's natural detoxification processes. Barbara discusses how herbs like Milk Thistle and Dandelion support liver function, helping the body to filter and eliminate toxins more efficiently. This support is crucial for maintaining overall health and well-being.

Balancing Hormones: Herbs can also play a role in balancing hormones. Barbara points out that herbs like Chaste Tree and Black Cohosh are used in traditional medicine to help regulate menstrual cycles and alleviate menopausal symptoms. These herbs work by interacting with hormone receptors and supporting the endocrine system.

Modulating Immune Response: Some herbs help modulate the immune system, either by boosting it or calming it down. For instance, Echinacea is known for its immune-boosting properties, while Licorice Root can help regulate the immune response. Barbara explains that this modulation helps the body maintain a balanced immune function.

Enhancing Digestive Health: Herbs can promote digestive health by supporting digestion and reducing inflammation. Ginger, for example, aids digestion and can reduce nausea, while Slippery Elm helps soothe the digestive tract. Barbara emphasizes the importance of these herbs in maintaining a healthy digestive system.

Promoting Mental Clarity: Some herbs are known for their cognitive benefits. Ginkgo Biloba and Rosemary are two examples that Barbara discusses, highlighting their ability to improve memory and focus. These herbs work by enhancing blood flow to the brain and supporting mental function.

Safe and Effective Use: Barbara underscores the importance of using herbs safely and effectively. Understanding the correct dosage and potential interactions with other medications is crucial. Consulting with a knowledgeable herbalist or healthcare provider can help ensure that you're using herbs in a way that supports your health goals.

Common Herbs for Everyday Ailments

Herbs are like nature's medicine cabinet, offering natural remedies for a range of everyday ailments. Barbara O'Neill explores some of the most common herbs that can be used to address common issues, providing practical tips on how to incorporate them into your daily life.

Peppermint for Digestive Comfort: Peppermint is a versatile herb known for its soothing effects on the digestive system. Barbara highlights its use in easing indigestion, bloating, and nausea. Peppermint tea or a few drops of peppermint oil can provide quick relief for digestive discomfort.

Ginger for Nausea and Inflammation: Ginger is another go-to herb with powerful benefits. It's widely used to relieve nausea, whether from motion sickness or morning sickness. Ginger also has anti-inflammatory properties, making it useful for soothing sore muscles and joint pain. Try ginger tea or add fresh ginger to your meals for its health benefits.

Chamomile for Relaxation and Sleep: Chamomile is well-loved for its calming effects, making it a perfect herb for reducing stress and promoting better sleep. Barbara suggests sipping chamomile tea in the evening to help unwind and prepare for restful sleep.

Echinacea for Immune Support: Echinacea is renowned for its immune-boosting properties. Barbara explains that it's often used to help prevent or reduce the duration of colds and flu. Echinacea supplements or teas can be a great addition to your wellness routine, especially during cold and flu season.

Lavender for Stress Relief and Sleep: Lavender is not only a fragrant herb but also a powerful tool for managing stress and improving sleep quality. Barbara recommends using lavender essential oil in a diffuser or adding a few drops to a warm bath to help you relax after a long day.

Turmeric for Inflammation: Turmeric contains curcumin, a compound with strong anti-inflammatory properties. Barbara notes that turmeric can be beneficial for conditions like arthritis and muscle pain. Incorporate turmeric into your cooking or take it as a supplement to help manage inflammation.

Lemon Balm for Anxiety and Digestive Health: Lemon balm is a gentle herb known for its calming effects on the nervous system. Barbara suggests using lemon balm tea to alleviate anxiety and improve digestion. It's a soothing choice for promoting a sense of calm and relaxation.

Thyme for Respiratory Health: Thyme has antimicrobial and expectorant properties, making it useful for respiratory issues like coughs and colds. Barbara points out that thyme tea or steam inhalation with thyme can help clear congestion and soothe the throat.

Garlic for Immune and Cardiovascular Health: Garlic is not only a flavorful addition to meals but also a potent herb for supporting immune and cardiovascular health. Barbara discusses its use in reducing blood pressure and cholesterol levels. Incorporate garlic into your diet for its heart-healthy benefits.

Aloe Vera for Skin Irritations: Aloe vera is well-known for its soothing effects on the skin. Barbara highlights its use in treating minor burns, cuts, and sunburns. Apply aloe vera gel directly to the affected area for quick relief and healing.

Anti-Inflammatory Herbs and Their Benefits

Inflammation is a natural response by the body to injury or infection, but when it becomes chronic, it can lead to various health issues. Fortunately, many herbs offer natural anti-inflammatory properties that can help manage and reduce inflammation. Barbara O'Neill delves into some of these powerful herbs and their benefits, providing insights on how they can support your health.

Turmeric: Turmeric is perhaps the most well-known anti-inflammatory herb. Barbara explains that its active compound, curcumin, has strong anti-inflammatory and antioxidant effects. Turmeric can help reduce pain and swelling associated with conditions like arthritis. Incorporate turmeric into your diet through curries, teas, or supplements for its potent benefits.

Ginger: Ginger is another herb with notable anti-inflammatory properties. Barbara points out that ginger can help relieve pain and inflammation, particularly in the joints. It's also beneficial for digestive inflammation. Enjoy ginger in your meals, teas, or as a supplement to harness its healing potential.

Boswellia: Boswellia, also known as frankincense, is an herb used in traditional medicine for its anti-inflammatory effects. Barbara highlights its role in reducing symptoms of inflammatory conditions such as arthritis and asthma. Boswellia supplements can be a helpful addition to support overall inflammation management.

Green Tea: Green tea contains polyphenols, which are powerful antioxidants with anti-inflammatory properties. Barbara discusses how regular consumption of green tea can help reduce inflammation and support overall health. Enjoy a cup of green tea daily to benefit from its soothing effects.

Willow Bark: Willow bark has been used historically for its pain-relieving and anti-inflammatory properties. Barbara explains that it contains salicin, which is similar to aspirin. Willow bark can help alleviate pain and inflammation, especially in cases of chronic pain. It's available in supplement form or as a tea.

Devil's Claw: Devil's claw is an herb native to Southern Africa, known for its anti-inflammatory and pain-relieving properties. Barbara points out that it's often used to treat arthritis and other inflammatory conditions. Devil's claw supplements can be an effective way to manage inflammation and support joint health.

Rosemary: Rosemary is not only a fragrant herb but also one with anti-inflammatory benefits. Barbara explains that its antioxidant compounds can help reduce inflammation and improve circulation. Use rosemary in cooking or as a herbal tea for its beneficial effects.

Cat's Claw: Cat's claw is a vine native to the Amazon rainforest with notable anti-inflammatory properties. Barbara highlights its use in treating inflammatory conditions and boosting immune function. Cat's claw is available in supplement form and can be a valuable addition to your health regimen.

Cayenne Pepper: Cayenne pepper contains capsaicin, which has anti-inflammatory and pain-relieving effects. Barbara discusses how cayenne pepper can help reduce inflammation and support digestive health. Add a pinch of cayenne pepper to your meals or use it in topical preparations for its soothing benefits.

Echinacea: While primarily known for its immune-boosting properties, echinacea also has anti-inflammatory effects. Barbara notes that it can help reduce inflammation related to respiratory infections and support overall immune health. Echinacea tea or supplements can be useful for managing inflammation.

Herbal Treatments for the Digestive System

The digestive system plays a crucial role in our overall health, and maintaining its balance is essential for well-being. Barbara O'Neill explores a variety of herbs that can support digestive health and alleviate common digestive issues. Here's a guide to some effective herbal treatments for the digestive system:

Peppermint: Peppermint is well-known for its soothing effects on the digestive tract. Barbara highlights its ability to relieve symptoms of indigestion, bloating, and gas. Peppermint tea is a simple and effective way to calm an upset stomach and improve digestion. For additional relief, try peppermint oil capsules.

Ginger: Ginger is a versatile herb that has been used for centuries to aid digestion. Barbara explains that ginger can help alleviate nausea, motion sickness, and digestive discomfort. Fresh ginger or ginger tea can be particularly soothing after meals. It also has anti-inflammatory properties that support overall digestive health.

Chamomile: Chamomile is famous for its calming effects, not just for the mind but also for the digestive system. Barbara notes that chamomile tea can help reduce bloating, cramping, and indigestion. Its gentle nature makes it a great choice for soothing digestive issues and promoting relaxation.

Fennel: Fennel seeds have been traditionally used to ease digestive discomfort. Barbara points out that fennel can help relieve gas, bloating, and indigestion. Chewing on fennel seeds after meals or drinking fennel tea can aid in digestion and provide relief from common digestive complaints.

Licorice Root: Licorice root is known for its soothing properties on the digestive tract. Barbara explains that it can help with symptoms of heartburn, gastritis, and ulcers. Licorice root tea or supplements can provide relief, but it's important to use it in moderation and consult with a healthcare provider if you have high blood pressure.

Slippery Elm: Slippery elm has a unique ability to coat and soothe the digestive tract. Barbara highlights its use in treating conditions like acid reflux and irritable bowel syndrome (IBS). Slippery elm powder can be mixed with water to create a soothing drink that helps calm the digestive lining.

Dandelion: Dandelion is often overlooked but has beneficial properties for digestive health. Barbara points out that dandelion root can support liver function and stimulate digestion. Dandelion tea or supplements can aid in detoxifying the liver and improving overall digestive efficiency.

Marshmallow Root: Marshmallow root is known for its mucilaginous properties, which help to soothe and protect the digestive lining. Barbara explains that it can be beneficial for conditions like gastritis and ulcers. Marshmallow root tea or capsules can provide relief from irritation and inflammation.

Coriander: Coriander seeds have digestive benefits that Barbara highlights, including their ability to relieve bloating and gas. Coriander can be added to dishes or brewed into a tea to aid digestion and support gastrointestinal health.

Aloe Vera: Aloe vera is often associated with skincare, but it also has benefits for the digestive system. Barbara discusses how aloe vera juice can help soothe the digestive tract and support healthy bowel movements. It's a gentle way to improve digestion and reduce inflammation in the gut.

Immune-Boosting Herbs for Preventative Care

Maintaining a strong immune system is key to preventing illness and staying healthy. Barbara O'Neill emphasizes the power of herbs in supporting immune function and providing a natural boost to your body's defenses. Here's a look at some of the top immune-boosting herbs that can enhance your preventative care routine:

Echinacea: Echinacea is widely recognized for its immune-supportive properties. Barbara explains that it can help stimulate the immune system and increase resistance to infections. Whether taken as a tea, tincture, or supplement, echinacea is a great herb to include during cold and flu season for its preventative benefits.

Elderberry: Elderberry is celebrated for its antiviral properties. Barbara highlights that it can help reduce the duration and severity of colds and flu. Elderberry syrup or capsules are commonly used as a preventative measure to support immune health and fend off illness.

Astragalus: Astragalus is an adaptogenic herb known for its ability to strengthen the immune system. Barbara points out that it helps the body adapt to stress and enhances overall immune function. Astragalus can be taken in tea or supplement form to provide ongoing support for your immune system.

Garlic: Garlic isn't just a flavorful addition to meals—it's also a powerful immune booster. Barbara explains that garlic has antimicrobial and antiviral properties, making it effective in preventing infections. Incorporate garlic into your diet or take it as a supplement to support immune health.

Ginger: Ginger is well-known for its anti-inflammatory and immune-boosting effects. Barbara discusses how ginger can help combat infections and strengthen the immune system. Enjoy ginger in teas, smoothies, or as a culinary spice to harness its immune-supportive benefits.

Reishi Mushroom: Reishi mushroom is revered in traditional medicine for its immune-enhancing properties. Barbara notes that it can help regulate and support the immune system. Reishi is commonly available in supplement form and can be a valuable addition to your preventative health regimen.

Shiitake Mushroom: Shiitake mushrooms are not only delicious but also beneficial for immune health. Barbara highlights their role in boosting immune function and supporting overall well-being. Shiitake mushrooms can be enjoyed in soups, stir-fries, or taken as a supplement.

Licorice Root: Licorice root has immune-boosting and anti-inflammatory properties. Barbara explains that it can support the immune system and help reduce symptoms of respiratory infections. Licorice root tea or supplements can be used to enhance immune function and overall health.

Holy Basil (Tulsi): Holy basil, also known as tulsi, is an adaptogen that supports immune health and reduces stress. Barbara points out that it helps balance the body's systems and enhance overall vitality. Tulsi tea or supplements can be a great addition to your daily routine for immune support.

Oregano: Oregano is more than just a culinary herb; it also has powerful immune-boosting properties. Barbara discusses how oregano oil contains compounds that support immune function and fight infections. Use oregano in your cooking or take it as an oil supplement for its preventative benefits.

How to Grow and Harvest Medicinal Herbs

Growing your own medicinal herbs can be incredibly rewarding, both for their healing properties and for the joy of tending to a garden. Barbara O'Neill provides practical tips and advice on how to cultivate and harvest these beneficial plants, making it easier for you to enjoy their full potential.

Choosing the Right Herbs: Start by selecting herbs that are suited to your climate and soil conditions. Barbara recommends beginning with hardy herbs like peppermint, lavender, and chamomile, which are relatively easy to grow and maintain. Research the specific needs of each herb to ensure they thrive in your garden.

Preparing the Soil: Healthy soil is essential for growing medicinal herbs. Barbara suggests enriching the soil with organic matter such as compost or well-rotted manure. Ensure the soil is well-draining and has a pH level suited to the herbs you plan to grow. Testing the soil can help you make any necessary adjustments.

Planting Herbs: When planting herbs, Barbara advises spacing them according to their mature size to avoid overcrowding. Follow the planting instructions on seed packets or plant labels, as each herb has its own requirements for depth and spacing. Planting herbs at the right time of year is also crucial—some herbs prefer cool weather, while others thrive in warmer conditions.

Watering and Care: Regular watering is important, but Barbara emphasizes the need to avoid overwatering. Most medicinal herbs prefer soil that is slightly dry between waterings. Mulching around the plants can help retain moisture and reduce weeds. Additionally, provide adequate sunlight, as most herbs require full sun to grow robustly.

Pruning and Harvesting: Pruning herbs not only keeps them healthy but also encourages new growth. Barbara suggests harvesting herbs just before they reach full maturity for the best flavor and medicinal properties. For most herbs, the leaves are the primary part used, and they should be harvested in the morning after the dew has dried.

Drying Herbs: Proper drying is essential to preserve the medicinal properties of herbs. Barbara recommends hanging herbs in small bunches in a cool, dry place with good airflow. Alternatively, use a dehydrator or an oven set to a low temperature. Once dried, store herbs in airtight containers away from light and moisture.

Harvesting Specific Herbs:

- Peppermint: Harvest the leaves just before the plant starts to flower for the strongest flavor and medicinal benefits.
- Lavender: Cut the flower spikes when the buds are just starting to open. Bundle and hang them to dry.
- Chamomile: Pick the flowers when they are fully open but before they start to wilt. Dry them gently to preserve their delicate properties.

Storing Herbs: Once dried, Barbara advises labeling your jars with the herb's name and the date of harvest. Store herbs in a cool, dark place to maintain their potency. Properly stored, dried herbs can retain their medicinal properties for up to a year.

Using Fresh vs. Dried Herbs: While dried herbs are convenient for long-term storage, Barbara notes that fresh herbs can offer a more vibrant flavor and medicinal potency. Use fresh herbs when possible, and consider growing a small supply of both fresh and dried herbs for various needs.

Making Herbal Preparations at Home

Creating your own herbal preparations is a wonderful way to harness the healing power of plants and ensure that you're using high-quality, natural remedies. Barbara O'Neill offers practical tips for making a variety of herbal preparations right in your kitchen. Here's a friendly guide to get you started on making herbal preparations at home:

Herbal Teas: Herbal teas are one of the simplest ways to enjoy the benefits of herbs. Barbara suggests using fresh or dried herbs to make your tea. To prepare:

- **Boil Water:** Start by boiling water and letting it cool slightly before pouring over your herbs.
- **Steep the Herbs:** Place 1-2 teaspoons of dried herbs or a handful of fresh herbs in a teapot or cup. Pour the hot water over the herbs and let them steep for 5-10 minutes.
- **Strain and Enjoy:** Strain the herbs out and enjoy your tea. You can add honey or lemon for extra flavor.

Infused Oils: Infused oils are great for making soothing topical treatments. Barbara explains that they are used in balms, salves, and massage oils. To make an infused oil:

- Choose Your Herb: Select herbs known for their skin benefits, like lavender or calendula.
- Combine Herbs and Oil: Place your dried herbs in a clean jar and cover with a carrier oil (such as olive oil or coconut oil). Seal the jar and let it sit in a warm, sunny place for 2-4 weeks, shaking it gently every few days.
- Strain and Store: After infusing, strain out the herbs using a fine mesh strainer or cheesecloth. Store the infused oil in a clean, dark bottle.

Herbal Tinctures: Tinctures are concentrated extracts of herbs that can be taken in small doses. Barbara notes that they are made by soaking herbs in alcohol or vinegar. To make a tincture:

- Prepare the Herbs: Chop dried or fresh herbs and place them in a jar.

- Add Alcohol or Vinegar: Cover the herbs with high-proof alcohol (like vodka) or apple cider vinegar. Seal the jar tightly.
- Infuse: Let the mixture sit in a cool, dark place for 4-6 weeks, shaking it daily.
- Strain and Bottle: Strain the herbs out and transfer the tincture to a dropper bottle. Take the recommended dose as needed.

Herbal Salves and Balms: Salves and balms are excellent for soothing skin issues and providing relief to sore muscles. Barbara provides a basic recipe for making them:

- Infuse the Oil: Start with an infused oil of your choice, as described above.
- Melt Beeswax: Gently melt beeswax in a double boiler (about 1 part beeswax to 4 parts infused oil).
- Combine and Pour: Once the beeswax is melted, mix it with the infused oil and pour into tins or jars. Let it cool and harden before using.

Herbal Syrups: Herbal syrups are tasty and effective for soothing sore throats and coughs. Barbara's method includes:

- Prepare an Herbal Infusion: Make a strong tea from your chosen herbs (like elderberry or ginger).
- Add Sweetener: Add honey or maple syrup to the warm infusion and stir until well combined. Use about 1 part honey for every 1 part herbal tea.
- Store and Use: Pour the syrup into a clean bottle and store in the refrigerator. Take a spoonful as needed.

Herbal Baths: Herbal baths can be incredibly relaxing and therapeutic. Barbara suggests:

- Prepare Herbal Sachets: Place dried herbs (like chamomile or lavender) in a muslin bag or cheesecloth. Tie it closed.
- Add to Bath: Place the sachet under the running water as the tub fills. Let it steep in the bathwater before soaking.

Tips for Success:

- Use Quality Herbs: Ensure you're using fresh or well-dried herbs to get the most out of your preparations.
- Label Everything: Clearly label your preparations with the date and contents.
- Consult Resources: For dosage and specific uses, refer to reliable herbal guides or consult with a herbalist.

Safety and Precautions with Herbal Use

Herbs can be powerful allies in promoting health and healing, but it's essential to use them safely to avoid potential risks. Barbara O'Neill emphasizes the importance of understanding how to use herbs responsibly and provides helpful tips for ensuring safe and effective herbal use.

Start Slow: When trying a new herb, Barbara recommends starting with a small dose to see how your body responds. This gradual approach allows you to monitor for any adverse reactions and gauge the herb's effectiveness before increasing the dosage.

Know Your Herbs: It's crucial to research any herb you plan to use. Barbara suggests familiarizing yourself with its benefits, potential side effects, and interactions with other medications or herbs. Reliable sources include herbal guides, reputable websites, and consultations with trained herbalists.

Consult with Healthcare Providers: If you're pregnant, nursing, or taking prescription medications, it's wise to consult with a healthcare professional before using herbal remedies. Barbara advises checking for any possible interactions or contraindications that might affect your health.

Quality Matters: Use high-quality herbs from reputable sources to ensure their safety and potency. Barbara cautions against using herbs from unknown or questionable sources, as they might be contaminated or incorrectly identified.

Understand Dosages: Herbal preparations vary in potency, and dosages can differ based on the form of the herb (tea, tincture, etc.). Barbara emphasizes following recommended dosages and guidelines, and if in doubt, seek advice from a knowledgeable herbalist.

Be Aware of Allergies: Just like with any substance, you may be allergic to certain herbs. Barbara suggests doing a patch test for topical preparations and starting with small amounts of herbal teas or tinctures to check for allergic reactions before using them regularly.

Avoid Overuse: More is not always better when it comes to herbs. Barbara advises against excessive use, which can lead to potential side effects or diminish the herb's effectiveness. Stick to recommended dosages and avoid using multiple herbs with similar effects simultaneously without guidance.

Pregnancy and Nursing: Certain herbs may not be safe during pregnancy or breastfeeding. Barbara recommends consulting with a healthcare provider to ensure the herbs you use are safe for you and your baby.

Children and Pets: When using herbs around children or pets, Barbara advises being cautious. Some herbs that are safe for adults may not be suitable for young children or animals. Always research and seek advice on appropriate herbal use for these groups.

Monitor and Adjust: Keep track of how you feel after using herbs and make adjustments as needed. Barbara suggests noting any changes in symptoms or side effects and discontinuing use if you experience any adverse effects.

Label and Store Properly: Ensure all your herbal preparations are clearly labeled with the name, date, and contents. Store them in a cool, dry place, away from direct sunlight, to maintain their potency and safety.

Seek Professional Advice: When in doubt, Barbara encourages seeking advice from a qualified herbalist or healthcare provider. They can provide personalized recommendations based on your individual health needs and circumstances.

Book 5: Natural Remedies for Women's Health

Hormonal Balance and Natural Approaches

Maintaining hormonal balance is crucial for overall well-being, and Barbara O'Neill offers insightful guidance on how natural approaches can help. Hormones influence many aspects of health, from mood and energy levels to reproductive health and metabolism. Here's a friendly guide to achieving hormonal balance using natural methods.

Understand Your Hormones: Hormones are chemical messengers that regulate various bodily functions. Barbara emphasizes the importance of understanding how different hormones, such as estrogen, progesterone, and cortisol, impact your body. Knowledge about your hormone levels can help you make informed choices for balancing them naturally.

Eat a Balanced Diet: A diet rich in whole foods can support hormonal health. Barbara suggests focusing on:

- Fruits and Vegetables: They provide essential vitamins, minerals, and antioxidants that support hormone production and regulation.
- Healthy Fats: Include sources like avocados, nuts, seeds, and fatty fish to support hormone synthesis.
- Lean Proteins: Foods such as poultry, beans, and legumes help stabilize blood sugar levels, which is crucial for hormonal balance.
- Whole Grains: Choose complex carbohydrates like oats and quinoa to provide steady energy and prevent insulin spikes.

Incorporate Phytoestrogens: Phytoestrogens are plant compounds that can mimic the effects of estrogen in the body. Barbara highlights foods such as flaxseeds, soy products, and legumes as great sources of phytoestrogens. They can help balance estrogen levels, especially during menopause or in cases of hormonal imbalance.

Manage Stress: Chronic stress can disrupt hormonal balance by increasing cortisol levels. Barbara recommends stress-reducing practices such as:

- Mindfulness and Meditation: Regular mindfulness exercises can help lower stress and improve emotional well-being.
- Exercise: Engaging in physical activity can reduce stress and promote overall health.
- Relaxation Techniques: Activities like yoga, deep breathing, and journaling can also help manage stress.

Get Regular Exercise: Regular physical activity supports hormonal balance by improving insulin sensitivity and reducing stress. Barbara suggests incorporating a mix of aerobic exercises, strength training, and flexibility exercises into your routine.

Prioritize Sleep: Quality sleep is essential for hormonal regulation. Barbara emphasizes the need for:

- Consistent Sleep Schedule: Go to bed and wake up at the same time every day.
- Sleep Environment: Create a restful environment by keeping your bedroom cool, dark, and quiet.

Herbal Support: Certain herbs are known for their ability to support hormonal balance. Barbara points out:

- Chaste Tree (Vitex): Often used to support progesterone levels and alleviate symptoms of PMS.
- Ashwagandha: Known for its adaptogenic properties, which help the body cope with stress.
- Red Clover: Contains phytoestrogens that may help manage menopause symptoms.

Avoid Endocrine Disruptors: Barbara advises reducing exposure to chemicals that can interfere with hormone function. These include:

- Plastic Products: Opt for glass or stainless steel instead of plastic containers.
- Personal Care Products: Choose natural or organic skincare and cosmetics.
- Pesticides: Wash fruits and vegetables thoroughly or choose organic options when possible.

Stay Hydrated: Proper hydration supports overall health, including hormonal function. Barbara suggests drinking plenty of water throughout the day and limiting caffeinated and sugary beverages.

Monitor Your Symptoms: Keeping track of your symptoms can help you identify patterns and make necessary adjustments. Barbara recommends using a journal or app to record your menstrual cycle, mood changes, and any other relevant symptoms.

Consult a Professional: If you have persistent hormonal issues, Barbara encourages seeking advice from a healthcare provider or a specialist in natural medicine. They can offer personalized recommendations and treatments based on your individual needs.

Herbs and Supplements for Menstrual Health

Menstrual health plays a significant role in overall well-being, and Barbara O'Neill advocates for natural remedies to support a healthy cycle. By incorporating certain herbs and supplements, you can manage symptoms and promote balance. Here's a friendly guide to some effective options for menstrual health.

Chaste Tree (Vitex): Chaste Tree is renowned for its ability to support hormonal balance and alleviate symptoms of premenstrual syndrome (PMS). Barbara highlights its role in regulating progesterone levels, which can help ease symptoms like mood swings, breast tenderness, and irregular cycles. It's usually taken as a tincture, capsule, or tea.

Red Clover: Known for its high content of phytoestrogens, Red Clover can be beneficial for managing symptoms of menopause and irregular periods. Barbara suggests using it as a tea or supplement to help balance estrogen levels and support overall reproductive health.

Evening Primrose Oil: This oil is rich in gamma-linolenic acid (GLA), an essential fatty acid that can help reduce PMS symptoms, including breast pain and mood swings. Barbara recommends taking it in capsule form for a few weeks before your menstrual cycle begins.

Ginger: Ginger has natural anti-inflammatory properties and can be very soothing for menstrual cramps. Barbara suggests drinking ginger tea or incorporating fresh ginger into your meals. It helps to reduce pain and improve digestion, which can be particularly beneficial during menstruation.

Turmeric: With its powerful anti-inflammatory and antioxidant properties, turmeric can help with menstrual cramps and overall menstrual health. Barbara recommends adding turmeric to your diet or taking it in supplement form to ease pain and support general wellness.

Dong Quai: Often referred to as the "female ginseng," Dong Quai is traditionally used in Chinese medicine to support menstrual health and alleviate symptoms like cramps and irregular periods. Barbara suggests taking it as a tea or in capsule form, but advises consulting with a healthcare provider before starting.

Magnesium: This mineral plays a key role in muscle relaxation and can help ease menstrual cramps. Barbara points out that magnesium supplements or magnesium-rich foods like leafy greens, nuts, and seeds can be particularly helpful during your period.

Calcium: Adequate calcium intake is essential for overall health and can help reduce PMS symptoms. Barbara recommends consuming calcium-rich foods like dairy products, fortified plant-based milks, or taking a supplement if needed.

Vitamin B6: This vitamin is crucial for hormone regulation and can help alleviate PMS symptoms such as mood swings and irritability. Barbara suggests incorporating foods high in Vitamin B6, like bananas, avocados, and poultry, or considering a supplement.

Peppermint: Peppermint tea is a soothing option for relieving menstrual cramps and digestive issues. Barbara notes its antispasmodic properties, which can help relax uterine muscles and reduce discomfort.

Cramp Bark: This herb is specifically known for its antispasmodic properties, which can help alleviate menstrual cramps. Barbara recommends using it in tincture or capsule form, especially if you experience intense cramping.

How to Use Herbs and Supplements Safely:

- Start Slowly: Introduce one herb or supplement at a time to gauge your body's response.
- Consult a Professional: Before starting any new supplement or herb, especially if you have underlying health conditions or are pregnant, Barbara advises consulting with a healthcare provider.
- Choose Quality Products: Opt for high-quality, reputable brands to ensure safety and effectiveness.

Natural Solutions for Menopause Symptoms

Navigating menopause can be a challenging time, but Barbara O'Neill offers a range of natural solutions to help manage symptoms and support overall well-being. Embracing these natural remedies can ease the transition and promote a healthier, more balanced life during this phase. Here's a friendly guide to some effective natural solutions for menopause symptoms.

Phytoestrogens: Phytoestrogens are plant compounds that can mimic estrogen in the body, helping to balance hormone levels. Barbara suggests incorporating foods like soy products, flaxseeds, and lentils into your diet. These can help alleviate symptoms like hot flashes and night sweats by providing a gentle, plant-based source of estrogen.

Black Cohosh: This herb is commonly used to manage menopausal symptoms, particularly hot flashes and mood swings. Barbara recommends taking Black Cohosh in supplement form or as a tea. It's important to consult with a healthcare provider before starting any new supplement, especially if you have other health conditions.

Red Clover: Rich in phytoestrogens, Red Clover can help with hot flashes and overall hormonal balance. Barbara suggests using it as a tea or supplement to support menopausal health. It's also known for its potential benefits in improving bone density and cardiovascular health.

Evening Primrose Oil: This oil contains gamma-linolenic acid (GLA), which can help reduce menopausal symptoms such as hot flashes, breast tenderness, and mood swings. Barbara advises taking Evening Primrose Oil in capsule form to experience its full benefits.

Dong Quai: Often used in Traditional Chinese Medicine, Dong Quai is believed to support hormonal balance and relieve menopausal symptoms like hot flashes and fatigue. Barbara suggests incorporating it into your routine as a tea or supplement, after consulting with a healthcare provider.

Ginseng: Ginseng is known for its adaptogenic properties, which can help manage stress and fatigue during menopause. Barbara highlights its potential to boost energy levels and improve mood. Ginseng can be taken as a supplement or enjoyed as a tea.

Vitamin E: This vitamin is thought to help reduce the frequency and severity of hot flashes. Barbara recommends including Vitamin E-rich foods like nuts, seeds, and green leafy vegetables in your diet or considering a supplement if needed.

Calcium and Vitamin D: Menopause can impact bone health, making calcium and Vitamin D essential. Barbara suggests consuming calcium-rich foods like dairy products or fortified plant-based milks and getting enough Vitamin D through sunlight exposure or supplements to support bone density and overall health.

Herbal Teas: Herbal teas such as chamomile, peppermint, and ginger can offer relief from menopausal symptoms. Barbara recommends drinking these teas to help with relaxation, digestion, and managing hot flashes.

Lifestyle Changes: Alongside herbal remedies, Barbara emphasizes the importance of lifestyle changes:

- Healthy Diet: Focus on a balanced diet rich in whole foods, including fruits, vegetables, whole grains, and lean proteins.
- Regular Exercise: Engage in regular physical activity to boost mood, manage weight, and improve overall health.
- Stress Management: Practice relaxation techniques like mindfulness, yoga, or deep breathing to reduce stress and support emotional well-being.

Hydration: Staying well-hydrated can help with dryness and other menopausal symptoms. Barbara advises drinking plenty of water throughout the day and limiting caffeine and alcohol, which can exacerbate symptoms.

Sleep Hygiene: Quality sleep is essential for managing menopause symptoms. Barbara suggests establishing a consistent sleep routine, creating a comfortable sleep environment, and avoiding stimulants before bedtime.

Fertility and Pregnancy: Safe Natural Remedies

When it comes to supporting fertility and a healthy pregnancy, Barbara O'Neill emphasizes the importance of natural remedies that are gentle and effective. These remedies can help enhance fertility, support a healthy pregnancy, and nurture both mother and baby. Here's a friendly guide to some safe and natural options:

Fertility-Boosting Herbs: Certain herbs are known for their potential to support reproductive health and enhance fertility.

- Red Clover: Rich in phytoestrogens, Red Clover can help balance hormones and support reproductive health. Barbara suggests using it as a tea or supplement to promote overall fertility.
- Chaste Tree (Vitex): This herb is renowned for its ability to regulate menstrual cycles and support progesterone levels, which can enhance fertility. Barbara recommends taking it in tincture or capsule form.

Nutrient-Rich Diet: A balanced diet is crucial for fertility and a healthy pregnancy.

- Leafy Greens: Foods like spinach, kale, and Swiss chard are high in folate, which is essential for preventing neural tube defects and supporting overall reproductive health.
- Whole Grains: Include whole grains like quinoa, brown rice, and oats to ensure a steady supply of energy and essential nutrients.
- Lean Proteins: Incorporate sources of lean protein such as chicken, fish, and legumes to support hormonal balance and overall health.

Omega-3 Fatty Acids: Omega-3s play a crucial role in hormone production and overall reproductive health. Barbara suggests including fatty fish like salmon, walnuts, and flaxseeds in your diet or considering an omega-3 supplement.

Hydration: Staying hydrated is vital for fertility and pregnancy health. Barbara recommends drinking plenty of water throughout the day to support bodily functions and maintain amniotic fluid levels.

Exercise: Regular, moderate exercise can support fertility and a healthy pregnancy. Barbara advises incorporating activities like walking, swimming, and prenatal yoga to enhance circulation, reduce stress, and promote overall wellness.

Stress Management: Managing stress is important for both fertility and pregnancy. Techniques like meditation, deep breathing exercises, and gentle yoga can help reduce stress and improve overall health. Barbara emphasizes the importance of finding relaxation methods that work best for you.

Avoiding Toxins: Reducing exposure to environmental toxins can support fertility and a healthy pregnancy. Barbara suggests opting for natural cleaning products, avoiding processed foods, and minimizing exposure to chemicals and pollutants.

Prenatal Vitamins: While focusing on a nutrient-rich diet is key, Barbara highlights the importance of taking a high-quality prenatal vitamin to ensure you're getting essential nutrients like folic acid, iron, and calcium, which are crucial for a healthy pregnancy.

Acupuncture: Some studies suggest that acupuncture may help improve fertility by balancing hormones and increasing blood flow to the reproductive organs. Barbara recommends consulting with a qualified acupuncturist for personalized treatment.

Herbal Teas for Pregnancy: Certain herbal teas can offer gentle support during pregnancy:

- Raspberry Leaf Tea: Known for its potential to tone the uterine muscles and support labor, Barbara suggests drinking raspberry leaf tea in the second trimester.
- Ginger Tea: Ginger can help with nausea and digestive issues, making it a comforting option during the early stages of pregnancy.

Healthy Sleep Habits: Adequate rest is essential for fertility and a healthy pregnancy. Barbara advises establishing a consistent sleep routine and creating a restful sleep environment to support overall well-being.

Regular Check-ups: While natural remedies can support fertility and pregnancy, Barbara emphasizes the importance of regular check-ups with a healthcare provider to monitor your health and ensure a safe and healthy pregnancy.

Breast Health and Cancer Prevention

Maintaining breast health and focusing on cancer prevention are crucial aspects of women's wellness. Barbara O'Neill advocates for natural approaches that support breast health and reduce the risk of cancer. Here's a friendly guide to some effective, natural strategies:

Balanced Diet: A nutritious diet is key to supporting overall breast health and reducing cancer risk.

- Fruits and Vegetables: Barbara recommends a diet rich in colorful fruits and vegetables, which are high in antioxidants and vitamins. Foods like berries, broccoli, and carrots help combat oxidative stress and support immune function.
- Whole Grains: Incorporate whole grains such as quinoa, brown rice, and oats into your meals to provide fiber and essential nutrients.
- Healthy Fats: Include sources of healthy fats like avocados, nuts, seeds, and olive oil. These fats support hormonal balance and overall cellular health.

Phytoestrogens: Phytoestrogens are plant compounds that can mimic estrogen in the body, potentially balancing hormone levels.

- Flaxseeds: Flaxseeds are rich in lignans, a type of phytoestrogen that may help protect against hormone-related cancers. Barbara suggests adding flaxseeds to smoothies or oatmeal.
- Soy Products: Foods like tofu and edamame contain isoflavones, another type of phytoestrogen. Including moderate amounts in your diet can support hormonal health.

Cruciferous Vegetables: Vegetables such as broccoli, Brussels sprouts, and cauliflower contain compounds that support detoxification and may help reduce cancer risk. Barbara emphasizes the importance of these veggies in your diet for their potential protective effects.

Regular Exercise: Physical activity plays a significant role in maintaining breast health and reducing cancer risk. Barbara advises engaging in regular exercise, such as walking, swimming, or strength training, to promote overall health and support a healthy weight.

Stress Management: Chronic stress can impact hormone levels and overall health. Barbara suggests practicing stress-reducing techniques like mindfulness, yoga, or deep breathing exercises to maintain emotional and physical well-being.

Regular Screenings: Early detection is crucial for effective cancer prevention. Barbara underscores the importance of regular mammograms, clinical breast exams, and self-breast exams to monitor breast health and catch any potential issues early.

Avoiding Toxins: Reducing exposure to environmental toxins can support breast health. Barbara recommends opting for natural personal care products, avoiding excessive exposure to plastics, and choosing organic foods when possible to minimize exposure to harmful chemicals.

Herbal Support: Certain herbs may offer additional support for breast health.

- Turmeric: Known for its anti-inflammatory and antioxidant properties, turmeric may help support overall breast health. Barbara suggests incorporating it into your diet or taking it as a supplement.
- Green Tea: Rich in antioxidants called catechins, green tea may help protect against cellular damage. Drinking green tea regularly can be a beneficial addition to your routine.

Healthy Weight Management: Maintaining a healthy weight is important for reducing breast cancer risk. Barbara advises focusing on a balanced diet and regular exercise to support a healthy weight and overall well-being.

Hydration: Staying well-hydrated supports overall health and detoxification. Barbara recommends drinking plenty of water throughout the day to help your body stay balanced and support breast health.

Sleep Hygiene: Quality sleep is essential for overall health. Barbara emphasizes the importance of establishing a consistent sleep routine and creating a restful sleep environment to support your body's natural repair processes.

Emotional Well-being: Maintaining emotional health is crucial for overall wellness. Barbara suggests finding activities that bring joy and relaxation, and seeking support if needed to manage stress and promote a positive outlook.

Managing Stress and Emotional Health in Women

Stress and emotional health are integral to overall well-being, and Barbara O'Neill offers valuable insights on managing these aspects naturally. For women, balancing daily demands with emotional and physical health can be challenging, but adopting a holistic approach can make a significant difference. Here's a friendly guide to managing stress and supporting emotional health:

Recognize Stress Triggers: Understanding what triggers stress in your life is the first step towards managing it effectively. Barbara suggests keeping a journal to identify patterns and triggers, which can help you address the root causes of stress.

Mindfulness and Meditation: Mindfulness practices can be incredibly effective for reducing stress and promoting emotional well-being. Barbara recommends incorporating mindfulness or meditation into your daily routine. Even just a few minutes each day can help calm the mind and reduce anxiety.

Deep Breathing Exercises: Deep breathing is a simple yet powerful tool for managing stress. Barbara suggests practicing deep breathing exercises, such as inhaling deeply through your nose for a count of four, holding for four, and exhaling slowly through your mouth for another count of four. This can help lower stress levels and improve mental clarity.

Regular Physical Activity: Exercise is a natural stress reliever and mood booster. Barbara advises engaging in regular physical activity that you enjoy, whether it's walking, dancing, swimming, or yoga. Exercise helps release endorphins, which can improve mood and reduce feelings of stress.

Healthy Diet: Eating a balanced diet plays a crucial role in managing stress and maintaining emotional health. Barbara recommends including plenty of fruits, vegetables, whole grains, and lean proteins in your diet. Foods rich in omega-3 fatty acids, such as salmon and flaxseeds, can also support brain health and mood stability.

Quality Sleep: Adequate and restful sleep is essential for managing stress and maintaining emotional balance. Barbara emphasizes the importance of establishing a consistent sleep routine, creating a relaxing bedtime environment, and aiming for 7-9 hours of sleep each night.

Supportive Relationships: Having a strong support network can make a big difference in managing stress. Barbara encourages nurturing positive relationships with family and friends, as social support provides comfort and helps alleviate feelings of isolation.

Relaxation Techniques: Finding relaxation techniques that work for you can help manage stress. Barbara suggests exploring options like progressive muscle relaxation, aromatherapy with essential oils, or taking a warm bath. These activities can promote relaxation and reduce stress levels.

Set Boundaries: Learning to set healthy boundaries is important for managing stress. Barbara advises being mindful of your limits and not overcommitting yourself. It's okay to say no when necessary and prioritize self-care.

Creative Outlets: Engaging in creative activities can be a great way to relieve stress and express emotions. Whether it's painting, writing, gardening, or playing a musical instrument, Barbara encourages finding a creative outlet that brings you joy and helps you unwind.

Seek Professional Help: If stress or emotional challenges become overwhelming, seeking professional help is a positive step. Barbara supports consulting with a therapist or counselor who can provide guidance and support tailored to your needs.

Self-Compassion: Practicing self-compassion involves being kind to yourself and acknowledging your efforts. Barbara highlights the importance of treating yourself with the same kindness and understanding that you would offer to a friend.

Engage in Enjoyable Activities: Make time for activities that bring you joy and relaxation. Barbara encourages finding hobbies or interests that you love, as they can provide a sense of fulfillment and help you manage stress.

Gratitude Practice: Cultivating a sense of gratitude can shift your focus from stressors to positive aspects of your life. Barbara suggests keeping a gratitude journal and noting things you're thankful for each day to boost your mood and perspective.

Detoxification for Women's Hormonal Health

Detoxification plays a key role in supporting hormonal health and overall well-being. Barbara O'Neill emphasizes that a well-functioning detoxification system helps balance hormones and maintain a healthy, vibrant body. Here's a friendly guide to understanding how detoxification can benefit women's hormonal health:

Understanding Hormonal Imbalance: Hormonal imbalances can affect various aspects of health, including mood, energy levels, and menstrual cycles. Barbara explains that detoxification helps eliminate excess hormones and toxins that may disrupt hormonal balance.

The Liver's Role: The liver is a central player in the body's detoxification process. Barbara highlights that a healthy liver is crucial for breaking down and eliminating excess hormones, such as estrogen, which can contribute to imbalances if not properly processed.

Supporting Liver Health: To support liver function, Barbara recommends incorporating liver-friendly foods into your diet:

- Leafy Greens: Spinach, kale, and dandelion greens are rich in nutrients that support liver health and aid in detoxification.
- Cruciferous Vegetables: Broccoli, Brussels sprouts, and cauliflower help boost liver enzymes and support the detoxification process.
- Beets: Beets are known for their detoxifying properties and can help improve liver function.

Hydration: Staying well-hydrated is essential for effective detoxification. Barbara advises drinking plenty of water throughout the day to help flush out toxins and support the body's natural detox processes.

Fiber-Rich Foods: Fiber helps the body eliminate waste and toxins effectively. Barbara recommends including fiber-rich foods such as fruits, vegetables, and whole grains in your diet to support healthy digestion and hormonal balance.

Herbal Support: Certain herbs can aid in detoxification and support hormonal health:

- Milk Thistle: Known for its liver-supportive properties, milk thistle helps protect and regenerate liver cells.
- Dandelion Root: Dandelion root supports liver function and acts as a gentle diuretic, promoting the elimination of excess fluids and toxins.
- Turmeric: With its anti-inflammatory properties, turmeric supports liver health and helps balance hormones.

Reducing Exposure to Toxins: Minimizing exposure to environmental toxins can support hormonal health. Barbara recommends opting for organic foods, using natural cleaning products, and avoiding plastics to reduce toxin exposure.

Balanced Diet: A balanced diet supports overall hormonal health. Barbara emphasizes the importance of eating a variety of nutrient-dense foods to provide essential vitamins and minerals that support detoxification and hormonal balance.

Regular Exercise: Physical activity promotes circulation and helps the body eliminate toxins through sweat. Barbara encourages incorporating regular exercise into your routine to support detoxification and overall health.

Quality Sleep: Adequate sleep is essential for the body's detoxification processes. Barbara highlights the importance of establishing a consistent sleep routine and creating a restful environment to support the body's natural repair processes.

Stress Management: Chronic stress can impact hormonal balance and detoxification. Barbara advises practicing stress-reducing techniques, such as mindfulness, yoga, or deep breathing exercises, to support hormonal health and overall well-being.

Detoxification Protocols: Periodic detoxification can help reset the body and support hormonal health. Barbara suggests gentle detox protocols, such as short-term detox diets or cleansing routines, to help eliminate accumulated toxins and support hormonal balance.

Consulting with a Healthcare Professional: Before starting any detoxification program, Barbara recommends consulting with a healthcare professional to ensure it's appropriate for your individual needs and health conditions.

Supporting Thyroid Function Naturally

The thyroid gland plays a crucial role in regulating metabolism, energy levels, and overall health. Barbara O'Neill offers practical and natural approaches to support thyroid function and maintain balance. Here's a friendly guide to nurturing your thyroid naturally:

Understanding Thyroid Health: The thyroid is a small but mighty gland located at the base of the neck. It produces hormones that regulate metabolism, energy, and growth. Barbara explains that supporting thyroid health is essential for overall well-being and vitality.

Balanced Diet: A nutrient-rich diet is vital for supporting thyroid function. Barbara recommends focusing on foods that are rich in key nutrients for thyroid health:

- Iodine: Essential for thyroid hormone production. Include iodine-rich foods like seaweed, fish, and dairy products.
- Selenium: Supports thyroid hormone synthesis and protects the thyroid gland. Good sources include Brazil nuts, sunflower seeds, and mushrooms.
- Zinc: Plays a role in thyroid hormone metabolism. Include zinc-rich foods such as pumpkin seeds, lentils, and chickpeas.

Avoiding Goitrogens: Goitrogens are substances that can interfere with thyroid function by inhibiting iodine uptake. Barbara suggests moderating the intake of raw cruciferous vegetables like broccoli, cauliflower, and cabbage, especially if you have thyroid concerns. Cooking these vegetables can reduce their goitrogenic effects.

Hydration: Staying well-hydrated supports overall health and helps the body function optimally. Barbara recommends drinking plenty of water throughout the day to aid in digestion and detoxification, which indirectly supports thyroid function.

Herbal Support: Certain herbs can help support thyroid health:

- Ashwagandha: Known for its adaptogenic properties, ashwagandha helps balance thyroid function and manage stress.
- Bladderwrack: A type of seaweed rich in iodine, bladderwrack supports thyroid health and hormone production.
- Guggul: This herb has been traditionally used to support thyroid function and promote healthy metabolism.

Regular Exercise: Physical activity helps maintain a healthy metabolism and supports thyroid function. Barbara encourages incorporating regular exercise, such as walking, jogging, or yoga, to keep your metabolism in check and support overall well-being.

Quality Sleep: Adequate sleep is crucial for hormonal balance and thyroid health. Barbara highlights the importance of establishing a consistent sleep routine and creating a restful sleep environment to support the body's natural repair processes.

Stress Management: Chronic stress can impact thyroid function and overall health. Barbara suggests practicing stress-reducing techniques such as mindfulness, meditation, or deep breathing exercises to help manage stress and support thyroid function.

Avoiding Environmental Toxins: Exposure to environmental toxins can affect thyroid health. Barbara advises reducing exposure to chemicals by using natural cleaning products, avoiding plastics, and opting for organic foods when possible.

Regular Health Check-ups: Regular check-ups with a healthcare provider can help monitor thyroid function and address any concerns. Barbara emphasizes the importance of staying informed about your thyroid health and working with a healthcare professional to ensure optimal function.

Detoxification: Periodic detoxification can support overall health and thyroid function. Barbara recommends gentle detox practices, such as consuming detoxifying foods, staying hydrated, and engaging in regular exercise to help support the body's natural detox processes.

Mindful Nutrition: Paying attention to how different foods affect your thyroid health can help you make informed dietary choices. Barbara suggests keeping a food journal to track how certain foods and nutrients impact your energy levels and overall well-being.

Embracing a Holistic Approach: Supporting thyroid function naturally involves a holistic approach that includes diet, lifestyle, and stress management. Barbara's advice emphasizes the importance of integrating these strategies to maintain a healthy thyroid and overall balance.

Osteoporosis Prevention and Natural Remedies

Osteoporosis is a condition that weakens bones, making them more susceptible to fractures and breaks. Barbara O'Neill offers a wealth of natural strategies to help prevent osteoporosis and maintain strong, healthy bones. Here's a friendly guide to supporting bone health and preventing osteoporosis naturally:

Understanding Osteoporosis: Osteoporosis is often called a "silent disease" because bone loss occurs without obvious symptoms until a fracture happens. Barbara explains that maintaining bone density is crucial for overall health and mobility.

Bone-Boosting Nutrients: A diet rich in bone-healthy nutrients is essential for osteoporosis prevention. Barbara recommends focusing on:

- Calcium: Vital for bone strength. Include calcium-rich foods like leafy greens (kale, bok choy), dairy products, and fortified plant-based milks.
- Vitamin D: Helps the body absorb calcium. Spend time in the sun and include vitamin D-rich foods like fatty fish (salmon, mackerel) and fortified foods.
- Magnesium: Supports bone health and helps regulate calcium levels. Good sources include nuts, seeds, whole grains, and legumes.

- Vitamin K: Essential for bone mineralization. Include vitamin K-rich foods such as spinach, broccoli, and Brussels sprouts.

Weight-Bearing Exercise: Regular weight-bearing exercises strengthen bones and improve bone density. Barbara recommends activities like:

- Walking: A simple yet effective exercise for bone health.
- Strength Training: Using weights or resistance bands helps build bone strength and muscle mass.
- Dancing: Fun and effective for maintaining bone density and balance.

Avoiding Bone-Damaging Habits: Certain habits can negatively impact bone health. Barbara suggests:

- Limiting Alcohol: Excessive alcohol consumption can lead to bone loss. Moderation is key.
- Avoiding Smoking: Smoking interferes with bone health and slows down the healing process. Quitting is crucial for maintaining strong bones.

Herbal Support: Some herbs can support bone health and reduce the risk of osteoporosis:

- Horsetail: Rich in silica, which helps strengthen bones and connective tissues.
- Red Clover: Contains compounds that may support bone density and overall bone health.
- Nettle Leaf: Provides a range of nutrients beneficial for bone health, including calcium and magnesium.

Bone-Healthy Lifestyle Choices: Integrating healthy lifestyle choices can further support bone health:

- Hydration: Drinking plenty of water supports overall health and helps maintain bone density.
- Balanced Diet: Eating a variety of nutrient-dense foods ensures you get essential vitamins and minerals for bone health.
- Stress Management: Chronic stress can impact bone health. Barbara recommends practices like mindfulness, yoga, or meditation to manage stress and support overall well-being.

Regular Bone Density Testing: Monitoring bone density helps assess bone health and prevent osteoporosis. Barbara emphasizes the importance of regular check-ups with your healthcare provider to keep track of bone health and address any concerns early.

Holistic Approach: Preventing osteoporosis involves a holistic approach that combines diet, exercise, and lifestyle choices. Barbara's advice highlights the importance of integrating these strategies to maintain strong and healthy bones.

Embracing a Nutrient-Rich Diet: Focusing on foods that support bone health helps build and maintain bone density. Barbara encourages making dietary choices that include plenty of calcium, vitamin D, magnesium, and vitamin K to support bone strength.

Positive Attitude and Consistency: Maintaining a positive attitude and staying consistent with bone-healthy habits are key to long-term success. Barbara believes that a proactive approach to bone health can make a significant difference in preventing osteoporosis and promoting overall well-being.

Building Long-Term Health and Wellness

Building long-term health and wellness is about creating a lifestyle that supports your well-being in every aspect—physically, mentally, and emotionally. Barbara O'Neill emphasizes that a holistic approach to health can lead to lasting benefits and a fulfilling life. Here's a friendly guide to building and maintaining long-term health and wellness:

Adopt a Balanced Diet: Nutrition is the cornerstone of long-term health. Barbara suggests focusing on a balanced diet that includes a variety of whole foods:

- Fruits and Vegetables: Rich in vitamins, minerals, and antioxidants that support overall health.
- Whole Grains: Provide essential nutrients and fiber for digestive health.
- Lean Proteins: Support muscle health and repair. Include options like fish, poultry, beans, and legumes.
- Healthy Fats: Found in nuts, seeds, avocados, and olive oil, these fats support heart health and brain function.

Stay Active: Regular physical activity is crucial for maintaining health and wellness. Barbara recommends:

- Consistency: Aim for at least 150 minutes of moderate aerobic activity or 75 minutes of vigorous activity per week.
- Variety: Incorporate different types of exercise, such as cardio, strength training, and flexibility exercises like yoga.

Prioritize Mental Health: Mental well-being is just as important as physical health. Barbara advises:

- Stress Management: Practice techniques like meditation, deep breathing, and mindfulness to manage stress effectively.
- Healthy Relationships: Surround yourself with supportive and positive people who contribute to your emotional well-being.
- Self-Care: Take time for activities that you enjoy and that help you relax and recharge.

Get Quality Sleep: Adequate sleep is essential for overall health and wellness. Barbara highlights:

- Establish a Routine: Go to bed and wake up at the same time each day to regulate your sleep cycle.
- Create a Restful Environment: Make your bedroom conducive to sleep by keeping it dark, quiet, and cool.

Stay Hydrated: Proper hydration supports all bodily functions. Barbara recommends drinking plenty of water throughout the day to keep your body well-hydrated and functioning optimally.

Regular Health Check-ups: Preventive care is key to long-term health. Barbara encourages:

- Routine Screenings: Schedule regular check-ups with your healthcare provider to monitor and address any potential health issues early.

- Vaccinations: Stay up-to-date with recommended vaccinations to protect yourself from preventable diseases.

Healthy Lifestyle Choices: Making mindful choices contributes to long-term wellness. Barbara suggests:

- Avoiding Harmful Substances: Limit alcohol consumption, avoid smoking, and steer clear of recreational drugs.
- Safe Practices: Follow safety guidelines to prevent accidents and injuries.

Embrace Lifelong Learning: Staying informed about health and wellness helps you make better choices. Barbara recommends:

- Education: Read books, attend workshops, and stay updated on health information to continually improve your well-being.
- Adaptability: Be open to adjusting your health strategies as needed to fit your evolving needs.

Cultivate Positive Habits: Developing and maintaining healthy habits is essential for long-term success. Barbara advises:

- Goal Setting: Set realistic and achievable health goals to stay motivated and track your progress.
- Consistency: Make small, sustainable changes to your lifestyle that you can stick with over time.

Find Joy and Purpose: Engaging in activities that bring you joy and a sense of purpose contributes to overall happiness and well-being. Barbara emphasizes:

- Passions: Pursue hobbies and interests that make you feel fulfilled.
- Volunteering: Helping others and contributing to your community can enhance your sense of purpose and satisfaction.

Book 6: The Immune System and Natural Defense

Understanding the Immune System

The immune system is your body's defense network, designed to keep you healthy by fighting off harmful invaders like bacteria, viruses, and other pathogens. Barbara O'Neill emphasizes the importance of a strong immune system for overall well-being. Here's a friendly guide to understanding how this remarkable system works:

What is the Immune System? The immune system is a complex network of cells, tissues, and organs that work together to protect the body from illness and infection. Think of it as your body's built-in security system, always on the lookout for potential threats.

Key Components of the Immune System: The immune system consists of several key players:

- White Blood Cells: These are the body's primary defense fighters. Different types of white blood cells, such as lymphocytes and macrophages, work to identify and destroy invaders.
- Lymphatic System: This includes lymph nodes, spleen, and tonsils. It helps filter harmful substances from the blood and supports immune cell function.
- Bone Marrow: This is where many immune cells are produced. It's like the factory where immune cells are made and then sent out to do their job.
- Thymus: Located in the chest, the thymus is where T-cells mature and learn to distinguish between harmful invaders and the body's own cells.

How the Immune System Works: The immune system uses a multi-layered approach to defend against threats:

- Barrier Defenses: Your skin and mucous membranes act as the first line of defense, preventing pathogens from entering your body.
- Innate Immunity: This is the body's immediate response to invaders. It includes inflammation, which helps to isolate and eliminate threats.
- Adaptive Immunity: This is a more specialized response. It involves recognizing specific pathogens and creating a memory of them to respond more effectively if they show up again.

Immune Response Process: When the immune system detects an invader, it goes through several steps:

- Detection: Immune cells identify harmful pathogens through receptors that recognize specific markers on the invaders.
- Response: Immune cells then attack and neutralize the invaders. They might release chemicals to destroy the pathogens or tag them for other cells to remove.
- Memory Formation: After an attack, the immune system remembers the invader. This helps it respond faster and more effectively if the same pathogen invades again.

Maintaining a Healthy Immune System: To support your immune system, Barbara advises:

- Balanced Diet: Eat a variety of nutrient-rich foods to provide the vitamins and minerals your immune system needs. Key nutrients include vitamin C, vitamin D, zinc, and antioxidants.
- Regular Exercise: Physical activity helps to boost overall immune function and circulation.
- Adequate Sleep: Quality sleep is essential for a well-functioning immune system. Aim for 7-9 hours each night.
- Stress Management: Chronic stress can weaken the immune system. Incorporate stress-reducing practices like mindfulness, relaxation exercises, and hobbies you enjoy.
- Hydration: Drinking plenty of water supports all bodily functions, including immune health.

Common Immune System Issues: Sometimes, the immune system can malfunction:

- Autoimmune Disorders: The immune system mistakenly attacks the body's own tissues.
- Immunodeficiency: The immune system is weakened, making it harder to fight off infections.

Supporting Your Immune System Naturally: Barbara suggests natural remedies to enhance immune health:

- Herbal Teas: Herbs like echinacea, ginger, and garlic have been traditionally used to support immune function.
- Probiotics: These beneficial bacteria can support gut health, which is closely linked to immune function.

Strengthening the Immune System with Nutrition

Nutrition plays a crucial role in keeping your immune system strong and ready to fend off illnesses. Barbara O'Neill highlights how the right nutrients can support and enhance your body's natural defenses. Here's a friendly guide on how to use nutrition to boost your immune system:

The Role of Nutrition in Immunity: Good nutrition provides the building blocks your immune system needs to function optimally. A well-balanced diet helps ensure that your body has the vitamins, minerals, and other nutrients required to maintain a strong defense system.

Key Immune-Boosting Nutrients: Incorporating a variety of nutrient-rich foods into your diet can help strengthen your immune system:

- Vitamin C: Found in citrus fruits, strawberries, and bell peppers, vitamin C is essential for the production and function of white blood cells, which are crucial for fighting infections.
- Vitamin D: Essential for immune health, vitamin D can be obtained from fatty fish, fortified dairy products, and sunlight exposure. It helps regulate immune responses and may reduce inflammation.
- Zinc: This mineral, present in nuts, seeds, and whole grains, supports immune cell function and helps heal wounds.
- Vitamin A: Found in carrots, sweet potatoes, and leafy greens, vitamin A helps maintain the health of your skin and mucous membranes, which are the first line of defense against pathogens.

- Antioxidants: Foods rich in antioxidants, like berries, green tea, and dark chocolate, help protect your cells from damage caused by free radicals, which can weaken the immune system.

Incorporating Immune-Boosting Foods:

- Citrus Fruits: Oranges, grapefruits, and lemons are packed with vitamin C, which is known for its immune-enhancing properties.
- Leafy Greens: Spinach, kale, and Swiss chard provide vitamins A and C, as well as antioxidants that support overall health.
- Garlic and Ginger: These herbs have natural anti-inflammatory and antimicrobial properties that can help the body combat infections.
- Yogurt and Probiotics: Probiotics found in yogurt and fermented foods can support gut health, which is closely linked to immune function.

Hydration Matters: Drinking plenty of water helps your body function properly and supports all of its systems, including the immune system. Staying hydrated ensures that your body can effectively flush out toxins and maintain healthy mucous membranes.

Balancing Your Diet: Aim for a diet that includes a wide range of foods to cover all your nutritional bases. Barbara recommends focusing on:

- Whole Grains: Oats, brown rice, and quinoa provide fiber and essential nutrients.
- Lean Proteins: Include sources like chicken, fish, legumes, and tofu to support immune cell production and repair.

Avoiding Nutrient Deficiencies: Certain dietary habits can lead to nutrient deficiencies that may weaken your immune system:

- Minimize Processed Foods: Highly processed foods often lack essential nutrients and may contain unhealthy fats and sugars.
- Moderate Alcohol Intake: Excessive alcohol can impair immune function and deplete essential nutrients.

The Power of a Healthy Diet: By making mindful food choices and incorporating a variety of nutrient-rich foods into your meals, you can provide your immune system with the support it needs. Barbara's approach to nutrition emphasizes balance and variety, which are key to maintaining optimal health and immune function.

The Role of Probiotics in Immune Health

Probiotics, often referred to as "good" bacteria, play a significant role in maintaining a healthy immune system. Barbara O'Neill emphasizes their importance in supporting overall health and enhancing the body's natural defenses. Here's a friendly guide to understanding how probiotics benefit your immune system:

What Are Probiotics? Probiotics are live microorganisms that, when consumed in adequate amounts, offer health benefits. They are primarily found in fermented foods and supplements and help maintain a healthy balance of gut bacteria.

The Gut-Immune Connection: A large portion of your immune system is housed in the gut, often referred to as the "gut-associated lymphoid tissue" (GALT). This means that the health of your gut directly impacts your immune function. Probiotics help support a balanced gut microbiome, which is essential for a robust immune response.

How Probiotics Support Immune Health:

- Balancing Gut Flora: Probiotics help maintain a healthy balance of beneficial bacteria in the gut. This balance can prevent the overgrowth of harmful bacteria and support overall immune function.
- Enhancing Immune Responses: Probiotics can stimulate the production of antibodies and enhance the activity of immune cells, such as macrophages and T-cells, which play a crucial role in defending against infections.
- Reducing Inflammation: Some probiotic strains have anti-inflammatory properties that can help reduce inflammation in the gut and throughout the body, supporting a healthier immune response.
- Supporting Gut Barrier Function: Probiotics help strengthen the gut lining, which acts as a barrier to prevent harmful substances from entering the bloodstream. A strong gut barrier is essential for preventing immune system overreactions.

Sources of Probiotics:

- Fermented Foods: Incorporate foods like yogurt, kefir, sauerkraut, kimchi, and miso into your diet. These foods naturally contain beneficial probiotic strains.
- Probiotic Supplements: If you're not a fan of fermented foods, probiotic supplements are a convenient option. They come in various forms, including capsules, tablets, and powders.

Choosing the Right Probiotics:

- Strain Matters: Different probiotic strains offer various benefits. Look for strains with proven benefits for immune health, such as Lactobacillus rhamnosus and Bifidobacterium lactis.
- Quality Counts: Choose high-quality supplements with live, active cultures. Ensure they are stored properly to maintain their effectiveness.

Integrating Probiotics into Your Routine:

- Start Gradually: Introduce probiotics into your diet slowly to allow your gut to adjust. This can help avoid digestive discomfort.
- Consistency Is Key: For the best results, incorporate probiotics regularly into your diet or supplement routine. Consistency helps maintain a healthy balance of gut bacteria.

Possible Side Effects and Considerations: While probiotics are generally safe for most people, some might experience mild digestive symptoms, such as bloating or gas, initially. If you have underlying health conditions or are on medication, consult with a healthcare professional before starting probiotics.

The Holistic Approach: Barbara's holistic approach to health emphasizes that while probiotics are beneficial, they should be part of a broader lifestyle that includes a balanced diet, regular exercise, adequate sleep, and stress management.

Herbal Immune Boosters and Adaptogens

Herbal remedies have long been used to support the immune system and promote overall well-being. Barbara O'Neill highlights the power of certain herbs known for their immune-boosting and adaptogenic properties. Let's explore how these natural allies can help you stay healthy and resilient.

Understanding Immune Boosters and Adaptogens:

- Immune Boosters: These herbs support the body's defense mechanisms, helping to strengthen and regulate immune responses.
- Adaptogens: Adaptogens are herbs that help the body adapt to stress and maintain balance. They can support overall health and enhance the body's resilience to various stressors.

Popular Herbal Immune Boosters:

- Echinacea: Often used to prevent or shorten the duration of colds, Echinacea is known for its ability to stimulate the immune system. It can increase the production of white blood cells and improve the body's response to infections.
- Elderberry: Elderberry is rich in antioxidants and has been shown to support immune function. It can help reduce the severity and duration of colds and flu.
- Astragalus: This herb is known for its immune-enhancing properties. It can help strengthen the body's defenses, improve energy levels, and support overall vitality.
- Ginger: Ginger has natural anti-inflammatory and antioxidant properties. It can help support immune health by reducing inflammation and enhancing circulation.

Effective Adaptogens for Stress and Wellness:

- Ashwagandha: Ashwagandha is a powerful adaptogen that helps the body cope with stress. It supports immune function by reducing stress-induced immune suppression and improving overall vitality.
- Rhodiola: Rhodiola is known for its ability to enhance mental and physical endurance. It helps the body adapt to stress, which can, in turn, support immune function and overall well-being.
- Holy Basil (Tulsi): Holy Basil is revered for its stress-reducing and immune-supportive properties. It helps balance stress hormones and promotes a healthy immune response.
- Reishi Mushroom: Often called the "mushroom of immortality," Reishi is known for its immune-modulating effects. It can help enhance the immune system's ability to fight infections and improve overall health.

Incorporating Herbs into Your Routine:

- Teas and Tinctures: Herbal teas and tinctures are popular ways to enjoy the benefits of immune-boosting herbs. Sipping on a cup of Echinacea or Elderberry tea can be soothing and beneficial.
- Supplements: Herbal supplements are available in various forms, including capsules, tablets, and powders. Choose high-quality supplements from reputable sources to ensure effectiveness.
- Cooking and Recipes: Incorporate herbs like ginger and turmeric into your meals. They not only add flavor but also provide health benefits.

Precautions and Considerations:

- Consult with a Professional: Before starting any new herbal regimen, especially if you have underlying health conditions or are on medication, consult with a healthcare provider.
- Quality Matters: Ensure that you use high-quality herbs from reliable sources to get the best benefits. Look for products that are organic and free from additives.

Combining Herbs for Enhanced Benefits: Many people find that combining different herbs can provide synergistic effects. For example, blending Echinacea with Elderberry may enhance overall immune support.

Natural Remedies for Autoimmune Disorders

Autoimmune disorders occur when the immune system mistakenly attacks the body's own tissues. Barbara O'Neill emphasizes a holistic approach to managing these conditions, focusing on natural remedies that can support overall health and balance the immune system. Here's a friendly guide to some effective natural strategies for managing autoimmune disorders:

Understanding Autoimmune Disorders:

- What They Are: Autoimmune disorders occur when the immune system becomes overactive and targets healthy cells. Common conditions include rheumatoid arthritis, lupus, and multiple sclerosis.
- Symptoms: Symptoms can vary widely but often include fatigue, joint pain, inflammation, and digestive issues.

Dietary Approaches:

- Anti-Inflammatory Diet: Adopting an anti-inflammatory diet can help reduce inflammation and support overall health. Focus on whole, nutrient-dense foods like fruits, vegetables, lean proteins, and healthy fats. Avoid processed foods, sugary snacks, and excessive amounts of red meat.
- Elimination Diet: Identifying and eliminating potential food triggers can be beneficial. Common triggers include gluten, dairy, and nightshade vegetables. An elimination diet helps pinpoint which foods may exacerbate symptoms.
- Bone Broth: Rich in nutrients like collagen and amino acids, bone broth supports gut health and may help reduce inflammation. It's a soothing and nutritious addition to your diet.

Herbal Remedies:

- Turmeric: Turmeric contains curcumin, a powerful anti-inflammatory compound. It can help reduce joint pain and inflammation associated with autoimmune disorders. Incorporate turmeric into your diet through cooking or as a supplement.
- Ginger: Ginger has natural anti-inflammatory properties and can help ease symptoms such as pain and swelling. Use fresh ginger in teas or add it to your meals.
- Licorice Root: Licorice root has immune-modulating properties and can help balance the immune system. However, it should be used cautiously, as it can affect blood pressure.

Supplements and Nutrients:

- Omega-3 Fatty Acids: Found in fish oil and flaxseed oil, omega-3 fatty acids have anti-inflammatory effects and support overall immune function.
- Vitamin D: Adequate levels of vitamin D are crucial for immune health. Consider getting your levels tested and supplementing if needed, especially if you have limited sun exposure.
- Probiotics: Probiotics support gut health, which is vital for a balanced immune system. A healthy gut can help modulate immune responses and reduce inflammation.

Lifestyle Modifications:

- Stress Management: Chronic stress can exacerbate autoimmune symptoms. Incorporate stress-reducing practices such as yoga, meditation, and deep-breathing exercises into your daily routine.
- Regular Exercise: Moderate, regular exercise can help manage symptoms and improve overall health. Activities like walking, swimming, or gentle yoga are often well-tolerated.
- Adequate Sleep: Ensure you get enough restorative sleep each night. Good sleep hygiene practices can support overall health and help manage autoimmune symptoms.

Detoxification:

- Gentle Detox: Supporting the body's natural detoxification processes can be beneficial. Focus on staying hydrated, eating a balanced diet, and incorporating detoxifying foods like leafy greens and cruciferous vegetables.

Consult with a Professional:

- Personalized Care: Work with a healthcare provider knowledgeable about autoimmune disorders to tailor natural remedies to your specific needs. They can help you create a balanced plan that complements your medical treatment.

Managing Allergies Naturally

Allergies can make everyday life challenging, causing discomfort from sneezing and itching to more severe reactions. Barbara O'Neill's holistic approach to managing allergies focuses on natural remedies that can help alleviate symptoms and support overall health. Here's a friendly guide to managing allergies naturally:

Understanding Allergies:

- What They Are: Allergies occur when the immune system overreacts to substances (allergens) such as pollen, pet dander, or certain foods. This reaction can cause symptoms like congestion, hives, and itchy eyes.
- Common Triggers: Common allergens include pollen, dust mites, mold, pet dander, and certain foods like nuts or shellfish.

Dietary Adjustments:

- Anti-Inflammatory Foods: Incorporate foods that help reduce inflammation, such as fruits, vegetables, nuts, and fatty fish. These can support overall immune health and reduce allergy symptoms.
- Local Honey: Consuming local honey may help your body gradually build tolerance to local pollen, potentially reducing seasonal allergy symptoms. Start with a small amount and see how you feel.
- Omega-3 Fatty Acids: Found in fish oil and flaxseeds, omega-3s have anti-inflammatory properties that can help manage allergy symptoms. Include sources like salmon, walnuts, and chia seeds in your diet.

Herbal Remedies:

- Butterbur: Butterbur is a herb known for its ability to reduce symptoms of hay fever and other allergies. It may help decrease inflammation and congestion. Consult with a healthcare provider for appropriate dosage and use.
- Nettle Leaf: Nettle leaf has natural antihistamine properties and can help reduce allergy symptoms. It can be taken as a tea or in supplement form.
- Peppermint: Peppermint tea or essential oil can help clear nasal congestion and soothe the throat. It's a refreshing and natural way to ease allergy symptoms.

Environmental Adjustments:

- Air Purifiers: Using air purifiers with HEPA filters can help reduce indoor allergens such as dust and pet dander. Keep your home environment as allergen-free as possible.
- Regular Cleaning: Regularly clean your home to reduce dust, mold, and pet dander. Vacuum with a HEPA filter and wash bedding frequently to minimize allergen exposure.
- Pollen Monitoring: During peak pollen seasons, keep windows closed and stay indoors during high pollen counts. Check local pollen forecasts to plan outdoor activities.

Hydration and Detoxification:

- Stay Hydrated: Drinking plenty of water helps keep mucous membranes hydrated and can alleviate congestion. Aim to drink at least 8 glasses of water a day.
- Gentle Detox: Supporting the body's natural detoxification processes can help manage allergies. Include detoxifying foods like leafy greens, lemon, and ginger in your diet.

Lifestyle Practices:

- Stress Management: Chronic stress can exacerbate allergy symptoms. Practice stress-reducing techniques such as yoga, meditation, and deep breathing to help manage your overall well-being.
- Regular Exercise: Moderate exercise can support a healthy immune system and help clear nasal congestion. Choose activities that you enjoy and that fit your fitness level.

Consult with a Professional:

- Personalized Advice: Work with a healthcare provider knowledgeable about allergies and natural remedies to create a plan that suits your specific needs. They can help you integrate these strategies safely and effectively.

How to Fight Infections with Natural Treatments

Infections can disrupt your daily life, but the good news is that there are natural ways to help your body fight back without relying on heavy pharmaceuticals. Nature offers an array of powerful remedies that not only treat infections but also support your immune system in staying strong.

Garlic is known as one of nature's most potent antibiotics. It contains a compound called allicin, which has been shown to have antibacterial, antiviral, and antifungal properties. You can eat garlic raw, mix it into meals, or even take garlic supplements to boost your infection-fighting power. It's a simple yet effective way to naturally ward off harmful microbes.

Echinacea is a popular herb often used to prevent or shorten the duration of colds and other respiratory infections. It stimulates the immune system, helping your body fight off bacteria and viruses more efficiently. Echinacea can be taken as a tea, in capsule form, or as a tincture. It's particularly helpful at the onset of infection when your immune system needs a quick boost.

Honey, especially raw or Manuka honey, is packed with antimicrobial properties. Not only does it help soothe a sore throat, but it can also be applied topically to wounds to prevent infection. Taking a spoonful of honey in tea or on its own can be an easy and effective remedy for bacterial infections.

Ginger has long been used in natural medicine to fight infections. Its anti-inflammatory and antioxidant properties help reduce pain, fever, and swelling, making it ideal for treating infections such as colds, flu, and even more severe illnesses. You can enjoy ginger as a tea, add it to smoothies, or incorporate it into meals for a natural healing boost.

Turmeric, with its active ingredient curcumin, is another powerful infection-fighter. Curcumin has antimicrobial, antiviral, and anti-inflammatory effects that help the body fend off infections. Consuming turmeric in meals, smoothies, or taking curcumin supplements can aid in battling infections naturally.

Apple cider vinegar has natural antibacterial properties that make it a great remedy for mild infections. It can help balance your body's pH, which is essential for keeping harmful bacteria at bay. Dilute it in water and drink it, or use it topically to treat skin infections.

Oregano oil is an incredibly strong natural antibiotic. It contains compounds like carvacrol and thymol, which have been shown to inhibit the growth of bacteria and viruses. Taking oregano oil in capsule form or adding a few drops to a glass of water can help combat infections, but be cautious as it is very potent.

Your gut plays a vital role in your immune system, and keeping it healthy can help prevent and fight infections. Probiotics, found in fermented foods like yogurt, sauerkraut, and kefir, help maintain a healthy balance of good bacteria in your gut, boosting your immune defenses against infections.

Herbal teas, such as chamomile, peppermint, and elderberry, can help fight infections while soothing symptoms. Elderberry tea is especially known for its antiviral properties, which can be effective against colds and flu. Drinking herbal teas also helps keep you hydrated, which is essential for flushing out toxins and supporting your immune system.

While these natural treatments can do wonders for fighting infections, never underestimate the power of rest and hydration. Your body needs time and energy to heal, and staying hydrated helps flush out toxins and keep your immune system functioning optimally.

Seasonal Illnesses: Cold, Flu, and Immunity

As the seasons change, many of us brace ourselves for the inevitable arrival of colds and flu. These seasonal illnesses can catch us off guard, but with the right approach, you can strengthen your immune system and reduce the risk of getting sick—or at least recover more quickly.

Why Do We Get Sick in Certain Seasons?

Colds and flu tend to spike during the colder months, and there's a reason for that. When the weather cools down, we spend more time indoors, often in close quarters with others, making it easier for viruses to spread. The colder air also dries out the mucous membranes in our nose and throat, weakening our first line of defense against infections. Plus, shorter days can mean less sun exposure, which affects our vitamin D levels—a key nutrient for immunity.

One of the best things you can do is to start preparing your immune system before cold and flu season arrives. A strong immune system is your best defense against seasonal illnesses. Here are some simple ways to boost your immunity naturally:

- Vitamin C: This well-known immune booster helps protect cells from damage and supports the production of white blood cells, which are crucial for fighting infections. You can get your vitamin C from foods like citrus fruits, bell peppers, and leafy greens, or through supplements.
- Vitamin D: Known as the "sunshine vitamin," vitamin D plays a key role in immune health. Since it's harder to get enough sun in the colder months, consider adding a supplement or eating vitamin D-rich foods like fatty fish and fortified dairy products.
- Zinc: Zinc is another powerful immune-supporting nutrient. It helps the body produce and activate T-cells, which fight off viruses. You can find zinc in foods like pumpkin seeds, nuts, and legumes.
- Probiotics: Your gut health is closely tied to your immune system, so keeping your gut flora in balance with probiotics can help prevent illness. Foods like yogurt, kefir, and fermented vegetables are great sources of these beneficial bacteria.

When cold and flu season hits, natural remedies can provide excellent support to keep illness at bay:

- Elderberry Syrup: Elderberries are packed with antioxidants and have been shown to help reduce the severity and duration of colds and flu. Elderberry syrup can be taken daily as a preventative measure or when symptoms first appear.
- Echinacea: This herb is widely used to help prevent colds and shorten their duration. Taking echinacea as a tea or in capsule form can boost your body's natural defenses.
- Hydration: Drinking plenty of fluids, especially warm teas like ginger or chamomile, can help soothe a sore throat and keep the body hydrated, which is essential for your immune system to function properly.

Though colds and flu are both viral illnesses, they have distinct symptoms. Colds generally come on slowly, starting with a sore throat, followed by sneezing, congestion, and mild fatigue. Flu, on the other hand, tends to hit hard and fast, with sudden fever, body aches, fatigue, and sometimes chills and cough. Knowing the difference can help you decide how to treat your symptoms.

Even with a strong immune system, sometimes we still catch a cold or the flu. When this happens, it's important to give your body the care it needs to recover:

- Rest: Your body uses a lot of energy to fight off infections, so rest is crucial. Don't push yourself—listen to your body and take it easy.
- Stay Hydrated: Drinking plenty of water, herbal teas, and broths helps thin mucus and prevent dehydration, which can worsen symptoms.
- Soothing Remedies: Warm saltwater gargles can help ease a sore throat, while steam inhalation (try adding eucalyptus oil) can relieve congestion. Honey is also a great remedy to soothe coughs and sore throats.

To keep your immune system strong all year round, focus on maintaining healthy lifestyle habits:

- Balanced Diet: A diet rich in whole foods, fruits, and vegetables ensures your body gets the nutrients it needs to keep your immune system in top shape.
- Regular Exercise: Moderate physical activity can boost your immune system and help it function more effectively.
- Adequate Sleep: Getting enough sleep is essential for your body's natural defenses. Aim for 7-9 hours a night to give your immune system the time it needs to recharge.
- Stress Management: Chronic stress can weaken your immune system, making you more susceptible to illness. Finding ways to manage stress—like meditation, yoga, or simply taking time to relax—can make a big difference in your overall health.

Daily Habits for Immune System Maintenance

Your immune system works tirelessly to protect you from illness, but it needs your support to stay strong and effective. By adopting some simple, healthy habits, you can boost your immune system's performance and help it function at its best every day.

The foundation of a strong immune system is the food you eat. A diet rich in whole, nutrient-dense foods gives your body the vitamins and minerals it needs to fight off infections and stay healthy. Aim to include the following in your daily meals:

- Fruits and Vegetables: These are packed with vitamins, antioxidants, and fiber that support immune health. Leafy greens, berries, citrus fruits, and bell peppers are great options to load up on.
- Healthy Fats: Fats found in foods like avocados, nuts, seeds, and olive oil help reduce inflammation and support cell health, both of which are essential for a strong immune response.
- Protein: Your body uses protein to build antibodies that fight off infections. Be sure to include lean meats, fish, eggs, beans, or plant-based protein sources in your diet.

Water plays a vital role in keeping your immune system functioning properly. It helps transport nutrients to your cells and flush out toxins from your body. Staying hydrated also supports your lymphatic system, which is crucial for filtering out harmful bacteria and viruses. Aim to drink plenty of water throughout the day, and consider adding herbal teas for extra immune support.

Your body heals and regenerates while you sleep, making rest one of the most important habits for maintaining a healthy immune system. During sleep, your immune system produces and releases proteins called cytokines, which are essential for fighting infections and inflammation. Aim for 7-9 hours of quality sleep each night to give your body the time it needs to recharge and stay strong.

Exercise isn't just good for your heart and muscles—it also strengthens your immune system. Regular, moderate exercise boosts circulation, allowing immune cells to move more freely throughout your body. Activities like walking, cycling, yoga, or even dancing can be great ways to stay active. Just be sure not to overdo it—extreme exercise without enough rest can actually weaken your immune defenses.

Chronic stress can suppress your immune system, making you more vulnerable to illness. Incorporating stress management techniques into your daily routine can have a positive impact on your immunity. Try to take time each day to relax and unwind, whether it's through meditation, deep breathing exercises, yoga, or simply spending time doing something you enjoy. Learning to manage stress can keep your immune system in balance.

Spending time outdoors has numerous health benefits, including boosting your immune system. Sunlight helps your body produce vitamin D, which is crucial for immune health. Even just 15-30 minutes of sunlight a day can make a difference. Fresh air can also improve circulation and oxygen levels, further supporting your immune function. Whether it's a walk in the park or gardening, getting outside daily is a great habit to maintain.

It may sound simple, but washing your hands regularly is one of the most effective ways to prevent infections. Make it a habit to wash your hands with soap and water before meals, after using the bathroom, and after coming into contact with public surfaces. This helps prevent the spread of germs and keeps your immune system from being overwhelmed.

Processed foods, refined sugars, and artificial additives can weaken your immune system over time. These foods promote inflammation and can disrupt the balance of healthy bacteria in your gut, which is vital for immune health. Reducing your intake of processed snacks, sugary drinks, and fast food, and focusing on whole, nourishing foods can make a big difference in keeping your immune system strong.

Your gut plays a major role in your immune system, with about 70% of your immune cells residing in your gut. Supporting your gut health through a diet rich in fiber, probiotics, and prebiotics helps promote a healthy balance of bacteria that strengthens your immune system. Foods like yogurt, kefir, sauerkraut, and other fermented foods are great for boosting gut health.

While it's always best to get nutrients from food, some supplements can provide extra immune support when needed. Common immune-boosting supplements include:

- Vitamin C: Helps boost the production of white blood cells.
- Vitamin D: Supports immune function, especially in winter when sunlight is limited.
- Zinc: A key mineral that helps fight infections and supports immune function.
- Probiotics: Promote a healthy gut microbiome, which in turn supports immune health.
- Elderberry: Known for its antiviral properties and ability to shorten cold and flu duration.

Book 7: Natural Remedies for Men's Health

Supporting Prostate Health Naturally

As men age, prostate health becomes an important aspect of overall well-being. While prostate issues are common, especially as you get older, there are natural ways to support and maintain a healthy prostate. By incorporating certain foods, lifestyle habits, and natural remedies into your routine, you can help reduce the risk of prostate-related problems and support long-term prostate health.

A healthy diet is key to maintaining prostate health, and certain foods are particularly beneficial:

- Tomatoes: These are rich in lycopene, an antioxidant that has been shown to support prostate health. Cooked tomatoes, like those in sauces and soups, offer even more bioavailable lycopene.
- Cruciferous Vegetables: Vegetables like broccoli, cauliflower, and Brussels sprouts contain compounds that may help reduce the risk of prostate issues. They're packed with nutrients that support detoxification and hormone balance.
- Healthy Fats: Omega-3 fatty acids, found in fatty fish like salmon, chia seeds, and flaxseeds, help reduce inflammation, which can benefit the prostate. On the other hand, try to limit unhealthy fats like those in processed foods and fried items.
- Green Tea: Green tea contains potent antioxidants, especially catechins, that can support prostate health. Drinking green tea regularly may help reduce the risk of developing prostate problems.

Proper hydration supports all bodily functions, including the health of the prostate. Drinking plenty of water helps flush toxins from your body and can reduce the risk of urinary problems, which are often linked to prostate issues. Aim for about 8 glasses of water a day, and try to limit caffeine and alcohol, which can irritate the bladder.

Staying active is not only good for your heart and muscles, but it can also promote prostate health. Regular physical activity helps to reduce inflammation, maintain healthy hormone levels, and improve circulation. Exercises like walking, swimming, or yoga can make a big difference in prostate health.

- Pelvic Floor Exercises: Strengthening the pelvic floor muscles through exercises like Kegels can support urinary function and improve prostate health. These exercises are simple to do and can help with common prostate issues like urinary incontinence.

Several herbs have been shown to support prostate health naturally. While they aren't a substitute for medical treatment, these natural remedies can be a great addition to your wellness routine:

- Saw Palmetto: One of the most well-known herbs for prostate health, saw palmetto has been used for centuries to support urinary function and reduce symptoms of an enlarged prostate (BPH). It's available in supplement form and can help balance hormones linked to prostate health.
- Pygeum: Derived from the African cherry tree, pygeum is another herbal remedy that has been traditionally used to treat urinary symptoms associated with prostate issues. It's thought to help reduce inflammation and improve urinary flow.

- Stinging Nettle: This herb has been used to support prostate health, especially in combination with saw palmetto. It can help reduce symptoms of an enlarged prostate and support overall urinary health.
- Pumpkin Seed Oil: Pumpkin seeds are rich in zinc and other nutrients that promote prostate health. Pumpkin seed oil is often used to help reduce urinary symptoms related to an enlarged prostate.

Hormones play a major role in prostate health, particularly testosterone and its byproducts. Keeping your hormone levels balanced can support a healthy prostate. You can do this by maintaining a healthy weight, exercising regularly, and eating a diet rich in vegetables, healthy fats, and lean protein. Limiting sugar and refined carbs can also help reduce the risk of hormone-related prostate issues.

While natural remedies and a healthy lifestyle are great for maintaining prostate health, it's also important to get regular check-ups as you age. Prostate screenings can help detect any issues early, before they become more serious. Talk to your healthcare provider about the right time to start screenings, especially if you have a family history of prostate problems.

Chronic stress can have a negative impact on your overall health, including your prostate. Stress increases inflammation and can affect hormone balance, which in turn can lead to prostate issues. Finding ways to manage stress, such as meditation, yoga, or spending time outdoors, can have a positive effect on your prostate health and overall well-being.

Natural Solutions for Erectile Dysfunction

Erectile dysfunction (ED) is a common issue for men, especially as they age, but it doesn't have to be a permanent part of life. While medications are available, many men prefer to explore natural solutions that address the root cause of the issue. By making certain lifestyle changes and using natural remedies, you can improve erectile function and boost overall sexual health.

Good circulation is key to healthy erectile function, and that starts with a healthy heart. Since ED is often related to poor blood flow, maintaining heart health can significantly improve your ability to achieve and sustain an erection.

- Eat Heart-Healthy Foods: A diet rich in whole foods like fruits, vegetables, whole grains, lean protein, and healthy fats supports circulation and reduces the risk of cardiovascular problems, which are often linked to ED.
- Limit Processed Foods: Processed and fried foods, along with excess sugar, can contribute to poor heart health and circulation issues, which in turn can affect erectile function.
- Stay Active: Regular physical activity improves blood flow, reduces stress, and supports heart health. Aim for at least 30 minutes of moderate exercise, like walking or swimming, each day.

Stress and anxiety can play a significant role in ED. When your mind is preoccupied with stress, it becomes harder for your body to relax and respond sexually. Learning to manage stress can have a positive impact on your sexual health.

- Practice Relaxation Techniques: Techniques like deep breathing, meditation, or yoga can help calm your mind and reduce stress levels. Even taking a few moments each day to focus on your breath can help alleviate tension.

- Consider Counseling: Sometimes, ED can be linked to emotional or psychological factors. Talking with a therapist can help address underlying issues and improve your mental and sexual well-being.

Testosterone plays a crucial role in sexual function, and low levels of testosterone can contribute to ED. Supporting your body's natural hormone balance is key to improving erectile function.

- Maintain a Healthy Weight: Being overweight can lower testosterone levels and increase the risk of ED. Maintaining a healthy weight through diet and exercise can support hormone balance.
- Get Enough Sleep: Poor sleep can reduce testosterone levels, so it's important to prioritize 7-9 hours of quality sleep each night to keep your hormones in balance.
- Consider Herbal Supplements: Certain herbs have been traditionally used to support testosterone levels and sexual function:

    Ashwagandha: Known for its stress-relieving properties, ashwagandha can also help support testosterone levels and improve sexual health.

    Tribulus Terrestris: This herb is often used to boost libido and testosterone levels, making it a popular choice for those looking to improve erectile function.

    Maca Root: Maca is an adaptogen that's been used for centuries to enhance libido and sexual performance. It may also support hormone balance.

Healthy blood flow is essential for erectile function. There are natural ways to improve circulation, which can help with ED.

- Eat Foods that Boost Nitric Oxide: Nitric oxide helps relax blood vessels, improving blood flow. Foods like beets, leafy greens, and citrus fruits can help boost your body's production of nitric oxide.
- Try L-Arginine: L-arginine is an amino acid that helps the body produce nitric oxide, which can improve circulation and erectile function. It's available as a supplement, but it's also found in foods like nuts, seeds, and lean meats.
- Ginkgo Biloba: This herb is known to improve circulation and may help with ED by increasing blood flow to the penis. It's available as a supplement and can be used alongside other natural remedies.

Smoking can damage blood vessels, reducing circulation and increasing the risk of ED. If you smoke, quitting is one of the most effective ways to improve erectile function and overall health. Similarly, while moderate alcohol consumption may not cause issues, excessive drinking can interfere with sexual performance. Limiting alcohol can help restore healthy erectile function.

Strengthening the pelvic floor muscles can improve erectile function by supporting the structures involved in achieving an erection. Pelvic floor exercises, also known as Kegel exercises, are simple to perform and can have a big impact on sexual health. Regular practice of these exercises can help improve both erectile function and urinary control.

Several herbs have been traditionally used to treat ED and improve sexual performance:

- Ginseng: Known as a natural aphrodisiac, ginseng is often used to enhance sexual function and improve erections. Studies have shown that it can help increase blood flow and reduce symptoms of ED.
- Horny Goat Weed: This herb has been used in traditional Chinese medicine to improve sexual function. It's thought to increase blood flow to the penis and enhance libido.
- Yohimbine: Derived from the bark of the African yohimbe tree, yohimbine is a natural supplement that has been used to treat ED. It works by increasing blood flow and supporting nerve function, although it's important to use this herb under guidance, as it can have side effects in some people.

Communication with your partner is key to addressing ED in a healthy and supportive way. Talking openly about the issue can reduce anxiety and help you find solutions together. Building emotional intimacy and maintaining a strong connection with your partner can enhance both your relationship and your sexual health.

Boosting Testosterone Levels Naturally

Testosterone plays a vital role in men's health, affecting everything from energy levels and mood to muscle mass and libido. As men age, testosterone levels naturally decline, but there are natural ways to support and boost your testosterone without the need for medications or treatments. By incorporating specific lifestyle habits, foods, and natural supplements, you can help maintain healthy testosterone levels and enhance overall well-being.

Physical activity is one of the most effective ways to naturally boost testosterone. Strength training and high-intensity interval training (HIIT) are particularly effective:

- Weightlifting: Lifting weights and engaging in resistance training stimulates testosterone production. Focus on compound movements like squats, deadlifts, and bench presses, which target large muscle groups.
- HIIT: Short bursts of intense activity followed by periods of rest can help increase testosterone levels. A quick 20-30 minute HIIT session can make a big difference.
- Avoid Overtraining: While exercise boosts testosterone, overtraining can have the opposite effect by raising stress hormone (cortisol) levels. Balance intense workouts with recovery periods.

Sleep is crucial for healthy testosterone production. Most of your body's testosterone is produced during sleep, especially deep sleep stages. To naturally boost your levels:

- Aim for 7-9 Hours: Try to get a full night's sleep consistently. Poor sleep can lead to lower testosterone, so creating a sleep-friendly environment—dark, cool, and quiet—can help.
- Manage Sleep Apnea: If you have sleep apnea or trouble breathing at night, this can lower testosterone. Getting treatment for sleep issues can help restore healthy hormone levels.

The food you eat has a direct impact on testosterone production. Focus on foods that support hormone balance and avoid those that may disrupt it:

- Healthy Fats: Good fats, like those found in avocados, olive oil, nuts, seeds, and fatty fish, are essential for testosterone production. Avoid trans fats and processed oils, which can lower testosterone.
- Protein and Carbs: A diet rich in protein supports muscle mass and hormone production. Carbohydrates are also important, especially for maintaining energy during workouts, but focus on whole grains, fruits, and vegetables rather than refined sugars and processed carbs.
- Zinc and Magnesium: Both minerals are vital for testosterone production. Foods like oysters, pumpkin seeds, spinach, and almonds are excellent sources of zinc and magnesium. Supplementing with these minerals can also help boost levels.

Being overweight or obese is often linked to lower testosterone levels, as excess fat tissue can convert testosterone into estrogen. By maintaining a healthy weight, you can naturally support better hormone balance.

- Focus on Fat Loss: Reducing excess body fat, particularly around the abdomen, can improve testosterone levels. A combination of strength training and a balanced diet can help.
- Avoid Crash Diets: Severe calorie restriction can lead to lower testosterone. Focus on sustainable, nutrient-rich eating habits for gradual fat loss.

Chronic stress increases the production of cortisol, a hormone that can interfere with testosterone levels. Managing stress effectively can help keep your testosterone levels healthy:

- Practice Relaxation Techniques: Meditation, deep breathing, or yoga can help reduce stress levels and balance hormones.
- Take Breaks: Ensure that you incorporate regular breaks and downtime into your day to avoid burnout. A balanced life leads to better hormone regulation.

While exercise is great for testosterone, excessive endurance exercise or long periods of cardio can reduce testosterone levels. It's essential to strike a balance:

- Strength Train More: Focus on weightlifting and resistance training to boost testosterone.
- Keep Cardio Moderate: Incorporate moderate cardio for heart health, but avoid long, exhaustive cardio sessions that can increase cortisol and decrease testosterone.

Certain herbs have been shown to naturally boost testosterone production:

- Ashwagandha: This adaptogenic herb helps reduce stress, increase energy, and support testosterone production. It has been shown to improve testosterone levels in men with low levels.
- Fenugreek: Often used to boost libido and testosterone, fenugreek can help improve strength and overall testosterone levels.
- Ginger: Ginger has long been used in natural medicine, and research suggests that it can boost testosterone and improve fertility in men.
- Tribulus Terrestris: A popular herb for boosting libido, Tribulus has also been linked to improved testosterone levels, especially in men with lower levels.

Excessive alcohol consumption and recreational drugs can negatively affect testosterone levels. While moderate alcohol consumption may not have a significant impact, regular heavy drinking can reduce testosterone production and impair hormone balance. Similarly, anabolic steroid use and recreational drug use can disrupt natural hormone production.

Vitamin D is essential for testosterone production, and spending time in the sun helps your body produce this crucial vitamin naturally:

- Get Sunlight: Aim for 15-30 minutes of sun exposure several times a week, especially during the morning or late afternoon when the sun is less intense.
- Supplement if Needed: If you live in a region with limited sun or can't get outside much, a vitamin D supplement can help maintain healthy testosterone levels.

Regular sexual activity is not only good for your relationship but also for maintaining healthy testosterone levels. Engaging in regular sexual activity can help stimulate the production of testosterone and other hormones related to sexual health.

Detoxification for Men's Hormonal Balance

Detoxification plays an essential role in maintaining hormonal balance, especially for men. Hormones like testosterone, cortisol, and insulin can be disrupted by the accumulation of toxins in the body, leading to fatigue, weight gain, low libido, and even mood swings. Fortunately, supporting your body's natural detoxification processes can help restore hormonal balance and improve overall health.

Here are some simple and effective ways to detox for better hormonal health:

The liver is your body's primary detox organ, responsible for filtering out toxins and metabolizing hormones. A healthy liver ensures that excess hormones are processed and eliminated effectively.

- Eat Liver-Friendly Foods: Foods like garlic, onions, beets, and leafy greens help support liver function. Incorporating these into your diet can assist in detoxification.
- Drink Plenty of Water: Staying hydrated helps the liver flush out toxins more efficiently. Aim for at least 8-10 glasses of water a day to support this natural process.

A diet high in processed foods, refined sugars, and unhealthy fats can introduce toxins that disrupt hormonal balance. Reducing or eliminating these from your diet is a crucial step toward detoxification.

- Avoid Processed Foods: Processed foods often contain chemicals and preservatives that can overload the liver and interfere with hormone function. Opt for whole, nutrient-dense foods instead.
- Limit Alcohol and Caffeine: Both alcohol and caffeine can stress the liver and disrupt hormonal regulation. While moderate consumption is fine, cutting back will help reduce the toxic load.

Herbs and natural remedies can support the body's detoxification processes and promote better hormonal health.

- Milk Thistle: Known for its liver-supporting properties, milk thistle can help detoxify and protect the liver, ensuring that it efficiently processes hormones like testosterone.
- Dandelion Root: This herb acts as a natural diuretic and liver tonic, helping to cleanse the body of toxins and improve hormonal balance.
- Turmeric: Turmeric's anti-inflammatory and liver-supporting benefits make it an excellent addition to any detox routine.

Fiber is essential for flushing out toxins from the digestive tract and keeping hormones in check. A lack of fiber can lead to reabsorption of excess estrogen, disrupting the balance of testosterone and other hormones.

- Eat Fiber-Rich Foods: Include foods like fruits, vegetables, whole grains, nuts, and seeds to ensure you're getting enough fiber in your diet.
- Consider Flaxseeds: Flaxseeds are particularly beneficial for hormonal detoxification, as they contain lignans that help bind and eliminate excess estrogen.

Exercise not only boosts testosterone levels but also aids in detoxification by promoting circulation and sweating, which helps eliminate toxins through the skin.

- Sweat It Out: Engage in regular physical activity, such as strength training or cardio, to encourage sweating and improve the body's natural detox process.
- Balance Intensity: Avoid overtraining, which can increase cortisol levels and interfere with hormonal balance. Instead, focus on a balanced exercise routine that includes both strength and relaxation.

Sweating is one of the body's most efficient ways to eliminate toxins. Using a sauna or engaging in activities that cause you to sweat regularly can help detoxify the body and promote better hormonal health.

- Use Infrared Saunas: Infrared saunas are particularly effective at deep detoxification, helping to eliminate heavy metals and other toxins stored in fat cells.
- Hydrate After Sweating: Be sure to drink plenty of water before and after sweating to replenish fluids and support kidney function.

Chronic stress leads to the overproduction of cortisol, which can throw your hormones out of balance. Stress management is a key part of detoxifying the body and maintaining healthy hormone levels.

- Practice Relaxation Techniques: Deep breathing, meditation, and yoga are all effective ways to reduce stress and support hormonal detoxification.
- Take Time for Yourself: Prioritize downtime to relax and unwind, ensuring that your body has a chance to restore balance.

Environmental toxins from air pollution, plastics, and chemicals in personal care products can build up in your body and disrupt hormonal balance. Taking steps to minimize your exposure can aid in detoxification.

- Choose Natural Products: Switch to natural, non-toxic cleaning products, skincare, and personal care items to reduce your exposure to harmful chemicals.

- Avoid BPA and Plastics: BPA and other chemicals found in plastics can mimic estrogen in the body, disrupting hormonal balance. Opt for glass or stainless steel containers whenever possible.

Intermittent fasting is a powerful tool for detoxification and can support hormonal balance by giving your digestive system time to rest and allowing your body to focus on eliminating toxins.

- Try the 16:8 Method: This involves fasting for 16 hours and eating within an 8-hour window each day. It's a simple way to encourage detoxification without drastically changing your diet.
- Listen to Your Body: While fasting can be beneficial, it's important to ease into it and find a method that works for your lifestyle and energy levels.

Sleep is a critical time for the body to detox and balance hormones. During deep sleep, your body repairs tissues and detoxifies cells, ensuring optimal hormone production.

- Prioritize 7-9 Hours of Sleep: Make sleep a priority to give your body the time it needs to cleanse and restore itself.
- Create a Sleep-Friendly Environment: Keep your bedroom dark, cool, and quiet to promote deeper, more restful sleep.

Cardiovascular Health: Natural Approaches

Taking care of your heart is crucial for long-term health and vitality. Cardiovascular disease remains one of the leading causes of illness, but the good news is that natural approaches can help you support your heart and maintain a healthy cardiovascular system. Through diet, lifestyle changes, and natural remedies, you can boost heart health and reduce the risk of heart disease.

Here are some natural ways to keep your heart strong and healthy:

A diet rich in whole, unprocessed foods is the foundation of good cardiovascular health. Certain foods are particularly beneficial for protecting the heart and improving circulation.

- Incorporate Omega-3 Fatty Acids: Foods like salmon, flaxseeds, walnuts, and chia seeds are high in omega-3 fatty acids, which help reduce inflammation and support heart health by lowering blood pressure and improving cholesterol levels.
- Embrace Leafy Greens: Vegetables such as spinach, kale, and broccoli are packed with vitamins, minerals, and antioxidants that can lower blood pressure and improve circulation.
- Eat Plenty of Fiber: Whole grains, fruits, and vegetables provide essential fiber, which helps to lower cholesterol levels and improve digestion.

Physical activity is one of the best things you can do for your heart. Exercise strengthens the heart muscle, improves circulation, and helps maintain healthy blood pressure.

- Cardio for the Heart: Aerobic exercises like walking, jogging, swimming, and cycling are particularly effective in boosting cardiovascular health. Aim for at least 30 minutes of moderate exercise most days of the week.

- Strength Training: Resistance exercises, such as weightlifting or bodyweight exercises, help improve overall fitness and support heart health by reducing body fat and improving muscle tone.

Chronic stress can negatively affect heart health by increasing blood pressure and contributing to inflammation. Managing stress is a key part of any heart-healthy lifestyle.

- Practice Mindfulness and Meditation: Techniques like deep breathing, meditation, and yoga can help reduce stress levels and improve overall mental and physical well-being.
- Take Time for Relaxation: Regularly making time for relaxation and hobbies you enjoy helps keep stress in check and supports your cardiovascular system.

High blood pressure is a significant risk factor for heart disease, but you can lower it through natural means without medication.

- Reduce Sodium Intake: Too much salt in your diet can raise blood pressure, so opt for fresh, whole foods and limit processed and salty foods.
- Increase Potassium: Potassium helps balance sodium levels in the body and can reduce the strain on the heart. Bananas, avocados, and sweet potatoes are excellent sources of potassium.

Certain herbs have been used for centuries to support heart health and improve circulation.

- Hawthorn Berry: Hawthorn is known for its ability to strengthen the heart muscle, improve blood flow, and lower blood pressure. It's available in teas, tinctures, or supplements.
- Garlic: Garlic is a natural blood thinner and can help lower cholesterol levels. Eating raw garlic or taking it in supplement form is an easy way to support cardiovascular health.
- Cayenne Pepper: Cayenne helps improve circulation and reduce the risk of blood clots. You can add cayenne to your meals or take it in supplement form.

Carrying excess weight, especially around the midsection, can strain your heart and increase your risk of cardiovascular disease. Maintaining a healthy weight is one of the most effective ways to protect your heart.

- Focus on Balanced Eating: Incorporate nutrient-dense foods into your meals, including fruits, vegetables, lean proteins, and healthy fats, while avoiding processed and sugary foods.
- Practice Portion Control: Being mindful of portion sizes can help prevent overeating and support healthy weight loss or maintenance.

Sleep is essential for heart health. When you don't get enough sleep, your body experiences more stress, leading to increased blood pressure and inflammation.

- Aim for 7-9 Hours of Sleep: Prioritize a full night's sleep to give your heart the rest it needs to function optimally.
- Create a Sleep-Friendly Environment: Keep your bedroom cool, dark, and quiet to promote better sleep quality.

Smoking is one of the most harmful habits for heart health, increasing the risk of heart attack, stroke, and other cardiovascular issues. Quitting smoking can dramatically improve heart health, no matter how long you've been a smoker.

- Seek Support if Needed: There are many resources available to help quit smoking, from counseling to nicotine replacement therapies. The sooner you quit, the better your heart will thank you.

Proper hydration is vital for maintaining healthy blood pressure and supporting overall cardiovascular function.

- Drink Plenty of Water: Aim to drink at least 8 glasses of water a day to keep your heart and blood vessels functioning smoothly.
- Limit Sugary Drinks: Sugary sodas and energy drinks can raise blood pressure and lead to weight gain, so opt for water, herbal teas, or infused water with lemon or cucumber for flavor.

High cholesterol can lead to plaque buildup in the arteries, increasing the risk of heart disease. Keeping cholesterol levels in check is crucial for heart health.

- Incorporate Healthy Fats: Include sources of healthy fats in your diet, such as avocados, olive oil, and nuts. These fats can help raise good cholesterol (HDL) while lowering bad cholesterol (LDL).
- Avoid Trans Fats: Trans fats found in processed and fried foods can increase bad cholesterol and should be minimized or avoided.

Maintaining Vitality and Longevity

Maintaining vitality and longevity is about keeping your energy levels high and supporting your health as you age. A combination of a balanced diet, regular exercise, stress management, and natural remedies can help you stay vibrant and healthy throughout your life. Here's how you can enhance your vitality and support a long, active life:

Eat a Nutrient-Dense Diet: Focus on consuming whole, unprocessed foods that are rich in essential vitamins and minerals. Incorporate fruits, vegetables, lean proteins, and healthy fats into your daily meals. Antioxidants found in foods like berries and leafy greens help combat oxidative stress and promote overall health. Omega-3 fatty acids from sources such as fatty fish and flaxseeds support heart health and reduce inflammation.

Stay Physically Active: Regular exercise is crucial for maintaining energy and strength. Engage in cardiovascular activities like walking, jogging, or swimming to boost heart health and endurance. Strength training exercises help preserve muscle mass, which naturally declines with age. Don't forget to include flexibility and balance exercises like yoga or tai chi to enhance overall fitness and mobility.

Prioritize Quality Sleep: Aim for 7-9 hours of restful sleep each night to allow your body to repair and rejuvenate. Establish a calming bedtime routine, avoid screens before bed, and create a comfortable sleep environment to improve sleep quality.

Manage Stress Effectively: Chronic stress can deplete your energy and impact your health. Practice mindfulness, meditation, or deep-breathing exercises to reduce stress levels. Spend time in nature, connect with loved ones, and engage in activities you enjoy to help manage stress and boost your mood.

Support Hormonal Balance: Maintaining balanced hormones is essential for vitality. Boost testosterone levels naturally by including zinc-rich foods in your diet, such as pumpkin seeds and oysters. Adaptogenic herbs like ashwagandha can help balance hormones and reduce stress.

Promote Brain Health: Keep your mind sharp by engaging in mentally stimulating activities such as puzzles, reading, or learning new skills. Include brain-boosting foods like omega-3-rich fish and antioxidant-rich berries in your diet. Staying socially active also supports cognitive function.

Regular Detoxification: Help your body remove toxins through regular detoxification. Support liver health with herbs like milk thistle and turmeric, drink plenty of water, and consume fiber-rich foods to aid digestion and waste removal.

Consider Natural Supplements: Supplements can enhance vitality and overall health. Ginseng can help combat fatigue, CoQ10 supports cellular energy production, and Vitamin D is important for immune function and energy levels.

Maintain a Positive Mindset: Cultivating a positive attitude contributes to your overall well-being. Practice gratitude, find purpose in your activities, and embrace laughter to improve your mood and vitality.

Book 8: Gut Health and Digestion

The Gut-Brain Connection and Its Importance

Hey there! Let's dive into a fascinating topic that's gaining a lot of attention lately: the gut-brain connection. It might sound a bit sciencey, but stick with me—this is really cool stuff!

Imagine your gut and brain are chatting away like old friends. It's not just a metaphor; they actually do communicate through something called the gut-brain axis. This is a bidirectional communication system that links your digestive system (your gut) with your central nervous system (your brain). Think of it as a superhighway of signals and messages between the two.

So, why is this connection so important? Well, it turns out that your gut health can have a big impact on your mental well-being. For instance, your gut houses a huge portion of your body's serotonin, a chemical that helps regulate mood, sleep, and appetite. When your gut is happy and healthy, it's like a cheerleader for your brain, helping to keep you feeling good and balanced.

But it's not just about feeling good. Research has shown that an imbalance in gut bacteria, known as dysbiosis, can contribute to mood disorders like anxiety and depression. This is because certain gut bacteria can produce or consume neurotransmitters, which are crucial for brain function. So, if your gut flora is out of whack, it might affect how you feel emotionally.

Another interesting point is how stress impacts the gut. When you're stressed, your gut can become more permeable, allowing toxins and bad bacteria to leak into your bloodstream. This can lead to inflammation and digestive issues, which in turn might make you feel even more stressed. It's a bit of a vicious cycle!

So, what can you do to keep this connection in tip-top shape? First, focus on a balanced diet rich in fiber, which helps nourish the good bacteria in your gut. Foods like fruits, vegetables, whole grains, and fermented foods (like yogurt and sauerkraut) are great for gut health. Additionally, managing stress through techniques like mindfulness, exercise, and adequate sleep can also support both your gut and brain.

In summary, taking care of your gut isn't just about digestion—it's about nurturing your overall well-being. A happy gut can lead to a happier, healthier you, so let's give this amazing connection the attention it deserves!

Healing Leaky Gut Syndrome Naturally

Hey there! Let's talk about something that might sound a bit alarming but is actually quite manageable with the right approach: leaky gut syndrome. It's not as scary as it sounds, and the good news is that you can support your gut's healing naturally.

So, what exactly is leaky gut syndrome? Well, think of your gut lining as a super-smart filter, designed to let nutrients pass through while keeping harmful substances out.

In leaky gut syndrome, this filter becomes more porous than it should be, allowing toxins, undigested food particles, and even bacteria to escape into your bloodstream. This can lead to inflammation and a range of symptoms, from digestive issues to fatigue and skin problems.

The first step in healing leaky gut syndrome is to focus on what you're eating. A diet that supports gut health is key. Here's what you can do:

Go for Gut-Friendly Foods: Load up on foods rich in fiber, like fruits, vegetables, and whole grains. These help nourish your good gut bacteria. Also, include fermented foods like yogurt, kefir, and sauerkraut. They're packed with probiotics, which are beneficial bacteria that help maintain a healthy gut flora.

Cut Out the Culprits: Some foods can contribute to gut inflammation and exacerbate leaky gut. Common culprits include refined sugars, processed foods, and gluten. You might want to experiment with reducing these and see how your body responds.

Embrace Bone Broth: This might sound a bit old-fashioned, but bone broth is a fantastic healing food. It's rich in gelatin and amino acids that can help repair the gut lining. Try sipping on it or using it as a base for soups and stews.

Support Your Gut with Supplements: Certain supplements can be beneficial for gut health. Look into options like L-glutamine, which is known for its role in gut repair, and zinc, which can help support the gut lining. Always check with a healthcare provider before starting any new supplements.

Stay Hydrated: Drinking plenty of water helps keep your digestive system moving smoothly and supports overall gut health.

Manage Stress: Stress can take a toll on your gut health, so finding ways to relax and unwind is crucial. Activities like yoga, meditation, or even just taking a few deep breaths can make a big difference.

Get Enough Sleep: Your body does a lot of healing while you sleep, so aim for 7-9 hours of restful sleep each night. Good sleep supports your gut health and overall well-being.

Probiotics and Digestive Health

Hey there! Let's chat about probiotics and how they can be a game-changer for your digestive health. If you've ever heard about "good bacteria" and wondered what the fuss is all about, you're in for a treat!

Probiotics are live microorganisms that, when taken in adequate amounts, offer a range of health benefits, especially for your digestive system. Think of them as the friendly neighborhood bacteria that help keep things running smoothly in your gut.

So, what do these probiotics do for you? Here's a quick rundown:

> Balancing the Gut Flora: Your gut is home to a diverse community of bacteria, and maintaining the right balance is crucial for good health. Probiotics help replenish and support the beneficial bacteria, which can be especially helpful if your gut flora has been disrupted by antibiotics, poor diet, or stress.
>
> Improving Digestion: Probiotics can aid in breaking down food and absorbing nutrients more effectively. They help with the fermentation of fiber, which produces short-chain fatty acids that nourish your gut cells and support digestion.
>
> Boosting the Immune System: A healthy gut flora plays a key role in supporting your immune system. Probiotics can help strengthen your gut barrier, making it more effective at keeping out harmful pathogens and reducing inflammation.
>
> Relieving Digestive Issues: If you're dealing with conditions like irritable bowel syndrome (IBS) or diarrhea, probiotics might be able to help. They can assist in reducing symptoms and restoring balance in your digestive system.
>
> Supporting Mental Health: Believe it or not, your gut and brain are connected through the gut-brain axis. Probiotics can positively influence this connection, potentially improving mood and reducing stress.

So, how can you get these beneficial bacteria into your diet? Here are some tasty and effective ways:

> Yogurt: Look for plain, unsweetened yogurt with live cultures. It's a delicious way to add probiotics to your daily routine.
>
> Kefir: This fermented milk drink is packed with probiotics and is a great alternative if you're not a fan of yogurt.
>
> Sauerkraut: Fermented cabbage is not only tangy and flavorful but also rich in probiotics. Just be sure to choose the unpasteurized variety to get the live cultures.
>
> Kimchi: This spicy Korean side dish is made from fermented vegetables and is another fantastic source of probiotics.
>
> Kombucha: This fermented tea is fizzy and refreshing, offering a dose of probiotics with every sip.

Herbal Remedies for Digestive Disorders

Hello! If you're looking for some natural ways to soothe digestive troubles, herbal remedies might be just what you need. Nature has provided us with a wealth of herbs that can support and improve digestive health. Let's explore some of the top herbal remedies that can help ease common digestive disorders.

Peppermint: This cool and refreshing herb is fantastic for calming an upset stomach and alleviating symptoms like bloating and gas. Peppermint tea is a popular choice, but you can also use peppermint oil capsules if you prefer. Just be mindful if you have acid reflux, as peppermint can sometimes make symptoms worse for some people.

Ginger: Ginger has been used for centuries to aid digestion and reduce nausea. It's great for soothing an upset stomach and can help with indigestion and motion sickness. You can enjoy ginger in many forms—fresh ginger tea, ginger ale (make sure it's made with real ginger), or even ginger chews.

Chamomile: Chamomile is well-known for its calming effects and is also a gentle aid for digestive issues. It can help with indigestion, bloating, and even mild diarrhea. A warm cup of chamomile tea before bed can also promote relaxation and better sleep.

Fennel Seeds: These little seeds are a powerhouse for digestive health. They can help reduce bloating, gas, and cramps. You can chew on a small amount of fennel seeds after meals or brew them into a tea.

Slippery Elm: Slippery elm is known for its soothing properties, making it helpful for digestive discomfort, including heartburn and inflammatory bowel conditions. It's often used in tea or lozenge form. It creates a protective coating in the digestive tract, which can ease irritation.

Dandelion: Dandelion is more than just a weed! It's a wonderful herb for supporting liver function and digestion. Dandelion root tea can stimulate appetite, help with digestion, and support liver health.

Licorice Root: Licorice root is beneficial for soothing the digestive tract and can help with conditions like gastritis and acid reflux. It's best used in moderation and under the guidance of a healthcare professional, as excessive use can have side effects.

Marshmallow Root: Not to be confused with the sugary treats, marshmallow root has a soothing effect on the digestive system. It helps reduce inflammation and irritation and is often used for conditions like gastritis and heartburn. Marshmallow root tea or supplements can be quite effective.

Managing Food Intolerances and Sensitivities

Hey there! If you've been feeling a bit off after meals or suspect you might have a food intolerance or sensitivity, don't worry—you're not alone, and there are plenty of ways to manage it naturally. Let's break down what you need to know about handling food intolerances and sensitivities, and how you can make adjustments to feel your best.

First, it's helpful to know the difference between food intolerances and food sensitivities. Food intolerances often involve difficulty digesting certain foods, which can lead to symptoms like bloating, gas, or diarrhea. Food sensitivities, on the other hand, can trigger more subtle reactions like headaches, fatigue, or mood changes, and they might not always involve the digestive system.

The first step in managing food intolerances or sensitivities is figuring out which foods are causing the trouble. Keeping a food diary can be incredibly helpful. Write down what you eat and any symptoms you experience. Over time, patterns might emerge that point to specific foods or ingredients.

Once you've identified potential culprits, try eliminating them from your diet for a few weeks. Then, gradually reintroduce them one at a time while monitoring your symptoms. This can help you pinpoint which foods you can tolerate and which ones you need to avoid.

Food labels can be a lifesaver when managing intolerances and sensitivities. Many processed foods contain hidden ingredients that might trigger your symptoms. Get into the habit of checking labels for allergens, additives, or ingredients you know you need to avoid.

There are plenty of delicious substitutes available if you need to avoid certain foods. For example, if you're lactose intolerant, try lactose-free dairy products or plant-based milk like almond or oat milk. If gluten is the issue, there are many gluten-free grains and flours to explore.

Eating a diet rich in whole foods—like fruits, vegetables, lean proteins, and whole grains—can help minimize the impact of food intolerances. These foods are less likely to contain hidden allergens or additives and can be gentler on your digestive system.

Believe it or not, stress can exacerbate food intolerances and sensitivities. Finding ways to manage stress, such as through relaxation techniques, exercise, or hobbies you enjoy, can help your digestive system stay balanced.

If you're having trouble managing your symptoms or if you're unsure about which foods to avoid, it's a good idea to consult with a healthcare professional. A dietitian or nutritionist can help you create a balanced eating plan that works for your unique needs.

For some people, digestive enzymes can help break down problematic foods more effectively, reducing symptoms. There are various enzyme supplements available, so talk to your healthcare provider about whether this could be a good option for you.

Natural Approaches for IBS and Colitis

Hello! If you're dealing with IBS (Irritable Bowel Syndrome) or colitis, you know how challenging these conditions can be. The good news is there are natural approaches that can help manage symptoms and support your gut health. Let's explore some friendly, effective strategies to find relief and improve your well-being.

Diet plays a huge role in managing IBS and colitis. Consider focusing on:

- Low-FODMAP Diet: For IBS, the Low-FODMAP diet can be a game-changer. FODMAPs are certain types of carbohydrates that can trigger symptoms. By identifying and avoiding high-FODMAP foods, you might find significant relief. Foods like bananas, rice, and oats are typically well-tolerated, while garlic, onions, and certain dairy products may need to be limited.

- Anti-Inflammatory Foods: For colitis, incorporating anti-inflammatory foods can help soothe the gut. Think leafy greens, fatty fish like salmon, berries, and turmeric. These foods can help reduce inflammation and support overall gut health.
- Hydration: Drinking plenty of water is crucial. Staying hydrated helps maintain healthy digestion and can ease symptoms of both IBS and colitis.

Probiotics, the beneficial bacteria that support gut health, can be especially helpful. They might help balance your gut flora and reduce symptoms. Look for high-quality probiotic supplements or enjoy fermented foods like yogurt, kefir, and sauerkraut.

Stress can significantly impact IBS and colitis symptoms. Finding ways to manage stress can make a big difference. Activities like yoga, meditation, and deep breathing exercises can help calm your mind and support digestive health.

Certain herbs can be soothing for digestive issues. For example:

- Peppermint: Peppermint tea or capsules can help relax the muscles of the gastrointestinal tract, reducing symptoms of IBS like cramping and bloating.
- Chamomile: Chamomile tea is gentle on the stomach and can help with inflammation and relaxation.
- Turmeric: With its anti-inflammatory properties, turmeric can support gut health. You can add it to your meals or take it as a supplement.

Eating smaller, more frequent meals rather than large meals can help reduce symptoms. This approach can be easier on your digestive system and help prevent overloading your gut.

Tracking what you eat and how you feel can help identify trigger foods. Note any symptoms you experience and see if there are patterns related to specific foods or meals. This can guide you in making dietary adjustments.

Fiber is important, but the type of fiber matters. Soluble fiber, found in foods like oats, apples, and carrots, is generally easier on the digestive system and can help manage symptoms. If fiber aggravates your symptoms, try adjusting the amount and type you consume.

Certain supplements can support digestive health:

- L-Glutamine: This amino acid supports the gut lining and can be beneficial for colitis.
- Slippery Elm: Known for its soothing properties, slippery elm can help with inflammation and digestive discomfort.

Supporting the Liver for Better Digestion

Hi there! If you're looking to boost your digestive health, don't overlook the importance of a well-functioning liver. This hardworking organ plays a crucial role in digestion, so giving it some extra love can have a big impact on how you feel. Let's explore some friendly ways to support your liver and enhance your digestive wellness.

Your liver thrives on a diet rich in nutrients. Here's what you can include:

- Leafy Greens: Foods like spinach, kale, and arugula are packed with antioxidants and nutrients that support liver function.
- Cruciferous Vegetables: Broccoli, Brussels sprouts, and cauliflower help boost liver detoxification processes and are great for overall health.
- Beets: Beets are fantastic for liver health. They contain betaine, which helps the liver process fats and improve detoxification.
- Fruits: Citrus fruits like oranges, lemons, and grapefruits are rich in vitamin C and antioxidants, which help the liver detoxify and function optimally.

Drinking plenty of water is essential for liver health. Water helps flush out toxins and supports the liver in its detoxification role. Aim for at least 8 glasses of water a day to keep your system well-hydrated.

Certain herbs can be incredibly supportive for your liver:

- Milk Thistle: This herb is renowned for its liver-protective properties. It helps protect liver cells from damage and supports detoxification.
- Dandelion Root: Dandelion root is excellent for liver health. It acts as a diuretic and helps stimulate bile production, aiding in digestion.
- Turmeric: Turmeric contains curcumin, a compound with powerful anti-inflammatory and antioxidant properties. It can support liver function and overall digestive health.

Your liver works hard to process and eliminate toxins, so it's important to avoid adding extra strain:

- Limit Alcohol: Excessive alcohol consumption can damage liver cells and impair its function. If you choose to drink, do so in moderation.
- Cut Down on Processed Foods: Processed foods often contain high levels of unhealthy fats, sugars, and additives that can burden the liver. Opt for whole, nutrient-dense foods whenever possible.

Physical activity supports liver health by helping maintain a healthy weight and promoting proper digestion. Aim for at least 30 minutes of moderate exercise most days of the week. Activities like walking, cycling, and swimming can all be beneficial.

Chronic stress can negatively affect liver function and digestion. Find ways to manage stress, such as through relaxation techniques, hobbies, or spending time with loved ones. Reducing stress can help your liver function more efficiently.

Getting enough restful sleep is vital for liver health. During sleep, your liver works on detoxifying and repairing itself. Aim for 7-9 hours of quality sleep each night to support overall health and well-being.

Incorporate foods known for their detoxifying properties:

- Garlic: Garlic contains sulfur compounds that aid in detoxification and support liver function.
- Green Tea: Rich in antioxidants, green tea helps protect the liver from damage and supports its detoxification processes.

Balancing the Microbiome for Optimal Health

Hey there! Let's dive into the fascinating world of the microbiome and how balancing it can lead to better overall health. Your microbiome is the community of microorganisms—bacteria, viruses, fungi, and other microbes—that live in and on your body, especially in your gut. Keeping this balance in check is crucial for your well-being. Here's how you can support a healthy microbiome and enjoy its many benefits.

Your microbiome thrives on variety, so try to include a range of foods in your diet. Different types of fibers and nutrients feed different types of beneficial microbes. Here's what to focus on:

- Fruits and Vegetables: Aim for a colorful variety. Different colors often mean different nutrients and fibers, which can support various microbes.
- Whole Grains: Foods like oats, barley, and quinoa provide prebiotics, which are like food for your good bacteria.
- Legumes: Beans, lentils, and chickpeas are great sources of fiber and can help nourish your microbiome.

Fermented foods are natural sources of probiotics, which are beneficial bacteria that can enhance the health of your microbiome. Try incorporating these into your diet:

- Yogurt: Choose plain yogurt with live cultures for a boost of good bacteria.
- Kefir: This fermented milk drink is rich in probiotics and can be a great addition to your diet.
- Sauerkraut and Kimchi: These fermented vegetables are not only delicious but also packed with probiotics.
- Kombucha: This fermented tea is fizzy and can be a refreshing way to add probiotics to your routine.

High amounts of processed foods and added sugars can negatively impact your microbiome by promoting the growth of harmful bacteria. Instead, focus on whole, nutrient-dense foods.

Drinking plenty of water helps maintain a healthy environment for your gut microbes. Aim for at least 8 glasses a day to keep things flowing smoothly.

Fiber is a superstar when it comes to microbiome health. It acts as food for beneficial bacteria and helps them thrive. Incorporate high-fiber foods like fruits, vegetables, whole grains, and legumes into your meals.

Chronic stress can disrupt the balance of your microbiome. Finding ways to manage stress—through relaxation techniques, physical activity, or hobbies—can have a positive impact on your gut health.

Antibiotics can disrupt the balance of your microbiome by killing both harmful and beneficial bacteria. Only use antibiotics when prescribed by your healthcare provider, and always complete the full course if needed.

Physical activity supports a healthy microbiome by promoting the growth of beneficial bacteria. Aim for at least 30 minutes of moderate exercise most days of the week.

Good sleep is essential for a balanced microbiome. Aim for 7-9 hours of quality sleep each night to support overall health and well-being.

If you're struggling to get enough probiotics from food alone, supplements can be a helpful addition. Choose a high-quality probiotic supplement that includes a variety of strains to support diverse microbial health.

Book 9: Stress Relief and Emotional Well-Being

Understanding the Impact of Stress on the Body

Hello! Let's talk about stress and how it affects your body. Stress is something we all experience, but it can have a significant impact on our health if not managed properly. Understanding how stress works can help you find ways to manage it better and improve your overall well-being. Let's break it down!

When you encounter a stressful situation, your body activates its "fight-or-flight" response. This is a natural reaction designed to help you deal with immediate threats. Here's what happens:

- Adrenaline Surge: Your adrenal glands release adrenaline, a hormone that increases your heart rate, boosts your energy, and sharpens your focus.
- Cortisol Release: At the same time, your body produces cortisol, another hormone that helps you manage stress by increasing glucose levels in your blood for quick energy.
- Physical Changes: Your muscles tense up, your breathing becomes rapid, and your digestive system slows down. These changes prepare your body to either fight or flee from danger.

Short-term stress, like getting through a big presentation, can be motivating and help you perform better. However, chronic or long-term stress—such as ongoing work pressures or personal challenges—can take a toll on your health.

How Chronic Stress Affects Your Body

- Immune System: Prolonged stress can weaken your immune system, making you more susceptible to illnesses and infections.
- Digestive System: Stress can disrupt your digestive system, leading to issues like indigestion, bloating, or even exacerbating conditions like IBS.
- Cardiovascular Health: Chronic stress can contribute to high blood pressure, increased risk of heart disease, and other cardiovascular issues.
- Mental Health: Stress affects your mental health, potentially leading to anxiety, depression, and mood swings. It can also impact your sleep quality and cognitive functions.
- Musculoskeletal System: Stress can cause muscle tension and pain, leading to headaches, back pain, and general discomfort.

Ongoing stress can upset your hormone balance. Elevated cortisol levels over time can interfere with other hormones, affecting everything from your metabolism to reproductive health.

Understanding the impact of stress is the first step toward managing it. Here are some friendly ways to cope:

- Practice Relaxation Techniques: Techniques like deep breathing, meditation, and yoga can help calm your mind and reduce stress.
- Get Moving: Regular physical activity helps release endorphins, which are natural stress relievers. Find an activity you enjoy, whether it's walking, dancing, or swimming.

- Connect with Others: Talking to friends, family, or a therapist can provide support and help you manage stress more effectively.
- Prioritize Self-Care: Make time for activities that make you feel good and help you unwind. Whether it's reading a book, taking a bath, or pursuing a hobby, self-care is essential.
- Set Realistic Goals: Break tasks into smaller, manageable steps and set realistic expectations to avoid feeling overwhelmed.
- Maintain a Balanced Diet: Eating a nutritious diet supports your body's ability to handle stress. Incorporate plenty of fruits, vegetables, whole grains, and lean proteins into your meals.

If stress feels overwhelming or persistent, don't hesitate to seek professional help. A mental health professional can offer strategies and support tailored to your needs.

Herbal Adaptogens for Stress Management

Hi there! If you're looking for natural ways to manage stress, herbal adaptogens might be just what you need. These incredible herbs help your body adapt to stress and restore balance, making them perfect allies in your journey toward better emotional well-being. Let's dive into some of the top adaptogens and how they can support you in handling stress more effectively.

Adaptogens are herbs that help your body cope with stress by regulating the adrenal system and supporting your body's ability to adapt to various stressors. They work by enhancing your resilience and helping you maintain balance, even when life gets hectic.

Here are some fantastic adaptogens you might want to consider:

- Ashwagandha: Often referred to as "Indian ginseng," ashwagandha is known for its ability to reduce cortisol levels and support the adrenal glands. It can help improve sleep, enhance mood, and boost overall energy levels. You can take it as a supplement or enjoy it in tea form.
- Rhodiola: Rhodiola is excellent for increasing mental and physical stamina. It helps combat fatigue and improves your body's ability to handle stress. It's particularly useful if you're feeling drained or overwhelmed. Rhodiola is typically available in capsule or extract form.
- Holy Basil (Tulsi): Holy basil, or tulsi, is a revered herb in Ayurvedic medicine. It helps reduce stress, support immune function, and promote a sense of calm. You can enjoy it as a soothing tea or in supplement form.
- Siberian Ginseng (Eleuthero): Despite its name, Siberian ginseng is not the same as true ginseng but offers similar benefits. It helps improve physical endurance, mental clarity, and stress resilience. Eleuthero is available as a tincture, capsule, or tea.
- Licorice Root: Licorice root supports adrenal function and helps balance cortisol levels. It also has anti-inflammatory properties. It's often used in herbal teas or supplements. However, be mindful of potential effects on blood pressure, and consult with a healthcare provider if you have any concerns.
- Schisandra: Schisandra berries are known for their ability to support liver health and overall vitality. They help the body adapt to stress, improve mental performance, and enhance physical endurance. Schisandra can be found in tincture, capsule, or powdered form.

How to Use Adaptogens

- In Tea: Many adaptogens can be brewed into calming and beneficial teas. Try incorporating them into your daily routine for a soothing, stress-reducing ritual.
- In Supplements: Adaptogen supplements are available in various forms, including capsules, tablets, and tinctures. Follow the recommended dosage on the packaging or as advised by a healthcare professional.
- In Smoothies: Add powdered adaptogens to your smoothies for a nutritious and stress-fighting boost. They blend well with fruits and vegetables and can be a tasty way to incorporate them into your diet.

Things to Keep in Mind

- Consult with a Professional: Before starting any new herbal regimen, it's a good idea to consult with a healthcare provider, especially if you're pregnant, nursing, or taking other medications.
- Listen to Your Body: Adaptogens are generally safe, but everyone's body responds differently. Start with a small amount and see how you feel before increasing your intake.
- Be Patient: Herbal adaptogens work gradually, so give them time to show their full benefits. Consistency is key to experiencing their positive effects.

While herbal adaptogens are a fantastic tool, remember that managing stress effectively often requires a holistic approach. Combine adaptogens with other stress-relief techniques like relaxation practices, regular exercise, and a balanced diet for the best results.

Nutrition for Mental Clarity and Stress Reduction

Hey there! Feeling a bit overwhelmed or foggy? Believe it or not, the foods you eat can play a big role in how clear-headed and calm you feel. Let's explore how you can use nutrition to boost your mental clarity and reduce stress, so you can feel your best every day.

Focus on Brain-Boosting Foods

Eating the right foods can support brain function and help keep stress at bay. Here are some top picks:

- Fatty Fish: Think salmon, mackerel, and sardines. These fish are rich in omega-3 fatty acids, which are great for brain health and can help reduce anxiety and depression.
- Blueberries: These tiny berries are packed with antioxidants that support brain function and may improve memory and cognitive performance. They also help fight inflammation, which can contribute to stress.
- Walnuts: Walnuts are loaded with omega-3s and antioxidants. They're fantastic for brain health and can help keep your mood balanced.
- Dark Chocolate: Enjoy a small amount of dark chocolate to boost your mood. It contains flavonoids that can improve brain function and reduce stress levels.

Stay Hydrated

Dehydration can affect your mood and cognitive function. Make sure to drink plenty of water throughout the day to keep your brain and body hydrated. Aim for at least 8 glasses of water a day. If you find plain water boring, try adding a splash of lemon or cucumber for a refreshing twist.

Complex carbohydrates provide a steady source of energy and help stabilize blood sugar levels. This can prevent mood swings and keep you feeling balanced. Opt for:

- Whole Grains: Foods like oats, quinoa, and brown rice provide long-lasting energy and support brain health.
- Sweet Potatoes: These are a great source of vitamins and minerals that help maintain stable blood sugar levels and boost mental clarity.

Proteins are essential for brain function and help regulate your mood. Incorporate these into your meals:

- Chicken and Turkey: These lean meats provide protein and tryptophan, an amino acid that can help regulate mood and sleep.
- Legumes: Beans, lentils, and chickpeas are excellent plant-based protein sources that also provide fiber to keep you feeling full and steady your energy levels.

Healthy fats are crucial for brain health and can help reduce stress:

- Avocados: Rich in healthy monounsaturated fats, avocados support brain function and can help keep your stress levels in check.
- Chia Seeds and Flaxseeds: These seeds are high in omega-3 fatty acids and fiber, which support mental clarity and reduce inflammation.

While a morning coffee or sugary treat might seem like a quick fix, too much caffeine and sugar can lead to crashes and heightened stress. Try to:

- Limit Caffeine: Too much caffeine can increase anxiety and disrupt your sleep. Opt for herbal teas or limit your coffee intake to one or two cups a day.
- Cut Back on Sugar: High sugar intake can lead to mood swings and energy crashes. Choose natural sweeteners like honey or maple syrup in moderation.

Skipping meals can lead to irritability and poor concentration. Aim to eat balanced meals and snacks throughout the day to keep your energy levels steady and your mood stable.

Certain herbs can also support mental clarity and stress reduction. Try:

- Green Tea: Contains L-theanine, an amino acid that promotes relaxation and helps improve focus.
- Chamomile Tea: Known for its calming effects, chamomile can help reduce stress and improve sleep quality.

How you eat can be just as important as what you eat. Take time to enjoy your meals without distractions, chew thoroughly, and listen to your body's hunger and fullness cues. Mindful eating can help you feel more satisfied and less stressed.

Managing Anxiety and Depression Naturally

Hi there! Feeling anxious or down can be really challenging, but there are natural ways to manage these feelings and help improve your overall well-being. Let's explore some gentle, effective strategies that might help you feel more balanced and uplifted.

What you eat can have a significant impact on your mood and mental health. Here are some dietary tips:

- Eat Mood-Boosting Foods: Incorporate foods rich in omega-3 fatty acids (like salmon and walnuts), antioxidants (such as blueberries and dark chocolate), and vitamins (like leafy greens and citrus fruits) to support your mental health.
- Regular Meals: Skipping meals or having irregular eating patterns can affect your mood. Aim for balanced meals and snacks throughout the day to keep your energy and mood stable.

Exercise isn't just good for your body; it's great for your mind too. Here's how staying active can help:

- Boosts Endorphins: Physical activity releases endorphins, which are natural mood lifters. Even a short walk can help improve your mood.
- Reduces Stress: Exercise helps lower cortisol levels, which can reduce feelings of stress and anxiety.
- Improves Sleep: Regular exercise can help improve the quality of your sleep, which is crucial for managing anxiety and depression.

Mindfulness and meditation are fantastic tools for calming your mind and reducing anxiety. Here's how you can get started:

- Mindfulness: Try focusing on the present moment without judgment. Techniques like mindful breathing or mindful eating can help bring you into the present and reduce anxiety.
- Meditation: Spend a few minutes each day practicing meditation to clear your mind and reduce stress. Apps and guided meditations can be great resources if you're new to the practice.

Relaxation techniques can help soothe your nervous system and manage stress:

- Deep Breathing: Practice deep breathing exercises to calm your body and mind. Inhale deeply through your nose, hold for a few seconds, and exhale slowly through your mouth.
- Progressive Muscle Relaxation: Tense and then relax different muscle groups in your body to help release physical tension and promote relaxation.

Talking to someone can provide relief and perspective. Consider:

- Therapy: Speaking with a mental health professional can help you explore and manage your feelings. Therapy can provide you with tools and strategies for coping with anxiety and depression.

- Support Groups: Joining a support group can connect you with others who understand what you're going through. Sharing experiences and receiving support can be incredibly comforting.

Certain herbs may support mental well-being:

- Chamomile: Known for its calming effects, chamomile can help reduce anxiety and promote relaxation.
- Lavender: Lavender, often used in aromatherapy, can help soothe anxiety and improve mood. You might use lavender essential oil in a diffuser or bath.
- St. John's Wort: This herb is traditionally used to support mood. However, it can interact with other medications, so consult a healthcare professional before using it.

Creating consistent, healthy routines can provide structure and stability:

- Sleep: Aim for 7-9 hours of quality sleep each night. Establish a calming bedtime routine and maintain a consistent sleep schedule.
- Daily Rituals: Incorporate daily rituals that bring you joy and relaxation, whether it's enjoying a cup of tea, reading a book, or taking a relaxing bath.

Doing things you enjoy can help lift your spirits and provide a sense of fulfillment:

- Pursue Hobbies: Engage in activities that make you happy, whether it's gardening, painting, or playing an instrument.
- Connect with Others: Spend time with friends and loved ones who make you feel supported and valued.

Focusing on what you're grateful for can shift your perspective and improve your mood:

- Gratitude Journal: Keep a journal where you write down things you're grateful for each day. This practice can help you focus on positive aspects of your life.

Sleep Hygiene for Stress Relief

Sleep is a cornerstone of well-being, but in our busy lives, it can often take a back seat. When it comes to managing stress, prioritizing good sleep hygiene is essential. Let's explore some friendly tips to help you achieve a restful night's sleep and tackle stress more effectively.

Your body thrives on routine. Try to go to bed and wake up at the same time every day, even on weekends. This consistency helps regulate your internal clock, making it easier to fall asleep and wake up feeling refreshed.

Wind down before bed with calming activities. Whether it's reading a book, taking a warm bath, or practicing gentle stretches, a soothing routine signals to your body that it's time to relax. Avoid stimulating activities like watching TV or scrolling through your phone right before bed.

Your bedroom should be a sanctuary for sleep. Keep it cool, dark, and quiet. Invest in a comfortable mattress and pillows, and remove any distractions like bright lights or noisy devices. Consider using blackout curtains or a white noise machine if needed.

The blue light from phones, tablets, and computers can interfere with your ability to fall asleep. Try to avoid screens at least an hour before bedtime. Instead, opt for activities that don't involve screens, like reading a physical book or practicing mindfulness.

What you eat and drink can affect your sleep. Avoid heavy meals, caffeine, and alcohol close to bedtime. Opt for a light snack if you're hungry before bed, such as a banana or a small handful of nuts, which can help promote better sleep.

Regular physical activity can improve your sleep quality. Aim for at least 30 minutes of moderate exercise most days of the week, but try to finish any vigorous activity a few hours before bedtime to avoid being too energized to sleep.

Incorporate relaxation techniques into your daily routine to manage stress and improve sleep. Practices like deep breathing exercises, meditation, or progressive muscle relaxation can help calm your mind and prepare you for a restful night.

If you find that you're still struggling with sleep despite trying these tips, it may be worth consulting a healthcare professional. They can help identify any underlying issues and provide tailored advice for improving your sleep hygiene.

Emotional Detoxification Practices

Just like we need to clear out physical toxins to stay healthy, our emotional well-being also benefits from a little detox now and then. Emotional detoxification helps us release negative feelings, reset our mindset, and cultivate a more positive outlook. Here are some friendly practices to help you cleanse your emotional palate and find a sense of peace.

Mindfulness and meditation are fantastic tools for emotional detox. By focusing on the present moment and observing your thoughts without judgment, you can create space between yourself and your emotions. Regular practice helps reduce stress and enhances your ability to manage emotions more effectively.

Writing down your thoughts and feelings can be incredibly cathartic. Journaling helps you process and understand your emotions, and it can be a great way to release pent-up feelings. Set aside a few minutes each day to jot down what's on your mind, and you'll likely find it easier to manage emotional stress.

Focusing on what you're grateful for can shift your mindset from negativity to positivity. Take a moment each day to reflect on the things you appreciate in your life. Whether it's through a gratitude journal or a simple mental note, recognizing the positives can help counterbalance the negative emotions.

Creativity is a powerful way to express and release emotions. Whether you enjoy painting, playing music, dancing, or crafting, engaging in creative activities allows you to channel your feelings into something positive and fulfilling.

Spending time in nature can be incredibly soothing for your mind and emotions. A walk in the park, a hike in the woods, or simply sitting outside and enjoying the fresh air can help you feel more grounded and connected, reducing emotional clutter.

It's important to protect your emotional space by setting boundaries with people and situations that drain your energy. Learning to say no when needed and prioritizing your own well-being can prevent emotional overload and promote a healthier emotional state.

Talking to friends, family, or a therapist about your feelings can provide relief and perspective. Sharing your thoughts with someone you trust can lighten the emotional load and offer valuable support and advice.

Exercise isn't just for physical health—it's great for your emotional well-being too. Activities like jogging, yoga, or even a brisk walk can release endorphins, boost your mood, and help you process and release emotions more effectively.

Holding onto grudges or unresolved conflicts can weigh heavily on your emotional state. Practicing forgiveness, whether it's forgiving others or yourself, can release negative feelings and promote inner peace.

Sometimes, the best way to detox emotionally is to simply take a break and relax. Whether it's a weekend getaway, a cozy night in, or a spa day, giving yourself time to unwind and recharge is crucial for emotional health.

Building Emotional Resilience

Building emotional resilience is like developing a mental muscle that helps you bounce back from life's challenges. It's about strengthening your ability to handle stress, adapt to change, and stay positive even when things get tough. Here's a friendly guide to help you build and maintain emotional resilience:

Focusing on the positive aspects of life can help you navigate through difficulties with a brighter outlook. Practice seeing challenges as opportunities for growth rather than setbacks. Celebrate small victories and keep a mental list of things you're grateful for to help maintain a positive perspective.

Having a support network is crucial for emotional resilience. Surround yourself with people who uplift and support you. Build and nurture relationships with friends, family, or support groups where you can share experiences and receive encouragement.

Taking care of yourself physically and emotionally is key to resilience. Ensure you're getting enough sleep, eating a balanced diet, and engaging in regular physical activity. Self-care also includes setting aside time for activities you enjoy and relaxation practices that recharge your energy.

Flexibility is a hallmark of emotional resilience. Embrace change as a natural part of life and focus on adapting rather than resisting it. When faced with new situations, approach them with an open mind and a willingness to learn.

Being able to tackle problems effectively boosts your confidence and resilience. Break down challenges into manageable steps, brainstorm possible solutions, and take proactive steps toward resolving issues. This approach helps you feel more in control and prepared for future obstacles.

Mindfulness techniques, such as deep breathing, meditation, or yoga, can help you manage stress and stay grounded. By staying present and focused, you can better handle stress and maintain emotional balance.

Setting and working toward achievable goals gives you a sense of purpose and accomplishment. Break larger goals into smaller, manageable tasks and celebrate your progress along the way. Realistic goal-setting helps build confidence and resilience.

Sometimes, building emotional resilience might require professional guidance. Don't hesitate to seek help from a therapist or counselor if you're struggling. They can offer valuable tools and strategies to help you develop resilience and cope with challenges more effectively.

Being kind to yourself during tough times is essential. Practice self-compassion by acknowledging your feelings without judgment and treating yourself with the same kindness you'd offer a friend. Recognize that everyone faces difficulties and that it's okay to seek support and take time to heal.

Take time to reflect on past challenges and how you handled them. Consider what worked well and what you might do differently next time. Learning from your experiences helps you grow and build stronger resilience for the future.

Book 10: Cancer Prevention and Natural Healing

Understanding the Body's Natural Defenses Against Cancer

Our bodies are equipped with a remarkable defense system designed to protect us from various health threats, including cancer. Understanding how these natural defenses work can give you insight into how to support and enhance your body's ability to ward off cancer. Let's explore how these defenses function and how you can help them stay strong.

Your immune system is like a dedicated team of soldiers patrolling your body, looking out for harmful invaders like viruses and cancerous cells. It consists of various components, including white blood cells, antibodies, and specialized organs like the spleen and lymph nodes. These elements work together to identify and destroy abnormal cells before they can cause harm.

Our cells are constantly exposed to damage from everyday activities and environmental factors. Luckily, cells have built-in repair mechanisms to fix this damage. Proteins called repair enzymes recognize and correct mistakes in our DNA, helping to prevent mutations that could lead to cancer. Keeping these repair mechanisms functioning well is key to reducing cancer risk.

Apoptosis is a process where damaged or abnormal cells undergo a controlled self-destruction. This "cell suicide" is a crucial defense mechanism that prevents damaged cells from multiplying and potentially forming tumors. A healthy body uses apoptosis to keep cell growth in check and maintain balance.

Your body has its own detoxification systems, primarily the liver, kidneys, and intestines. These organs work to eliminate toxins and waste products from the body. By supporting these systems through a healthy diet and adequate hydration, you help ensure they function effectively, which can aid in cancer prevention.

Chronic inflammation can contribute to cancer development. Fortunately, your body has anti-inflammatory responses that help manage and reduce inflammation. Eating a diet rich in anti-inflammatory foods like fruits, vegetables, nuts, and fatty fish can support these natural processes and lower your risk of cancer.

Hormones play a role in regulating cell growth and function. Maintaining a balance in hormone levels is important for preventing hormone-related cancers, such as breast or prostate cancer. Lifestyle factors like a balanced diet, regular exercise, and managing stress can help keep your hormonal systems in check.

Certain vitamins and minerals have protective effects against cancer. For example, antioxidants like vitamins C and E help neutralize harmful free radicals that can damage cells. Ensuring you get a variety of nutrients through a balanced diet can support your body's natural defenses and overall health.

Exercise is known to enhance immune function and reduce the risk of cancer. Engaging in regular physical activity helps maintain a healthy weight, reduces inflammation, and supports detoxification processes. Aim for a mix of aerobic and strength-training exercises to boost your body's defense systems.

Chronic stress can impact your immune system and overall health. Managing stress through techniques like meditation, yoga, or deep breathing can help maintain your body's natural defenses. A balanced emotional state supports a healthy immune response and overall resilience.

Minimizing exposure to known carcinogens—such as tobacco smoke, excessive alcohol, and certain chemicals—can reduce the risk of cancer. By making healthier choices and avoiding harmful substances, you support your body's natural ability to protect itself.

Nutrition and Lifestyle Changes for Cancer Prevention

When it comes to cancer prevention, what we put into our bodies and how we live our lives can make a significant difference. Embracing a healthy lifestyle isn't just about feeling good today; it's about setting the stage for long-term wellness. Let's dive into some nutrition and lifestyle changes that can help reduce your cancer risk and promote overall health.

Eating more fruits, vegetables, nuts, seeds, and whole grains is a cornerstone of cancer prevention. These foods are packed with antioxidants, vitamins, and minerals that help protect your cells from damage. Cruciferous vegetables like broccoli, cauliflower, and Brussels sprouts are especially potent, containing compounds that can help detoxify your body and inhibit cancer cell growth.

Whole grains like brown rice, quinoa, and oats are rich in fiber, which aids digestion and helps maintain a healthy weight. High-fiber diets are associated with a lower risk of several types of cancer, including colorectal cancer. Plus, whole grains provide essential nutrients that refined grains often lack.

Red meats, such as beef and pork, and processed meats like bacon and sausages, have been linked to an increased risk of cancer. Try to limit your intake of these meats and opt for leaner proteins such as chicken, turkey, or plant-based alternatives like legumes and tofu.

Drinking plenty of water is crucial for maintaining overall health. It helps flush toxins from your body and keeps your cells functioning properly. Aim for at least 8 glasses of water a day, and remember that herbal teas and water-rich fruits like cucumbers and melons can also contribute to your hydration.

Maintaining a healthy weight is important in cancer prevention. Obesity is linked to an increased risk of several cancers, including breast, colorectal, and pancreatic cancer. Balancing your calorie intake with physical activity can help manage your weight and reduce your risk.

Not all fats are created equal. Replace saturated fats and trans fats with healthier fats found in avocados, nuts, seeds, and olive oil. Omega-3 fatty acids, found in fatty fish like salmon and in flaxseeds, have anti-inflammatory properties that can help reduce cancer risk.

Moderation is key when it comes to alcohol. Excessive drinking has been linked to an increased risk of several cancers, including breast and liver cancer. If you choose to drink, do so in moderation—this means up to one drink per day for women and up to two drinks per day for men.

Regular physical activity helps maintain a healthy weight, improves immune function, and reduces inflammation, all of which contribute to cancer prevention.

Aim for at least 30 minutes of moderate exercise most days of the week. Activities like walking, swimming, or cycling can be enjoyable and beneficial.

Good sleep and stress management are often overlooked but are crucial for cancer prevention. Chronic stress and poor sleep can negatively impact your immune system and overall health. Establish a regular sleep schedule and find stress-reducing activities that work for you, such as yoga, meditation, or spending time in nature.

Smoking is a major risk factor for various cancers, including lung cancer. If you smoke, seek support to quit. Also, try to limit your exposure to environmental toxins such as pesticides, heavy metals, and chemicals in household products by opting for natural or organic alternatives whenever possible.

Detoxification Protocols for Cancer Patients

Detoxifying your body can be an important part of supporting your health, especially when facing cancer. While it's crucial to follow your doctor's advice and treatment plan, incorporating gentle detoxification practices can help support your body's natural healing processes. Here's a friendly guide to some detoxification protocols that might benefit cancer patients:

Water is your body's best friend when it comes to detoxification. Staying well-hydrated helps flush out toxins through your kidneys and urinary system. Aim for at least 8 glasses of water a day. Herbal teas, like ginger or dandelion, can also support detoxification and offer additional benefits.

Fruits and vegetables are packed with antioxidants and vitamins that can help your body detoxify naturally. Leafy greens like spinach and kale, cruciferous vegetables like broccoli, and colorful fruits such as berries are all excellent choices. These foods can help combat free radicals and support overall health.

The liver is your body's primary detox organ, so keeping it in tip-top shape is essential. Foods like beets, garlic, and turmeric can support liver function. Consider adding these to your meals to give your liver a little extra help. A daily serving of lemon water in the morning can also aid liver detoxification.

When it comes to detoxification, gentle is usually best, especially if you're undergoing cancer treatment. Gentle methods like Epsom salt baths can help draw out toxins through your skin and relax your muscles. Just be sure to consult your healthcare provider before trying any new detox methods.

Fiber plays a key role in the detoxification process by aiding digestion and helping your body eliminate waste. Foods like whole grains, beans, and flaxseeds are rich in fiber and can support healthy bowel movements, which are crucial for toxin elimination.

Pay attention to what you eat and how it affects your body. Eating smaller, more frequent meals can help with digestion and prevent overloading your system. Avoiding heavy, greasy foods and opting for lighter, easily digestible options can also make a difference.

Certain herbs, like milk thistle, dandelion root, and green tea, are known for their detoxifying properties. These can help support liver function and overall detoxification. However, always consult with your healthcare provider before adding any supplements to your routine to ensure they're safe and appropriate for your condition.

A healthy gut is essential for effective detoxification. Probiotic-rich foods like yogurt, kefir, and fermented vegetables can support a balanced gut flora and improve digestion. A healthy gut can enhance your body's ability to eliminate toxins and support overall health.

Rest is an important component of detoxification. Adequate sleep allows your body to repair and regenerate. Ensure you're getting enough quality sleep each night and find time for relaxation techniques like deep breathing, meditation, or gentle yoga.

Minimizing your exposure to environmental toxins can support your detoxification efforts. Choose natural or organic products when possible, avoid smoking, and be cautious with chemicals in cleaning products and personal care items. Simple changes, like using a water filter, can also reduce your exposure to contaminants.

Herbal Support for Cancer Treatment

Herbs have been used for centuries to support health and healing, and many people find them to be a helpful complement to conventional cancer treatments. While herbs should never replace medical treatments, they can offer additional support and relief. Here's a friendly guide to some herbs that may be beneficial during cancer treatment:

Turmeric, with its active compound curcumin, is renowned for its anti-inflammatory and antioxidant properties. It can help support the immune system and may aid in reducing inflammation related to cancer. Adding turmeric to your meals or taking it as a supplement (with your doctor's approval) can be a great way to incorporate this powerful herb into your routine.

Ginger is another fantastic herb with anti-inflammatory and anti-nausea properties. It can help alleviate nausea and digestive issues often experienced during cancer treatments. You can enjoy ginger in teas, smoothies, or as a spice in your cooking. Fresh ginger or ginger supplements can both be effective.

Green tea is rich in antioxidants called catechins, which have been studied for their potential cancer-fighting properties. Drinking a few cups of green tea each day can support overall health and provide a gentle boost to your immune system. Just be sure to choose a high-quality green tea and consult with your healthcare provider if you're considering supplements.

Echinacea is often used to support the immune system and may help reduce the risk of infections. This herb can be taken as a tea, tincture, or capsule. It's important to discuss its use with your healthcare provider, especially if you're on other medications or treatments.

Astragalus is known for its immune-boosting properties and its potential to help your body adapt to stress. It can support overall vitality and may enhance the effects of conventional cancer treatments. Astragalus is commonly available in capsules or as a tea.

Milk thistle contains silymarin, which is believed to support liver function and detoxification. This can be particularly helpful during cancer treatment, as your liver works hard to process medications and toxins. Milk thistle can be taken in capsule or tincture form. Always consult with your doctor before starting any new supplement.

Dandelion root is often used to support liver health and improve digestion. It may help with detoxification and reduce some of the side effects of cancer treatments. Dandelion root can be enjoyed as a tea or taken in supplement form.

Reishi mushrooms are known for their immune-supportive and adaptogenic properties. They may help your body cope with stress and support overall wellness. Reishi can be found in capsules, powders, or teas. Always check with your healthcare provider before adding new herbs to your regimen.

Cat's Claw is an herb used traditionally for its immune-supporting and anti-inflammatory properties. It may help reduce inflammation and support overall health during cancer treatment. It's available in capsule, tincture, or tea form.

Ginseng is known for its adaptogenic properties, which can help your body manage stress and improve energy levels. It may also support immune function and overall health. Ginseng is available in various forms, including teas, capsules, and extracts.

Tips for Using Herbs Safely

- Consult with Your Healthcare Provider: Always talk to your doctor or a qualified herbalist before starting any new herbal supplements, especially if you're undergoing cancer treatment or taking other medications.
- Choose Quality Products: Opt for high-quality herbs from reputable sources. Look for standardized extracts to ensure consistent potency.
- Start Slowly: Introduce new herbs gradually and monitor how your body responds. This can help you identify any potential side effects or interactions.
- Stay Informed: Research each herb's benefits and potential side effects. Understanding how each herb works can help you make informed decisions about your health.

Immune System Boosters for Cancer Recovery

Supporting your immune system during cancer recovery is crucial. A strong immune system can help your body fight off infections, manage side effects, and potentially improve your overall well-being. Here's a friendly guide to some effective ways to boost your immune system and support your recovery journey:

Eating a balanced diet rich in vitamins and minerals can help strengthen your immune system. Focus on incorporating a variety of colorful fruits and vegetables into your meals. Foods high in vitamin C (like oranges and bell peppers), vitamin A (like sweet potatoes and spinach), and zinc (like nuts and seeds) are particularly beneficial for immune health.

Water is essential for overall health and helps keep your body's systems running smoothly. Staying hydrated supports every cell in your body, including those in your immune system. Aim for at least 8 glasses of water a day, and consider hydrating with herbal teas and broths to add variety.

Probiotics are beneficial bacteria that support gut health, which is closely linked to immune function. Adding probiotic-rich foods like yogurt, kefir, and fermented vegetables (like sauerkraut and kimchi) to your diet can help maintain a healthy balance of gut flora, which in turn supports your immune system.

Rest is crucial for recovery and immune function. Ensure you're getting adequate sleep each night, as this is when your body does much of its repair and regeneration. Aim for 7-9 hours of quality sleep each night and create a relaxing bedtime routine to improve sleep quality.

Moderate exercise can enhance your immune system by promoting healthy circulation and reducing inflammation. Activities like walking, swimming, or gentle yoga can be beneficial. Be sure to listen to your body and consult with your healthcare provider before starting a new exercise routine.

Chronic stress can weaken your immune system and affect your recovery. Finding ways to manage stress can help support your immune health. Techniques such as deep breathing, meditation, and mindfulness can help reduce stress and promote overall well-being. Finding enjoyable hobbies or spending time with loved ones can also be beneficial.

Certain supplements may help boost your immune system, but it's important to use them with guidance from your healthcare provider. Some popular options include:

- Vitamin D: Supports immune function and can be especially helpful if you have low levels of this vitamin.
- Elderberry: Known for its potential immune-boosting properties and may help reduce the duration of colds.
- Mushroom Extracts: Such as reishi and shiitake, which may support immune health.

Maintaining good hygiene is important for preventing infections, especially during cancer recovery. Regular hand washing, avoiding close contact with sick individuals, and keeping your environment clean can help reduce your risk of illness.

Smoking and excessive alcohol consumption can negatively impact your immune system. If you smoke, seek support to quit, and try to limit alcohol intake to moderate levels (if you choose to drink).

Social support can have a positive impact on your immune health. Connecting with support groups or communities where you can share experiences and receive encouragement can be uplifting and beneficial for your emotional and physical well-being.

Managing Side Effects of Conventional Cancer Treatments

Cancer treatments, while essential, can come with a range of side effects. Managing these side effects can make your journey more comfortable and help you maintain your quality of life. Here's a friendly guide to some common side effects and strategies for managing them:

Nausea and vomiting are common side effects of cancer treatments. To help manage these:

- Eat Small, Frequent Meals: Instead of three large meals, try eating smaller portions throughout the day. Gentle, bland foods like crackers, rice, and applesauce can be easier on your stomach.
- Stay Hydrated: Sip clear fluids, like water or ginger tea, to stay hydrated and soothe your stomach.
- Ginger and Peppermint: Ginger and peppermint can help reduce nausea. Consider ginger tea or peppermint candies to ease queasiness.

Feeling tired or fatigued is another common side effect. Here are some tips to help manage fatigue:

- Prioritize Rest: Make sure you're getting enough sleep and rest during the day. Listen to your body and take naps if needed.
- Balance Activity: Gentle exercise, like walking or stretching, can help boost your energy levels. Just be sure to pace yourself and avoid overexertion.
- Nutrition: Eating a balanced diet with plenty of fruits, vegetables, and whole grains can provide the energy your body needs.

Cancer treatments can sometimes affect your appetite. To manage these changes:

- Eat What You Enjoy: Focus on foods you find appealing and enjoyable. If your taste buds are affected, try experimenting with different flavors and seasonings.
- Nutrient-Dense Snacks: Choose snacks that are high in nutrients, like nuts, yogurt, and smoothies, to help maintain your nutritional intake.
- Small Meals: Eating smaller, more frequent meals can make it easier to consume enough calories and nutrients.

Mouth sores can be painful and make eating difficult. Here's how to manage them:

- Avoid Irritants: Stay away from spicy, acidic, or rough-textured foods that can irritate your mouth. Opt for soft, bland foods instead.
- Oral Care: Rinse your mouth with a mild, non-alcoholic mouthwash or a saltwater solution to soothe sores and keep your mouth clean.
- Stay Hydrated: Drink plenty of fluids to keep your mouth moist and help with healing.

Treatments can sometimes cause skin changes, like dryness or sensitivity. To take care of your skin:

- Moisturize: Use gentle, fragrance-free moisturizers to keep your skin hydrated and reduce dryness.
- Protect Your Skin: Wear protective clothing and use sunscreen if you're exposed to sunlight. Avoid hot showers and harsh soaps that can further irritate your skin.
- Gentle Products: Opt for gentle, hypoallergenic skin care products to minimize irritation.

Hair loss can be a challenging side effect. To manage this:

- Head Coverings: Consider wearing hats, scarves, or wigs if you feel comfortable. Many find these can provide both warmth and a sense of normalcy.
- Gentle Care: If you're experiencing thinning hair, use mild shampoos and avoid harsh treatments like coloring or heat styling.

Treatments may impact your digestive system, causing symptoms like diarrhea or constipation. To address these issues:

- Fiber Intake: For constipation, increase your intake of high-fiber foods like fruits, vegetables, and whole grains. Drink plenty of water to help with digestion.
- Manage Diarrhea: For diarrhea, eat bland, easily digestible foods like bananas, rice, and toast. Avoid caffeine and high-fat foods.

Cancer treatments can take a toll on your emotional health. To support your mental well-being:

- Seek Support: Connect with support groups or counseling services. Talking to others who understand what you're going through can be incredibly helpful.
- Practice Relaxation: Engage in relaxation techniques like meditation, deep breathing, or gentle exercise to help manage stress and improve your mood.

Cancer treatments can affect your immune system. To help support it:

- Follow Hygiene Practices: Practice good hygiene to reduce the risk of infections. Wash your hands regularly and avoid crowded places when your immune system is compromised.
- Consult Your Healthcare Team: If you have any concerns about infections or other immune-related issues, reach out to your healthcare provider for guidance and support.

Mental and Emotional Support for Cancer Patients

Facing cancer is not just a physical journey; it's an emotional and mental one as well. Navigating this challenging time with resilience and positivity can make a significant difference in your overall well-being. Here's a friendly guide to finding mental and emotional support during your cancer journey:

Talking to a mental health professional can be incredibly beneficial. Therapists and counselors who specialize in oncology can provide support tailored to your unique experience. They can help you manage anxiety, depression, or any emotional challenges you may be facing. Don't hesitate to reach out for help—there's no need to go through this alone.

Support groups offer a sense of community and understanding. Connecting with others who are going through similar experiences can provide comfort, practical advice, and encouragement. Whether in-person or online, support groups can be a valuable resource for sharing experiences and finding emotional support.

Your friends and family want to support you, but they might not always know how. Be open with them about your needs and feelings. Sharing your thoughts and emotions can help you feel less isolated and strengthen your relationships.

Mindfulness practices, such as meditation, deep breathing exercises, and yoga, can help reduce stress and improve your emotional well-being. These techniques can provide a sense of calm and help you stay grounded during challenging times.

Do things that bring you joy and relaxation. Whether it's reading a book, watching your favorite movies, gardening, or crafting, engaging in activities you love can lift your spirits and provide a positive distraction.

Having a daily routine can provide a sense of normalcy and stability. Try to maintain regular sleep patterns, meal times, and activities. A structured routine can help you manage stress and maintain a sense of control.

Expressing yourself through creative activities like painting, writing, or music can be therapeutic. Creative outlets provide a way to process your emotions and find joy in the midst of challenges.

Be kind to yourself. Cancer treatment can be physically and emotionally demanding, and it's important to acknowledge and accept your feelings. Practicing self-compassion means treating yourself with the same kindness and understanding you would offer to a friend.

Setting small, achievable goals can provide a sense of accomplishment and purpose. These goals don't have to be grand—simple things like taking a walk, trying a new recipe, or completing a small project can help you feel more empowered.

If spirituality is important to you, find ways to incorporate it into your life. This might include prayer, meditation, or participating in religious or spiritual communities. Spiritual support can provide comfort and a sense of connection during difficult times.

While there are many aspects of cancer treatment and recovery that are beyond your control, focusing on the things you can influence can help you feel more empowered. This might include your daily routines, your diet, or your engagement in supportive activities.

Stress can impact your emotional and physical health, so finding ways to manage it is essential. Techniques such as progressive muscle relaxation, guided imagery, or gentle stretching can help reduce stress and improve your overall sense of well-being.

Acknowledge and celebrate your progress, no matter how small it may seem. Whether it's completing a treatment cycle, managing a difficult day with grace, or simply getting through a challenging week, recognizing your achievements can boost your morale and motivation.

Book 11: Cardiovascular Health and Longevity

Understanding Heart Health from a Holistic Perspective

Taking care of your heart isn't just about managing cholesterol or blood pressure; it's about looking at your overall well-being and how all aspects of your life contribute to heart health. Here's a friendly guide to understanding heart health from a holistic perspective:

Eating a variety of nutrient-rich foods is key to maintaining heart health. Focus on:

- Fruits and Vegetables: These are packed with vitamins, minerals, and antioxidants that help protect your heart. Aim for a colorful plate with a variety of produce.
- Whole Grains: Foods like oats, brown rice, and whole wheat are great for heart health. They provide fiber, which can help lower cholesterol levels.
- Healthy Fats: Incorporate sources of healthy fats such as avocados, nuts, seeds, and olive oil. These fats can support heart function and reduce inflammation.
- Lean Proteins: Opt for lean meats, fish, and plant-based proteins like beans and lentils. Omega-3-rich fish, such as salmon, are particularly beneficial for heart health.

Regular physical activity is crucial for heart health. It helps improve circulation, lower blood pressure, and manage weight. Aim for:

- Cardiovascular Exercise: Activities like walking, jogging, cycling, and swimming get your heart pumping and can boost cardiovascular fitness.
- Strength Training: Incorporate strength training exercises, like lifting weights or doing bodyweight exercises, to build muscle and support overall health.
- Consistency: Find activities you enjoy and make them a regular part of your routine. Even short bursts of activity can have a positive impact.

Chronic stress can negatively affect your heart health. To manage stress effectively:

- Practice Relaxation Techniques: Techniques such as deep breathing, meditation, and yoga can help reduce stress and improve heart health.
- Connect with Loved Ones: Spending time with family and friends can provide emotional support and reduce stress levels.
- Engage in Hobbies: Doing things you love and finding time for relaxation can help alleviate stress and promote overall well-being.

Quality sleep is vital for heart health. To ensure you're getting restorative rest:

- Establish a Sleep Routine: Go to bed and wake up at the same time each day to regulate your body's internal clock.
- Create a Relaxing Environment: Make your bedroom a peaceful, comfortable space that promotes restful sleep. Consider factors like room temperature, noise levels, and lighting.
- Limit Screen Time: Reduce exposure to screens before bedtime to improve sleep quality.

Maintaining a healthy weight helps reduce the risk of heart disease and related conditions. To manage your weight:

- Focus on Nutrition: Eat a balanced diet and watch portion sizes to help maintain a healthy weight.
- Stay Active: Combine regular physical activity with a healthy diet to support weight management.
- Set Realistic Goals: Make gradual changes to your lifestyle that you can sustain in the long term.

Certain habits can negatively impact heart health. To protect your heart:

- Quit Smoking: Smoking is a major risk factor for heart disease. Seek support to quit if you smoke.
- Limit Alcohol: Drink alcohol in moderation. For most adults, this means up to one drink per day for women and up to two drinks per day for men.

Your mental well-being is closely linked to your heart health. To support your mental health:

- Seek Support: If you're struggling with anxiety or depression, talk to a mental health professional for guidance and support.
- Practice Self-Care: Make time for activities that promote relaxation and joy, and ensure you're taking care of your emotional needs.

Regular check-ups with your healthcare provider can help monitor your heart health and catch any potential issues early. Keep track of:

- Blood Pressure: Regularly monitor and manage your blood pressure levels.
- Cholesterol Levels: Get your cholesterol checked to ensure it's within a healthy range.
- Heart Rate: Keep an eye on your heart rate and discuss any concerns with your doctor.

Educate yourself about heart health and stay informed about the latest research and recommendations. Knowledge is empowering and can help you make informed decisions about your health.

Nutrition and Herbs for Healthy Blood Pressure

Maintaining healthy blood pressure is key to cardiovascular health and overall well-being. A balanced diet and certain herbs can play a significant role in keeping your blood pressure within a healthy range. Here's a friendly guide to nutrition and herbs that support healthy blood pressure:

A nutritious diet is foundational for managing blood pressure. Focus on these dietary choices:

- Fruits and Vegetables: These are rich in vitamins, minerals, and antioxidants. Aim for a colorful variety to get a broad spectrum of nutrients. Leafy greens like spinach and kale are particularly beneficial due to their high potassium content, which helps balance sodium levels.
- Whole Grains: Foods like brown rice, quinoa, and whole wheat bread are high in fiber, which supports cardiovascular health and helps maintain stable blood pressure.
- Lean Proteins: Include sources like skinless poultry, fish, and legumes. Fish, particularly those rich in omega-3 fatty acids like salmon, can be particularly helpful in supporting heart health.

- Low-Fat Dairy: Opt for low-fat or fat-free dairy products like yogurt and milk. These can provide important nutrients like calcium, which plays a role in maintaining healthy blood pressure.
- Healthy Fats: Incorporate sources of healthy fats such as avocados, nuts, seeds, and olive oil. These fats support overall cardiovascular health and can help manage blood pressure.

Excess sodium can lead to high blood pressure. To manage sodium intake:

- Read Labels: Check food labels for sodium content, and try to choose lower-sodium options when available.
- Cook at Home: Preparing meals at home allows you to control the amount of salt added to your food. Use herbs and spices to flavor your dishes instead of salt.

Potassium helps counteract the effects of sodium and supports healthy blood pressure. Include potassium-rich foods such as:

- Bananas: A great source of potassium, bananas can easily be added to your diet.
- Sweet Potatoes: Rich in potassium, they can be a nutritious addition to meals.
- Beans: Beans like lentils and black beans are excellent sources of potassium.

Magnesium helps regulate blood pressure. Foods high in magnesium include:

- Nuts and Seeds: Almonds, pumpkin seeds, and sunflower seeds are good sources.
- Legumes: Beans, chickpeas, and lentils provide magnesium as well as fiber.
- Whole Grains: Foods like brown rice and oats contribute magnesium to your diet.

Certain herbs can be beneficial for maintaining healthy blood pressure. Here are a few to consider:

- Garlic: Garlic has been shown to have a positive effect on blood pressure. Incorporate fresh garlic into your cooking or consider garlic supplements after discussing with your healthcare provider.
- Hibiscus: Hibiscus tea has been linked to lowering blood pressure. Enjoy a cup of this flavorful herbal tea regularly.
- Hawthorn: Hawthorn is often used in traditional medicine for heart health. It may help improve blood flow and reduce blood pressure. Consult with a herbalist or healthcare provider to determine if it's right for you.
- Olive Leaf: Olive leaf extract has been studied for its potential benefits in managing blood pressure. It's available in various forms, including capsules and teas.

Adequate hydration is important for overall health, including blood pressure management. Drink plenty of water throughout the day, and consider herbal teas that support cardiovascular health.

Excessive caffeine and alcohol can impact blood pressure. Aim to moderate your intake:

- Caffeine: While moderate coffee consumption is generally considered safe, excessive caffeine can raise blood pressure. Try to limit your intake if you're sensitive to caffeine.
- Alcohol: Drinking alcohol in moderation is key. For most adults, this means up to one drink per day for women and up to two drinks per day for men.

Reducing Cholesterol Levels Naturally

Keeping your cholesterol levels in check is important for heart health and overall well-being. Thankfully, there are several natural ways to manage and reduce cholesterol levels. Here's a friendly guide to help you take charge of your cholesterol through diet, lifestyle, and other natural methods:

A balanced diet can have a big impact on your cholesterol levels. Focus on:

- Fiber-Rich Foods: Foods high in soluble fiber can help lower LDL (bad) cholesterol. Incorporate plenty of oats, barley, beans, lentils, fruits (like apples and oranges), and vegetables into your meals.
- Healthy Fats: Choose unsaturated fats instead of saturated fats. Use olive oil, avocado oil, and canola oil for cooking. Include sources of omega-3 fatty acids, such as salmon, flaxseeds, and walnuts, which can help improve your cholesterol profile.
- Nuts and Seeds: Almonds, walnuts, chia seeds, and flaxseeds are great for heart health. They provide healthy fats and fiber, which can help lower cholesterol.
- Fruits and Vegetables: These are naturally low in fat and high in nutrients. Eating a wide variety of colorful fruits and veggies ensures you get plenty of antioxidants and fiber.

Minimize your intake of unhealthy fats that can raise cholesterol levels:

- Saturated Fats: Found in red meat, butter, and full-fat dairy products. Opt for lean meats, low-fat dairy options, and healthier cooking oils.
- Trans Fats: Often found in processed foods and baked goods. Check food labels and avoid items with "partially hydrogenated oils."

Whole grains are a great source of fiber and can help lower cholesterol:

- Brown Rice and Quinoa: These provide fiber and essential nutrients. They're good substitutes for refined grains.
- Whole Wheat Products: Choose whole wheat bread, pasta, and cereals over refined versions.

Losing excess weight can positively affect your cholesterol levels:

- Balanced Diet and Exercise: Combine a heart-healthy diet with regular physical activity to achieve and maintain a healthy weight.
- Portion Control: Be mindful of portion sizes to avoid overeating, which can contribute to weight gain.

Physical activity helps raise HDL (good) cholesterol and lower LDL (bad) cholesterol:

- Cardiovascular Exercise: Aim for at least 150 minutes of moderate aerobic exercise (like brisk walking or cycling) per week. Even short bursts of activity can make a difference.
- Strength Training: Incorporate strength training exercises a couple of times a week to support overall health and metabolism.

If you smoke, quitting can improve your HDL (good) cholesterol levels and benefit your heart health:

- Seek Support: Consider using resources like counseling, nicotine replacement therapy, or medications to help you quit.
- Stay Motivated: Remind yourself of the benefits of quitting, such as improved heart health and overall well-being.

Drinking alcohol in moderation can help manage cholesterol levels:

- Moderation Guidelines: For most adults, this means up to one drink per day for women and up to two drinks per day for men.

Certain foods can help lower cholesterol naturally:

- Oats and Barley: Rich in beta-glucan, a type of soluble fiber that can help lower LDL cholesterol.
- Avocados: High in monounsaturated fats and fiber, which can improve cholesterol levels.
- Legumes: Beans, lentils, and chickpeas are great for reducing cholesterol and improving heart health.

Drinking plenty of water supports overall health, including cardiovascular health. Aim to drink water throughout the day and limit sugary or high-calorie beverages.

Certain herbs and supplements may help support healthy cholesterol levels:

- Plant Sterols and Stanols: These compounds, found in some fortified foods and supplements, can help block cholesterol absorption.
- Psyllium: Found in fiber supplements, psyllium can help lower cholesterol when included in a balanced diet.

The Role of Stress in Cardiovascular Health

Stress isn't just an emotional challenge; it can also have a big impact on your heart and overall cardiovascular health. Understanding how stress affects your body and finding ways to manage it can help you maintain a healthier heart. Here's a friendly guide to how stress influences cardiovascular health and what you can do about it:

When you're stressed, your body releases stress hormones like cortisol and adrenaline. These hormones can trigger:

- Increased Heart Rate: Your heart may beat faster, which can put extra strain on it.
- Elevated Blood Pressure: Stress can cause your blood vessels to constrict, leading to higher blood pressure.
- Higher Blood Sugar Levels: Stress can increase your blood sugar levels, which may contribute to heart disease over time.

While short-term stress can be manageable, chronic stress—when you're stressed out for long periods—can have more serious effects:

- Higher Risk of Heart Disease: Chronic stress can contribute to inflammation, high blood pressure, and other risk factors for heart disease.
- Unhealthy Coping Mechanisms: Stress may lead to unhealthy habits like smoking, overeating, or drinking alcohol, which can further harm cardiovascular health.
- Weakened Immune System: Ongoing stress can weaken your immune system, making you more susceptible to illness.

It's important to recognize when you're stressed and how it might be affecting your body:

- Physical Symptoms: These can include headaches, muscle tension, or digestive issues.
- Emotional Symptoms: You might feel anxious, irritable, or overwhelmed.
- Behavioral Changes: Stress can lead to changes in sleeping or eating habits, or a lack of interest in activities you usually enjoy.

Managing stress effectively can help protect your heart and improve your overall health. Here are some strategies to consider:

- Practice Relaxation Techniques: Deep breathing exercises, meditation, and progressive muscle relaxation can help calm your mind and body. Try incorporating these into your daily routine to reduce stress levels.
- Get Regular Exercise: Physical activity is a great stress reliever. Aim for at least 30 minutes of moderate exercise most days of the week. Activities like walking, swimming, or yoga can boost your mood and improve cardiovascular health.
- Stay Connected: Building strong relationships with family and friends can provide emotional support and help you manage stress. Don't hesitate to reach out and talk about your feelings with someone you trust.
- Prioritize Sleep: Quality sleep is crucial for managing stress and maintaining heart health. Establish a consistent sleep schedule, create a relaxing bedtime routine, and ensure your sleep environment is comfortable.
- Engage in Hobbies: Taking time to do things you enjoy can be a great way to unwind and reduce stress. Whether it's reading, gardening, or crafting, make sure to set aside time for activities that bring you joy.
- Set Realistic Goals: Break tasks into manageable steps and set achievable goals to avoid feeling overwhelmed. Learn to say no when necessary and prioritize self-care.
- Practice Mindfulness: Mindfulness techniques, such as paying attention to the present moment without judgment, can help reduce stress and improve your overall sense of well-being.
- Seek Professional Help: If stress becomes overwhelming or persistent, consider talking to a mental health professional. Therapy or counseling can provide valuable tools and support for managing stress effectively.

A healthy lifestyle can help mitigate the effects of stress and support cardiovascular health:

- Eat a Balanced Diet: Focus on a diet rich in fruits, vegetables, whole grains, and lean proteins. This can help your body better cope with stress and maintain overall health.
- Avoid Unhealthy Coping Mechanisms: Stay away from smoking, excessive alcohol consumption, or overeating as ways to manage stress. Instead, focus on positive coping strategies and healthy habits.

Exercise and Its Role in Heart Health

Exercise isn't just about staying fit; it's a powerful ally for your heart health. Engaging in regular physical activity can have a profound impact on your cardiovascular system, helping to keep your heart and blood vessels in top shape. Here's a friendly guide to understanding the role of exercise in heart health and how to make it a part of your routine:

Regular exercise offers a range of benefits for your cardiovascular system:

- Improves Heart Efficiency: Exercise strengthens your heart muscle, allowing it to pump blood more efficiently. This means your heart doesn't have to work as hard during rest or physical activity.
- Lowers Blood Pressure: Engaging in physical activity helps relax blood vessels and improve blood flow, which can lead to lower blood pressure over time.
- Boosts HDL Cholesterol: Exercise can increase your levels of HDL (good) cholesterol, which helps to remove LDL (bad) cholesterol from your bloodstream.
- Supports Weight Management: Regular physical activity helps manage body weight, reducing the risk of obesity-related conditions that can strain your heart.
- Enhances Blood Circulation: Exercise improves circulation and promotes healthy blood vessel function, which supports overall cardiovascular health.

Incorporating a variety of exercises into your routine can maximize cardiovascular benefits:

- Aerobic Exercise: Activities like walking, jogging, swimming, or cycling get your heart rate up and improve cardiovascular endurance. Aim for at least 150 minutes of moderate aerobic exercise or 75 minutes of vigorous activity per week.
- Strength Training: Building muscle through exercises like weight lifting or bodyweight exercises (e.g., squats, lunges) supports overall fitness and helps with weight management. Include strength training exercises at least two days a week.
- Flexibility and Balance: Activities such as yoga or stretching improve flexibility and balance, which can support overall fitness and prevent injuries. While not directly related to heart health, they contribute to overall well-being.

Starting an exercise routine doesn't have to be daunting. Here are some tips to help you get moving:

- Choose Activities You Enjoy: Find exercises that you look forward to doing. Whether it's dancing, hiking, or playing a sport, enjoying your workout can make it easier to stick with it.
- Set Realistic Goals: Start with manageable goals and gradually increase the intensity and duration of your workouts. Even small amounts of exercise can have positive effects on your heart.
- Make it a Habit: Try to incorporate exercise into your daily routine. Consider scheduling your workouts like any other important activity to help ensure consistency.
- Stay Active Throughout the Day: If finding time for a full workout is challenging, look for opportunities to be active throughout the day. Take the stairs instead of the elevator, go for short walks during breaks, or engage in active hobbies.
- Find a Workout Buddy: Exercising with a friend or family member can provide motivation and make workouts more enjoyable.

- Listen to Your Body: Pay attention to how your body feels during and after exercise. It's normal to experience some soreness, but if you feel pain or discomfort, be sure to consult with a healthcare provider.

Regular exercise is most beneficial when it becomes a lasting part of your lifestyle. Here's how to make it a sustainable habit:

- Stay Flexible: Life can be unpredictable, so be open to adjusting your exercise routine as needed. Find alternative activities or shorter workouts if you're pressed for time.
- Celebrate Progress: Acknowledge and celebrate your achievements, no matter how small. Recognizing your progress can boost motivation and help you stay committed.
- Keep It Fun: Continuously explore new activities or variations of your current workouts to keep things interesting and prevent boredom.

Supporting Circulation with Natural Remedies

Good circulation is key to a healthy cardiovascular system. It ensures that oxygen and nutrients are delivered efficiently throughout your body, while waste products are carried away. If you're looking for natural ways to boost your circulation and keep your cardiovascular system in top shape, you're in the right place! Here's a friendly guide to some effective natural remedies for supporting healthy circulation:

What you eat can significantly impact your circulation:

- Fruits and Vegetables: Rich in vitamins, minerals, and antioxidants, fruits and veggies help support healthy blood vessels and improve circulation. Berries, oranges, and leafy greens are particularly beneficial.
- Beets: Beets are known for their ability to improve blood flow. They contain nitrates, which can help dilate blood vessels and lower blood pressure.
- Citrus Fruits: Oranges, grapefruits, and lemons are high in vitamin C, which supports the health of blood vessels and improves circulation.
- Spices and Herbs: Turmeric and ginger are known for their anti-inflammatory properties and can help improve blood flow. Adding these to your meals can offer a tasty and healthful boost.

Proper hydration is essential for good circulation:

- Drink Plenty of Water: Keeping hydrated helps maintain blood volume and fluid balance, which supports efficient circulation. Aim to drink water throughout the day.
- Herbal Teas: Herbal teas like green tea and hibiscus tea not only provide hydration but also offer additional benefits. Green tea contains antioxidants that can support vascular health, while hibiscus tea can help lower blood pressure.

Physical activity is a natural way to support circulation:

- Regular Exercise: Engaging in regular exercise, such as walking, jogging, or swimming, helps improve blood flow and strengthens the heart. Aim for at least 150 minutes of moderate exercise per week.

- Incorporate Movement Breaks: If you're sitting for long periods, take breaks to stretch or walk around. Simple activities like standing up and moving can help keep your blood flowing.

Certain supplements can help support circulation:

- Ginkgo Biloba: Known for its potential to enhance blood flow, ginkgo biloba may improve circulation and support cognitive function. Be sure to consult with a healthcare provider before starting any new supplement.
- Garlic: Garlic has been shown to have beneficial effects on circulation and blood pressure. It can be consumed raw, cooked, or in supplement form.
- Cayenne Pepper: Containing capsaicin, cayenne pepper may help improve blood flow by dilating blood vessels. It can be added to meals or taken as a supplement.

Stress can negatively impact circulation, so incorporating relaxation practices into your routine can be beneficial:

- Deep Breathing: Deep breathing exercises can help lower stress levels and improve circulation. Practice slow, deep breaths to promote relaxation.
- Meditation: Regular meditation can reduce stress and improve overall cardiovascular health. Even a few minutes a day can make a difference.

Managing your weight is important for supporting healthy circulation:

- Balanced Diet: Eating a diet rich in whole foods, lean proteins, and healthy fats can help you maintain a healthy weight.
- Regular Physical Activity: Combining exercise with a balanced diet supports weight management and promotes good circulation.

Smoking is harmful to your circulatory system and overall health:

- Quit Smoking: If you smoke, quitting is one of the best things you can do for your circulation and heart health. Seek support and resources to help you stop smoking.

If you experience poor circulation in your legs, elevating them can help:

- Leg Elevation: When resting, try elevating your legs to improve blood flow and reduce swelling. This can be especially helpful if you spend long periods sitting or standing.

Book 12: Natural Skin and Hair Care Remedies

Detoxifying Your Skin Naturally

Your skin is not only the largest organ in your body but also a reflection of your overall health. It can absorb toxins from the environment and sometimes needs a little extra help to stay clear and glowing. Detoxifying your skin naturally can help remove impurities and rejuvenate your complexion. Here's a friendly guide to some simple and effective natural remedies for detoxifying your skin:

Keeping your skin clean is the first step in detoxification:

- Cleansing Oils: Natural oils like coconut oil or olive oil can gently remove makeup and impurities without stripping your skin of its natural oils. Simply massage a small amount into your skin and wipe away with a warm, damp cloth.
- Herbal Cleansers: Look for cleansers with natural ingredients like chamomile or green tea. These can help soothe and detoxify your skin while providing gentle cleansing.

Exfoliation helps remove dead skin cells and promotes a fresh, radiant complexion:

- DIY Scrubs: Create your own exfoliating scrub using natural ingredients like oatmeal, honey, and yogurt. For example, mix finely ground oats with a bit of honey to create a gentle scrub that also hydrates your skin.
- Fruit Enzymes: Enzyme-rich fruits like papaya and pineapple can naturally exfoliate your skin. Apply mashed fruit to your face and leave it on for 10-15 minutes before rinsing off.

Face masks can provide a deep cleanse and deliver nutrients directly to your skin:

- Clay Masks: Clay, such as bentonite or kaolin, can help draw out impurities and toxins from your skin. Mix the clay with water or apple cider vinegar to form a paste and apply it to your face. Leave it on until it dries, then rinse off with warm water.
- Green Tea Mask: Green tea is packed with antioxidants that help fight free radicals and reduce inflammation. Brew a strong cup of green tea, let it cool, and then apply it to your face with a cotton pad.
- Avocado and Honey Mask: Avocado is rich in vitamins and healthy fats, while honey is a natural humectant. Combine mashed avocado with honey for a hydrating and detoxifying mask.

Hydration is essential for maintaining healthy, detoxified skin:

- Drink Plenty of Water: Aim to drink at least 8 glasses of water a day to help flush out toxins and keep your skin hydrated.
- Herbal Teas: Herbal teas like chamomile or peppermint can also aid in detoxification and provide added hydration.

What you eat can affect your skin's health and detoxification:

- Eat Fresh Fruits and Vegetables: Incorporate plenty of fruits and veggies into your diet. Foods like berries, leafy greens, and cucumbers are rich in antioxidants and help cleanse your system from the inside out.
- Include Healthy Fats: Avocados, nuts, and seeds provide essential fatty acids that support skin health and help detoxify.
- Avoid Processed Foods: Minimize your intake of processed foods, sugary snacks, and high-fat foods that can contribute to skin issues.

Exercise helps improve circulation and promotes the removal of toxins through sweating:

- Engage in Cardio Workouts: Activities like jogging, swimming, or cycling boost your heart rate and increase blood flow, which can help your skin detoxify.
- Incorporate Sweating: Use a sauna or steam room to encourage sweating, which helps expel toxins through your skin.

Stress can affect your skin's appearance and health:

- Practice Relaxation Techniques: Incorporate practices like yoga, meditation, or deep breathing exercises into your routine to help manage stress and support overall skin health.
- Get Enough Sleep: Quality sleep is crucial for skin repair and detoxification. Aim for 7-9 hours of restful sleep each night.

Essential Oils for Skincare

Essential oils are nature's little powerhouses, packed with concentrated plant goodness that can work wonders for your skin. Whether you're looking to boost hydration, balance oil production, or calm irritation, essential oils offer a range of benefits. Here's a friendly guide to incorporating essential oils into your skincare routine:

Different essential oils have unique properties that can address various skin concerns. Here are some popular choices and their benefits:

- Lavender: Known for its calming and soothing properties, lavender oil can help with acne, reduce redness, and promote overall skin healing. It's great for all skin types, especially sensitive skin.
- Tea Tree: With its powerful antibacterial and antifungal properties, tea tree oil is fantastic for treating acne and preventing breakouts. Just be sure to use it sparingly, as it can be quite potent.
- Rosehip: Rich in essential fatty acids and antioxidants, rosehip oil is excellent for reducing the appearance of scars, fine lines, and wrinkles. It's particularly beneficial for dry or mature skin.
- Geranium: This oil helps balance oil production and improve skin tone. It can be helpful for those with oily or combination skin and may also assist in reducing the appearance of acne scars.
- Frankincense: Often used for its anti-aging benefits, frankincense oil can help reduce the appearance of fine lines and promote healthy skin regeneration. It's suitable for most skin types.
- Chamomile: Known for its anti-inflammatory and soothing properties, chamomile oil can help calm irritated skin and reduce redness. It's great for sensitive or dry skin.

Essential oils are potent, so it's important to use them correctly:

- Dilution: Always dilute essential oils with a carrier oil before applying them to your skin. Carrier oils like jojoba, sweet almond, or coconut oil help to safely disperse the essential oil. A general guideline is to use 1-2 drops of essential oil per teaspoon of carrier oil.
- Patch Test: Before using a new essential oil, perform a patch test to ensure you don't have an adverse reaction. Apply a small amount of the diluted oil to a patch of skin and wait 24 hours to see if any irritation occurs.
- Avoid Sensitive Areas: Keep essential oils away from sensitive areas like the eyes and mucous membranes. They can cause irritation if they come into contact with these areas.

There are many ways to use essential oils to enhance your skincare regimen:

- Facial Cleansers: Add a few drops of essential oil to your favorite facial cleanser or mix it with a gentle cleansing oil. This can help target specific skin concerns while you cleanse.
- Toners: Infuse your toner with essential oils to enhance its effects. For example, add a drop or two of lavender or chamomile oil to your toner for added soothing benefits.
- Serums: Incorporate essential oils into your serum by adding a few drops to your serum or moisturizer. This allows you to benefit from the oils' properties while nourishing your skin.
- Face Masks: Enhance your DIY face masks with essential oils. Add a few drops to your homemade mask mixture for an extra boost of skincare benefits.
- Spot Treatments: For targeted treatment of blemishes or problem areas, mix a drop of tea tree oil with a carrier oil and apply it directly to the affected area.
- Baths: Add a few drops of your favorite essential oil to a warm bath for a relaxing and skin-soothing experience.

To get the most out of your essential oils:

- Consistency is Key: Incorporate essential oils into your routine regularly for the best results. Skin benefits often develop over time with consistent use.
- Choose Quality Oils: Opt for high-quality, pure essential oils from reputable sources. Look for oils that are labeled as 100% pure and free from synthetic additives.
- Personalize Your Blend: Feel free to experiment with different essential oil blends to find what works best for your skin. Creating your own custom blend can be a fun and rewarding way to address your specific skincare needs.

Herbal Hair Treatments

Herbal hair treatments are a wonderful way to nurture your locks with nature's best. Herbs have been used for centuries to promote hair health and address various scalp and hair concerns. Whether you're looking to boost shine, strengthen strands, or soothe a dry scalp, there's a herbal remedy for you. Here's a friendly guide to some popular herbal hair treatments:

Nourishing Herbs for Strong and Healthy Hair

- Rosemary: Known for its stimulating properties, rosemary can help promote hair growth and improve circulation to the scalp. You can use it in several ways:

Rosemary Rinse: Steep a few sprigs of fresh rosemary or a couple of tablespoons of dried rosemary in boiling water. Let it cool, strain, and use it as a final rinse after shampooing.

Rosemary Oil: Add a few drops of rosemary essential oil to your shampoo or conditioner, or dilute it with a carrier oil and massage it into your scalp.

- Nettle: Rich in vitamins and minerals, nettle is great for strengthening hair and reducing dandruff.

    Nettle Tea Rinse: Brew nettle tea, let it cool, and use it as a hair rinse. It helps to nourish the scalp and hair follicles.

- Horsetail: Packed with silica, horsetail can help strengthen hair and improve its elasticity.

    Horsetail Infusion: Prepare an infusion by steeping dried horsetail in hot water, then apply it to your hair and scalp as a rinse.

Herbal Treatments for Scalp Health

- Chamomile: Known for its soothing and anti-inflammatory properties, chamomile can help calm an irritated scalp.

    Chamomile Rinse: Brew chamomile tea, let it cool, and use it as a final rinse to soothe the scalp and add a natural shine to your hair.

- Peppermint: Peppermint oil has a cooling effect that can invigorate the scalp and help with dandruff.

    Peppermint Scalp Massage: Mix a few drops of peppermint essential oil with a carrier oil and massage it into your scalp. Leave it on for 15-20 minutes before rinsing out.

- Aloe Vera: Aloe vera is excellent for hydrating and soothing the scalp.

    Aloe Vera Gel: Apply fresh aloe vera gel directly to your scalp, leave it on for 20 minutes, then rinse thoroughly. It helps to moisturize and reduce itching.

Herbal Masks for Shine and Strength

- Henna: A natural conditioner, henna can add shine and strength to your hair.

    Henna Treatment: Mix henna powder with water to form a paste, apply it to your hair, and leave it on for a few hours. Rinse out thoroughly for shiny, strengthened hair.

- Basil: Basil can help control oil production and add a healthy shine to your hair.

Basil Infused Oil: Infuse basil leaves in a carrier oil (such as coconut or olive oil) and use it as a hair treatment. Apply to your scalp and hair, leave it on for 30 minutes, then rinse out.

- Yarrow: Yarrow can help improve scalp circulation and strengthen hair.

    Yarrow Infusion: Steep dried yarrow in hot water to make an infusion. After cooling, apply it to your scalp and hair as a final rinse.

Tips for Using Herbal Hair Treatments

1. Consistency is Key: For the best results, use herbal treatments regularly. Hair health improves over time with consistent care.
2. Patch Test: Before trying a new herbal remedy, do a patch test to ensure you don't have any adverse reactions. Apply a small amount of the treatment to a small area of skin and wait 24 hours.
3. Choose Quality Ingredients: Opt for high-quality, organic herbs whenever possible to ensure you're getting the best benefits for your hair.
4. Mix and Match: Feel free to experiment with different herbal combinations to find what works best for your hair type and concerns.

Nutrition for Radiant Skin and Hair

Eating well isn't just good for your overall health—it's also a key ingredient for glowing skin and luscious hair. What you put into your body has a direct impact on how your skin and hair look and feel. Here's a friendly guide to the best nutrients and foods that can help you achieve radiant skin and beautiful hair.

Essential Nutrients for Healthy Skin and Hair

- Vitamin A: This vitamin is crucial for skin repair and maintaining healthy skin cells. It helps keep your skin smooth and free of blemishes.

    Sources: Carrots, sweet potatoes, spinach, and kale are rich in beta-carotene, which the body converts to vitamin A.

- Vitamin C: Known for its powerful antioxidant properties, vitamin C helps protect your skin from damage and supports collagen production, which keeps your skin firm and youthful.

    Sources: Citrus fruits (like oranges and grapefruits), strawberries, bell peppers, and broccoli are excellent sources.

- Vitamin E: This vitamin helps protect your skin from oxidative stress and can improve skin texture and elasticity.

    Sources: Nuts, seeds, avocados, and leafy greens are great sources of vitamin E.

- Biotin: Also known as vitamin B7, biotin is essential for healthy hair growth and can help strengthen brittle hair.

    Sources: Eggs, nuts, seeds, and whole grains are packed with biotin.

- Omega-3 Fatty Acids: These healthy fats help maintain the skin's lipid barrier, which keeps it hydrated and supple. They also reduce inflammation, which can be beneficial for conditions like acne and eczema.

    Sources: Fatty fish (like salmon and mackerel), chia seeds, flaxseeds, and walnuts are rich in omega-3s.

- Zinc: This mineral supports skin healing and helps regulate oil production, which can reduce acne and improve skin texture.

    Sources: Pumpkin seeds, nuts, whole grains, and legumes are good sources of zinc.

Staying hydrated is crucial for maintaining the health and appearance of your skin and hair. When you're well-hydrated, your skin looks plump and youthful, and your hair feels soft and manageable.

- Drink Plenty of Water: Aim to drink at least 8 glasses of water a day to keep your skin and hair hydrated from the inside out.
- Eat Water-Rich Foods: Incorporate fruits and vegetables with high water content, like cucumbers, watermelon, and oranges, into your diet.

Foods for Glowing Skin and Strong Hair

- Avocados: Packed with healthy fats and vitamins, avocados nourish your skin and hair, promoting a healthy glow and preventing dryness.
- Nuts and Seeds: Almonds, walnuts, and flaxseeds are rich in essential fatty acids, vitamin E, and zinc, which help support healthy skin and hair.
- Berries: Blueberries, strawberries, and raspberries are high in antioxidants that protect your skin from damage and support collagen production.
- Leafy Greens: Spinach, kale, and Swiss chard are loaded with vitamins A and C, which help maintain healthy skin and support hair growth.
- Sweet Potatoes: Rich in beta-carotene, sweet potatoes help keep your skin smooth and can give your complexion a natural, healthy glow.

Tips for a Radiant Complexion and Beautiful Hair

- Balance Your Diet: Aim for a balanced diet that includes a variety of nutrients from whole foods to support overall health and beauty.
- Avoid Excess Sugar: High sugar intake can lead to inflammation and skin issues, so try to limit your consumption of sugary foods and drinks.
- Opt for Whole Foods: Choose whole, unprocessed foods over processed options to ensure you're getting the most nutrients for your skin and hair.
- Monitor Your Intake: Pay attention to how different foods affect your skin and hair, and make adjustments to your diet as needed.

Avoiding Toxins in Beauty Products

When it comes to beauty and skincare, the saying "you are what you eat" could easily be extended to "you are what you apply." The products you use on your skin and hair can have a big impact on your health. Many conventional beauty products contain harmful chemicals that can irritate your skin, cause allergic reactions, or even disrupt your hormones. Here's a friendly guide to help you avoid toxins in beauty products and choose safer, more natural alternatives.

Here are some common toxins to watch out for in beauty products:

- Parabens: Used as preservatives to extend shelf life, parabens can mimic hormones in the body, potentially leading to hormonal imbalances. Look for products labeled "paraben-free."
- Phthalates: Often found in fragrances, phthalates are linked to reproductive and developmental issues. Choose products with natural or no added fragrances.
- Sulfates: These are harsh detergents found in many shampoos and cleansers that can strip your skin and hair of their natural oils, causing dryness and irritation. Opt for sulfate-free formulas.
- Formaldehyde: This preservative can be irritating and is a known carcinogen. It's best to avoid products that list formaldehyde or formaldehyde-releasing ingredients.
- Synthetic Fragrances: These can contain a cocktail of hidden chemicals that may cause allergic reactions or sensitivities. Choose products with natural essential oils for fragrance or those labeled as "fragrance-free."
- Toluene: Common in nail polishes, toluene can affect the nervous system and cause respiratory issues. Look for toluene-free nail products.

Opt for natural and organic beauty products to avoid harmful chemicals. Here's what to look for:

- Natural Ingredients: Products made with natural ingredients like plant extracts, essential oils, and herbal infusions are less likely to contain harmful chemicals.
- Organic Certification: Organic beauty products are made from ingredients grown without synthetic pesticides or fertilizers, reducing your exposure to potentially harmful substances.
- Eco-Friendly Brands: Many brands are committed to creating products without toxins and are transparent about their ingredient lists. Look for brands that prioritize sustainability and safety.

DIY beauty products can be a fun and rewarding way to avoid toxins. Here are some simple ideas:

- Face Masks: Mix natural ingredients like honey, yogurt, and oatmeal to create nourishing face masks. These ingredients are gentle and free from synthetic additives.
- Hair Conditioners: Blend coconut oil with a few drops of essential oil for a moisturizing hair conditioner that's free from artificial chemicals.
- Body Scrubs: Combine sugar or salt with olive oil and a few drops of your favorite essential oil to make a natural body scrub.

Reading Labels and Doing Your Research

- Check Ingredients Lists: Familiarize yourself with common harmful ingredients and read labels carefully. If you can't pronounce an ingredient or it sounds like a chemical, it might be worth avoiding.

- Research Brands: Look for brands with a commitment to transparency and safety. Many reputable brands provide detailed ingredient lists and information about their sourcing practices.
- Look for Certifications: Certifications like USDA Organic, Ecocert, and COSMOS can help you identify products that meet higher safety and environmental standards.

Tips for a Safer Beauty Routine

- Patch Test New Products: Before using a new product, do a patch test to ensure you don't have a sensitivity or allergic reaction.
- Stay Informed: Keep up with the latest research and guidelines on cosmetic safety. New information can help you make more informed choices.
- Simplicity is Key: Often, less is more. Using fewer products with simpler, natural ingredients can reduce your exposure to potential toxins.

Book 13: Hormonal Health and Balance

Understanding the Endocrine System

The endocrine system might not be the star of the show like the heart or brain, but it plays a crucial role in keeping your body balanced and healthy. Think of it as the body's internal communication network, sending messages through hormones to regulate everything from growth to mood. Here's a friendly guide to help you understand this amazing system and how it keeps things running smoothly.

The endocrine system is a network of glands that produce and release hormones into the bloodstream. These hormones act as messengers, traveling to various organs and tissues to regulate essential functions. It's like having a team of tiny helpers constantly working behind the scenes to keep everything in check.

Key Components of the Endocrine System

- Pituitary Gland: Often called the "master gland," the pituitary gland is located at the base of the brain. It controls other endocrine glands and releases hormones that regulate growth, metabolism, and reproduction.
- Thyroid Gland: Located in the neck, the thyroid gland produces hormones that control metabolism, energy levels, and overall growth. Think of it as your body's speedometer, adjusting how fast or slow processes run.
- Parathyroid Glands: These tiny glands, located behind the thyroid, help regulate calcium levels in the blood, which is crucial for bone health and muscle function.
- Adrenal Glands: Positioned on top of the kidneys, the adrenal glands produce hormones like adrenaline and cortisol that help manage stress, regulate metabolism, and control blood pressure.
- Pancreas: The pancreas plays a key role in digestion and blood sugar regulation by producing insulin and glucagon. These hormones help keep blood sugar levels stable.
- Ovaries (in women) and Testes (in men): These glands are responsible for producing sex hormones like estrogen, progesterone, and testosterone, which regulate reproductive functions and secondary sexual characteristics.
- Pineal Gland: Located in the brain, the pineal gland produces melatonin, which helps regulate sleep-wake cycles and seasonal rhythms.

Hormones are like little messengers traveling through your bloodstream to deliver instructions to different parts of the body. Each hormone has a specific target, and it only affects cells that have the right receptors. This precise communication ensures that your body functions harmoniously.

- Feedback Loops: The endocrine system uses feedback loops to maintain balance. For example, if your thyroid hormone levels drop, the pituitary gland will release more thyroid-stimulating hormone (TSH) to boost thyroid hormone production until balance is restored.
- Hormone Release Triggers: Hormones can be released in response to various factors, including stress, changes in diet, or even light exposure. The system adjusts hormone levels based on what's needed at any given time.

Common Endocrine System Issues

- Thyroid Disorders: Conditions like hypothyroidism (underactive thyroid) or hyperthyroidism (overactive thyroid) can affect metabolism and energy levels.
- Diabetes: When the pancreas doesn't produce enough insulin or the body doesn't use insulin effectively, it can lead to diabetes, affecting blood sugar levels.
- Adrenal Fatigue: Chronic stress can lead to adrenal fatigue, where the adrenal glands become overworked and struggle to produce adequate hormones.
- Hormonal Imbalances: Conditions such as polycystic ovary syndrome (PCOS) or menopause can disrupt hormone levels, affecting menstrual cycles, mood, and overall well-being.

Supporting Endocrine Health

- Balanced Diet: Eating a diet rich in whole foods, healthy fats, and lean proteins supports hormone production and balance. Include foods high in vitamins and minerals, such as leafy greens, nuts, and seeds.
- Regular Exercise: Physical activity helps regulate hormones and improve overall endocrine function. Aim for a mix of cardiovascular, strength, and flexibility exercises.
- Stress Management: Chronic stress can disrupt hormone balance. Practice relaxation techniques like yoga, meditation, or deep breathing to keep stress levels in check.
- Adequate Sleep: Quality sleep is essential for hormonal regulation. Aim for 7-9 hours of restful sleep each night to support overall endocrine health.
- Stay Hydrated: Drinking enough water helps maintain proper hormone function and supports overall bodily functions.

Managing Hormonal Imbalances Naturally

Hormonal imbalances can feel like your body's internal system is out of sync. Whether it's mood swings, fatigue, or irregular periods, these imbalances can affect your quality of life. The good news is that there are natural ways to help bring your hormones back into balance. Here's a friendly guide to managing hormonal imbalances with natural approaches that support your body's well-being.

Hormonal imbalances can be caused by various factors, including:

- Stress: Chronic stress can disrupt your hormone levels, leading to imbalances.
- Diet: A poor diet lacking in essential nutrients can affect hormone production and regulation.
- Sleep: Inadequate or poor-quality sleep can impact hormone levels and overall balance.
- Lifestyle Factors: Excessive alcohol consumption, lack of exercise, and exposure to environmental toxins can also contribute to imbalances.

A well-rounded diet supports hormone health by providing essential nutrients that help regulate hormone production and balance:

- Healthy Fats: Incorporate sources of healthy fats like avocados, nuts, seeds, and olive oil. These fats support hormone production and help maintain hormone balance.
- Lean Proteins: Foods like chicken, fish, and legumes provide the building blocks for hormone production.

- Fiber-Rich Foods: Fruits, vegetables, and whole grains help regulate hormone levels by supporting digestion and elimination of excess hormones.
- Antioxidants: Berries, leafy greens, and colorful vegetables are rich in antioxidants that protect your cells from damage and support overall hormonal health.
- Limit Processed Foods: Reduce your intake of refined sugars, trans fats, and processed foods, as these can disrupt hormone balance.

Stress management is key to maintaining hormonal balance. High levels of stress can lead to the overproduction of cortisol, which can disrupt other hormones. Here are some stress-busting strategies:

- Mindfulness and Meditation: Practicing mindfulness or meditation can help reduce stress levels and promote hormonal balance.
- Regular Exercise: Physical activity helps regulate cortisol levels and boosts endorphins, which can improve your mood and stress levels.
- Relaxation Techniques: Activities like deep breathing, yoga, or spending time in nature can help lower stress and support overall hormonal health.

Getting enough restorative sleep is crucial for hormone regulation. Here's how to improve your sleep quality:

- Establish a Sleep Routine: Go to bed and wake up at the same time each day to regulate your body's internal clock.
- Create a Relaxing Environment: Make your bedroom a calming space with minimal noise and light. Consider using blackout curtains and a white noise machine if needed.
- Avoid Stimulants: Limit caffeine and electronic device use before bedtime, as these can interfere with your ability to fall asleep.

Certain herbs can help support hormonal balance and address specific imbalances:

- Ashwagandha: Known for its adaptogenic properties, ashwagandha helps manage stress and support adrenal health.
- Chaste Tree (Vitex): This herb is commonly used to regulate menstrual cycles and support hormone balance, particularly in women.
- Maca Root: Often used to boost energy and support hormonal balance, maca root can be particularly beneficial during menopause.
- Holy Basil: This herb helps regulate cortisol levels and supports overall hormonal health.

Proper detoxification helps eliminate excess hormones and toxins from your body:

- Hydrate: Drink plenty of water to support kidney function and flush out toxins.
- Eat Detoxifying Foods: Foods like cruciferous vegetables (broccoli, cauliflower), beets, and green tea support liver function and detoxification.
- Consider a Gentle Detox: Incorporate occasional gentle detox practices like herbal teas or a short-term clean-eating regimen to support your body's natural detox processes.

Exercise not only helps manage stress but also supports hormone balance by:

- Improving Insulin Sensitivity: Regular exercise helps regulate blood sugar levels and insulin sensitivity.
- Supporting Hormone Production: Physical activity promotes the release of hormones that support mood, energy levels, and overall health.
- Enhancing Mood: Exercise boosts endorphins, which can help balance mood-related hormones and reduce feelings of anxiety or depression.

Minimize exposure to chemicals that can interfere with your hormone levels:

- Choose Natural Products: Opt for personal care and cleaning products free from synthetic chemicals and fragrances.
- Be Mindful of Plastics: Reduce use of plastic containers and bottles, as certain chemicals in plastics can disrupt hormone balance.

Herbs for Adrenal and Thyroid Support

When it comes to maintaining a balanced and healthy endocrine system, your adrenal and thyroid glands play crucial roles. The adrenal glands help manage stress and energy levels, while the thyroid regulates metabolism and overall energy. Fortunately, nature provides a range of herbs that can support both of these vital glands. Here's a friendly guide to some of the best herbs for adrenal and thyroid support.

Your adrenal glands work hard to help you handle stress and maintain energy. Here are some herbs that can lend a hand:

- Ashwagandha: Often called the "king of adaptogens," ashwagandha helps your body adapt to stress and promotes overall resilience. It supports adrenal function and helps manage cortisol levels, which can be beneficial if you're dealing with chronic stress.
- Rhodiola: This powerful herb is known for its ability to enhance mental and physical endurance. Rhodiola helps combat fatigue, boosts mood, and supports adrenal health by reducing stress and enhancing energy levels.
- Holy Basil (Tulsi): Holy basil is revered for its adaptogenic properties, which help your body handle stress more effectively. It also supports overall adrenal function and can help reduce anxiety and improve emotional well-being.
- Licorice Root: Licorice root helps maintain healthy cortisol levels and supports adrenal function. It can be particularly useful for those experiencing adrenal fatigue. However, it should be used with caution and under the guidance of a healthcare provider, especially if you have high blood pressure.
- Schisandra: This adaptogenic herb helps improve energy, endurance, and mental clarity. Schisandra supports adrenal health by balancing cortisol levels and promoting overall resilience to stress.

The thyroid gland regulates your metabolism and energy. Here are some herbs that can support thyroid function:

- Ashwagandha: In addition to its benefits for adrenal health, ashwagandha also supports thyroid function. It helps regulate thyroid hormones and can be beneficial for those dealing with hypothyroidism (underactive thyroid).
- Bladderwrack: This seaweed is a rich source of iodine, which is essential for thyroid hormone production. Bladderwrack supports thyroid function and can be particularly useful if you have low iodine levels.
- Guggul: Derived from the gum resin of the Commiphora wightii tree, guggul supports thyroid health by promoting healthy hormone levels. It can be helpful for managing symptoms of hypothyroidism.
- Siberian Ginseng (Eleutherococcus): This herb is known for its adaptogenic properties and supports thyroid function by helping to regulate energy levels and balance hormones.
- Kelp: Like bladderwrack, kelp is another seaweed high in iodine. It supports thyroid health by providing the necessary nutrients for thyroid hormone production.

How to Use These Herbs

- Tinctures: Liquid extracts of herbs can be taken daily as directed. They are absorbed quickly and can be an easy way to incorporate these herbs into your routine.
- Capsules and Tablets: Herbal supplements are available in capsule or tablet form for convenient dosing. Be sure to choose high-quality products from reputable brands.
- Teas: Some herbs, like holy basil and licorice root, can be brewed into soothing teas. Drinking herbal tea can be a relaxing way to support your adrenal and thyroid health.
- Powders: Herbs like ashwagandha can be added to smoothies or other beverages in powdered form for an easy health boost.

Tips for Using Herbs Safely

- Consult a Healthcare Provider: Before starting any new herbal regimen, it's always a good idea to consult with a healthcare provider, especially if you have existing health conditions or are taking other medications.
- Start Slowly: Introduce new herbs gradually and monitor how your body responds. This helps to ensure you're not experiencing any adverse effects.
- Quality Matters: Choose high-quality herbs from reputable sources. Organic and sustainably sourced herbs are often preferable for purity and effectiveness.
- Listen to Your Body: Pay attention to how you feel as you incorporate these herbs into your routine. If you notice any unusual symptoms or side effects, consult with a healthcare professional.

Supporting Women's Hormonal Health

Women's hormonal health is a vital aspect of overall well-being, influencing everything from mood and energy levels to reproductive health and bone density. Supporting your hormonal balance naturally can help you feel more balanced, energetic, and healthy. Here's a friendly guide to maintaining and nurturing your hormonal health.

Eating a varied and nutritious diet is foundational for hormonal health. Here's what to focus on:

- Healthy Fats: Include sources of healthy fats like avocados, nuts, seeds, and olive oil in your diet. These fats are crucial for hormone production and balance.
- Lean Proteins: Incorporate lean proteins such as chicken, fish, tofu, and legumes. Proteins help regulate blood sugar levels and support hormone synthesis.
- Fiber-Rich Foods: Fruits, vegetables, and whole grains are packed with fiber, which helps regulate hormones by supporting digestion and detoxification.
- Phytoestrogens: Foods like flaxseeds, soy products, and legumes contain phytoestrogens, which can help balance estrogen levels in the body.
- Limit Sugar and Processed Foods: Reducing your intake of refined sugars and processed foods can help prevent blood sugar spikes and support hormonal balance.

Stress is a major disruptor of hormonal balance. Here are some stress management techniques:

- Mindfulness and Meditation: Practices like mindfulness, meditation, and deep breathing can help lower stress levels and promote hormonal balance.
- Regular Exercise: Physical activity boosts endorphins and reduces cortisol levels, supporting both mood and hormonal balance.
- Relaxation Techniques: Incorporate relaxation practices like yoga, tai chi, or spending time in nature to help manage stress.

Good sleep is essential for hormonal health:

- Establish a Sleep Routine: Aim for 7-9 hours of quality sleep per night. Go to bed and wake up at the same time each day to regulate your internal clock.
- Create a Sleep-Friendly Environment: Make your bedroom a calm and relaxing space. Consider using blackout curtains, a white noise machine, or calming scents like lavender.
- Avoid Stimulants: Limit caffeine and electronic screen use before bedtime to improve sleep quality.

Certain herbs can offer valuable support for hormonal health:

- Vitex (Chaste Tree): This herb is often used to support menstrual health and balance estrogen levels. It can help regulate cycles and alleviate PMS symptoms.
- Dong Quai: Known as "female ginseng," dong quai supports menstrual health and can help balance hormones. It's often used in traditional medicine for menstrual and menopausal issues.
- Red Clover: This herb contains phytoestrogens and can support hormonal balance, particularly during menopause.
- Evening Primrose Oil: Rich in gamma-linolenic acid (GLA), evening primrose oil helps manage symptoms of PMS and supports overall hormonal balance.

Maintaining a healthy weight is important for hormonal health:

- Balance Calories: Eat a balanced diet that supports a healthy weight. Avoid extreme diets or sudden weight changes, which can disrupt hormonal balance.
- Regular Exercise: Engage in regular physical activity to support a healthy weight and overall hormonal function. Aim for a mix of cardiovascular, strength, and flexibility exercises.

Proper hydration supports overall health, including hormonal balance:

- Drink Water: Aim to drink plenty of water throughout the day to stay hydrated and support your body's detoxification processes.
- Limit Sugary Drinks: Avoid excessive consumption of sugary beverages, which can affect blood sugar levels and hormonal balance.

Minimize exposure to substances that can interfere with hormonal balance:

- Choose Natural Products: Opt for personal care and cleaning products that are free from synthetic chemicals and fragrances.
- Be Mindful of Plastics: Reduce the use of plastic containers and bottles, as certain chemicals in plastics can disrupt hormonal function.
- Filter Water: Consider using a water filter to reduce exposure to contaminants that might affect hormonal health.

Regular health check-ups can help monitor and support hormonal health:

- Routine Exams: Schedule regular visits with your healthcare provider to discuss any concerns and monitor hormone levels if needed.
- Blood Tests: Periodic blood tests can help identify any imbalances and guide appropriate interventions.

Natural Approaches to PMS and Menopause

Navigating the changes of PMS (premenstrual syndrome) and menopause can be challenging, but embracing natural approaches can help ease these transitions with greater ease and comfort. Here's a friendly guide to managing both PMS and menopause naturally, focusing on holistic practices and lifestyle changes that can make a positive difference.

PMS can bring a range of symptoms from mood swings and bloating to fatigue and cramps. Here's how you can naturally alleviate these symptoms:

- Balanced Diet: Eating a well-rounded diet rich in whole foods can help reduce PMS symptoms. Focus on:

    Complex Carbohydrates: Whole grains, fruits, and vegetables help stabilize blood sugar levels and can alleviate mood swings.

    Leafy Greens: Spinach, kale, and other greens are high in magnesium, which can help reduce cramps and irritability.

    Omega-3 Fatty Acids: Found in fatty fish, flaxseeds, and walnuts, these can help ease inflammation and improve mood.

- Stay Hydrated: Drinking plenty of water can help reduce bloating and keep you feeling more comfortable.

- Regular Exercise: Engage in regular physical activity to help boost endorphins and reduce symptoms like mood swings and fatigue. Even a daily walk can make a big difference.
- Herbal Teas: Herbal teas like chamomile, ginger, and peppermint can soothe digestive issues and help with cramps and bloating.
- Magnesium and Calcium: These minerals play a role in reducing PMS symptoms. Consider adding magnesium-rich foods like nuts and seeds, and calcium-rich foods like yogurt and leafy greens to your diet.
- Stress Management: Techniques like mindfulness, yoga, and deep breathing can help manage stress and improve overall well-being during PMS.

Menopause is a significant life transition that can bring various symptoms, from hot flashes and night sweats to mood changes and fatigue. Here's how you can support your body through this change:

- Healthy Diet: Eating a nutrient-dense diet can help manage menopause symptoms:

    Phytoestrogens: Foods like soy, flaxseeds, and lentils contain plant compounds that can help balance hormones and reduce hot flashes.

    Calcium and Vitamin D: Important for bone health, include foods like fortified plant milks, leafy greens, and fatty fish, or consider supplements if needed.

    Whole Foods: Focus on whole grains, fruits, vegetables, and lean proteins to support overall health and energy levels.

- Regular Exercise: Exercise is key to managing menopausal symptoms. It helps with weight management, improves mood, and boosts energy. Incorporate a mix of cardio, strength training, and flexibility exercises into your routine.
- Hydration: Drinking plenty of water can help with symptoms like dry skin and help manage hot flashes.
- Herbal Support: Certain herbs can offer relief from menopause symptoms:

    Black Cohosh: Often used to help reduce hot flashes and night sweats.

    Red Clover: Contains phytoestrogens that may help balance hormones and reduce menopausal symptoms.

    Dong Quai: Known as "female ginseng," it can support overall reproductive health and help with menopause symptoms.

- Mind-Body Practices: Practices like yoga, tai chi, and meditation can help with managing stress, improving mood, and supporting overall well-being.
- Adequate Sleep: Prioritize good sleep hygiene to combat insomnia and night sweats. Create a calming bedtime routine and keep your bedroom cool and comfortable.
- Avoid Triggers: Identify and avoid triggers for hot flashes, such as spicy foods, caffeine, and alcohol.

Additional Tips for Both PMS and Menopause

- Listen to Your Body: Pay attention to how different foods, activities, and supplements affect you. Personalizing your approach can lead to better results.
- Seek Support: Join support groups or talk to others who are going through similar experiences. Sharing tips and experiences can be comforting and helpful.
- Consult Healthcare Providers: If symptoms are severe or persistent, consult with a healthcare provider to explore additional options or treatments.

Boosting Fertility Naturally

Whether you're planning to start a family or looking to enhance your reproductive health, supporting fertility naturally can be a wonderful way to nurture your body and create the ideal environment for conception. Here's a friendly guide to boosting fertility with natural approaches that promote overall wellness and reproductive health.

What you eat plays a crucial role in your reproductive health. Here are some dietary tips to support fertility:

- Whole Foods: Focus on a diet rich in fruits, vegetables, whole grains, and lean proteins. These foods provide essential nutrients that support reproductive health and hormone balance.
- Healthy Fats: Include sources of healthy fats like avocados, nuts, seeds, and olive oil. These fats support hormone production and overall reproductive function.
- Lean Proteins: Opt for lean proteins such as chicken, fish, and plant-based proteins like legumes and tofu. Protein helps regulate blood sugar levels and supports hormonal balance.
- Folate and Iron: Foods high in folate (like leafy greens, beans, and citrus fruits) and iron (like spinach, lentils, and red meat) are essential for reproductive health and preparing the body for pregnancy.
- Limit Processed Foods: Reduce your intake of refined sugars, processed foods, and excessive caffeine, which can disrupt hormone balance and impact fertility.

Your weight can affect fertility, so maintaining a healthy weight is key:

- Balanced Diet: Eat a balanced diet to support a healthy weight. Extreme weight loss or gain can affect your menstrual cycle and hormone levels.
- Regular Exercise: Engage in regular physical activity to support a healthy weight and improve overall reproductive health. Aim for a mix of cardiovascular, strength, and flexibility exercises.

High stress levels can impact your fertility, so finding ways to manage stress is important:

- Relaxation Techniques: Incorporate practices like deep breathing, meditation, or yoga to help manage stress and promote relaxation.
- Mindfulness and Self-Care: Taking time for self-care and mindfulness can help reduce stress levels and improve your overall well-being.

Hormonal balance is crucial for fertility, and there are natural ways to support it:

- Herbal Supplements: Certain herbs can help balance hormones and support reproductive health:

    Vitex (Chaste Tree): Often used to support menstrual health and balance hormones.

    Red Clover: Contains phytoestrogens that can help balance hormone levels.

    Maca Root: Known for its ability to enhance energy, balance hormones, and support reproductive health.

- Regular Sleep: Prioritize quality sleep to support hormone production and overall health. Aim for 7-9 hours of restful sleep each night.

Reducing exposure to environmental toxins can help support fertility:

- Choose Natural Products: Opt for personal care and cleaning products that are free from synthetic chemicals and fragrances.
- Filter Water: Consider using a water filter to reduce exposure to contaminants that might affect reproductive health.
- Be Mindful of Plastics: Limit the use of plastic containers and bottles, as certain chemicals in plastics can disrupt hormonal function.

Proper hydration supports overall health and reproductive function:

- Drink Plenty of Water: Aim to drink plenty of water throughout the day to stay hydrated and support bodily functions.
- Limit Caffeine and Alcohol: Reducing or eliminating caffeine and alcohol can improve reproductive health and increase fertility.

Acupuncture has been used to support fertility and overall health for centuries:

- Fertility Support: Acupuncture may help improve blood flow to the reproductive organs, balance hormones, and reduce stress, potentially enhancing fertility.

Regular health check-ups can help monitor and support fertility:

- Routine Exams: Schedule regular visits with your healthcare provider to discuss any concerns and monitor reproductive health.
- Preconception Counseling: Consider preconception counseling to address any underlying health issues and create a plan for a healthy pregnancy.

Nutrition and Lifestyle for Hormonal Balance

Maintaining hormonal balance is key to feeling your best and supporting overall health. When hormones are in harmony, you might experience better mood stability, improved energy levels, and a more regulated menstrual cycle. Here's a friendly guide to using nutrition and lifestyle changes to help achieve and maintain hormonal balance.

Your diet plays a major role in hormone regulation. Focus on incorporating these dietary principles:

- Whole Foods: Opt for whole, unprocessed foods that provide essential nutrients. Fresh fruits, vegetables, whole grains, and lean proteins are great choices.
- Healthy Fats: Include sources of healthy fats, such as avocados, nuts, seeds, and olive oil. These fats are essential for hormone production and can help keep your hormones balanced.
- Lean Proteins: Eat lean proteins like chicken, fish, tofu, and legumes. Protein helps regulate blood sugar levels and supports hormone function.
- Fiber-Rich Foods: High-fiber foods like vegetables, fruits, and whole grains help maintain stable blood sugar levels and support healthy digestion, which is linked to hormonal balance.
- Phytoestrogens: Foods like flaxseeds, soy products, and legumes contain phytoestrogens that may help balance estrogen levels in the body.

Proper hydration is crucial for maintaining hormonal balance:

- Drink Plenty of Water: Aim to drink at least 8 glasses of water a day to keep your body hydrated and support various bodily functions, including hormone regulation.
- Limit Sugary Drinks: Reduce consumption of sugary drinks and caffeine, which can impact blood sugar levels and hormone balance.

Chronic stress can throw your hormones out of balance. Here's how to manage stress effectively:

- Relaxation Techniques: Incorporate stress-relief techniques into your daily routine. Deep breathing exercises, meditation, and yoga are excellent ways to reduce stress and support hormonal health.
- Mindfulness: Practice mindfulness and take time for activities you enjoy. Managing stress helps prevent the overproduction of stress hormones like cortisol, which can disrupt your hormonal balance.

Exercise helps regulate hormones and supports overall health:

- Find Activities You Enjoy: Whether it's walking, jogging, swimming, or dancing, choose activities that you enjoy and can do regularly.
- Balance Your Routine: Incorporate a mix of cardiovascular exercise, strength training, and flexibility exercises to support overall well-being and hormone regulation.

Adequate sleep is essential for hormonal balance:

- Establish a Sleep Routine: Aim for 7-9 hours of quality sleep each night. Try to go to bed and wake up at the same time every day to regulate your body's internal clock.

- Create a Relaxing Environment: Make your bedroom a calm and restful space. Avoid screens before bedtime and create a soothing bedtime routine to improve sleep quality.

A healthy gut can positively impact hormone levels:

- Include Probiotics: Foods like yogurt, kefir, and fermented vegetables contain probiotics that support gut health and can influence hormone regulation.
- Eat Fiber-Rich Foods: Consuming fiber-rich foods helps promote healthy digestion and regular bowel movements, which is important for hormone detoxification.

Minimizing exposure to substances that can disrupt hormonal balance is important:

- Choose Natural Products: Opt for personal care and cleaning products that are free from synthetic chemicals and fragrances.
- Reduce Plastic Use: Limit the use of plastic containers and bottles, as chemicals in plastics can interfere with hormone function.

Routine health check-ups can help monitor and support hormonal health:

- Consult Healthcare Providers: Regular visits with your healthcare provider can help address any hormonal issues and provide guidance on maintaining balance.
- Consider Testing: If you have symptoms of hormonal imbalance, your healthcare provider may suggest hormone testing to identify any imbalances and guide treatment options.

Preventing Hormonal Disruptions from Environmental Toxins

Our modern environment is filled with chemicals and toxins that can potentially disrupt our hormonal balance. Fortunately, there are steps you can take to minimize exposure and protect your hormonal health. Here's a friendly guide to preventing hormonal disruptions from environmental toxins.

The products you use on your skin and in your home can contain chemicals that may affect hormone levels:

- Personal Care Products: Opt for natural or organic personal care products like shampoos, lotions, and deodorants. Look for items labeled as free from parabens, phthalates, and synthetic fragrances.
- Cleaning Supplies: Use natural cleaning products or make your own using ingredients like vinegar, baking soda, and essential oils. These alternatives are often free from harsh chemicals that can affect hormonal health.

Certain chemicals in plastics, such as bisphenol A (BPA) and phthalates, can mimic hormones and disrupt endocrine function:

- Use Glass or Stainless Steel: Whenever possible, choose glass or stainless steel containers instead of plastic. These materials are less likely to leach harmful chemicals.
- Avoid Heating Plastics: Don't heat food in plastic containers, as heat can cause chemicals to leach into your food. Opt for microwave-safe glass or ceramic dishes instead.

- Minimize Use of Plastic Wrap: Try to limit the use of plastic wrap and other disposable plastic products in your kitchen.

Contaminants in tap water can include substances that may impact hormonal balance:

- Use a Water Filter: Invest in a high-quality water filter to remove common contaminants like chlorine, lead, and other chemicals that may affect your hormones.
- Avoid Bottled Water: Many bottled waters come in plastic bottles that can contain hormone-disrupting chemicals. Opt for filtered tap water or water stored in glass containers.

Pesticides used in agriculture can contain chemicals that might interfere with hormonal health:

- Choose Organic: Whenever possible, select organic fruits and vegetables. Organic produce is grown without synthetic pesticides and fertilizers.
- Wash Produce Thoroughly: Even if you can't always buy organic, washing fruits and vegetables thoroughly can help reduce pesticide residues.

Indoor air can be contaminated with chemicals from products, furnishings, and other sources:

- Ventilate Your Home: Open windows regularly to allow fresh air to circulate and reduce indoor pollutants.
- Use Air Purifiers: Consider using air purifiers with HEPA filters to help remove airborne toxins and improve indoor air quality.
- Choose Non-Toxic Paints: When painting or renovating, select non-toxic, low-VOC (volatile organic compound) paints and finishes to minimize exposure to harmful chemicals.

Certain foods may contain chemicals that impact hormonal balance:

- Limit Processed Foods: Processed and packaged foods can contain additives and preservatives that might affect your hormones. Focus on whole, unprocessed foods.
- Watch for Hormone-Injected Meats: Opt for hormone-free meats and dairy products to avoid exposure to synthetic hormones used in animal farming.

Helping your body detoxify can aid in reducing the impact of environmental toxins:

- Stay Hydrated: Drinking plenty of water helps your body flush out toxins more effectively.
- Eat Detoxifying Foods: Incorporate foods that support detoxification, such as leafy greens, cruciferous vegetables (like broccoli and cauliflower), and citrus fruits.
- Get Regular Exercise: Physical activity supports detoxification by promoting circulation and sweating, which helps eliminate toxins.

Staying informed about potential toxins and their sources can help you make better choices:

- Read Labels: Pay attention to ingredient lists and labels on personal care products, cleaning supplies, and food packaging.
- Research Brands: Look for brands that are transparent about their ingredients and committed to reducing harmful chemicals.

Book 14: Respiratory Health and Natural Remedies

Understanding the Respiratory System

Our respiratory system is a marvel of engineering, working tirelessly to keep us breathing easy and feeling good. Let's take a friendly dive into how this incredible system operates and why it's so important for our overall health.

At its core, the respiratory system's job is to bring oxygen into the body and expel carbon dioxide, a waste product. This process involves several key players:

- Nose and Mouth: Breathing starts here! Air enters the body through the nose or mouth, where it's warmed, filtered, and moistened before moving deeper into the system.
- Trachea: The trachea, or windpipe, is the main airway that directs air down to the lungs. Think of it as a major highway for airflow.
- Bronchi and Bronchioles: The trachea branches into two main bronchi, which then split into smaller bronchioles within the lungs. These bronchioles are like the smaller roads that deliver air to every corner of the lungs.
- Lungs: The lungs are the workhorses of the respiratory system. Inside them, the bronchioles end in tiny air sacs called alveoli. This is where the magic happens—oxygen passes through the walls of the alveoli into the blood, while carbon dioxide moves from the blood into the alveoli to be exhaled.

Breathing is both automatic and controlled. Here's how it typically goes:

- Inhalation: When you breathe in, the diaphragm (a dome-shaped muscle under your lungs) contracts and moves downward, creating a vacuum that pulls air into the lungs. The intercostal muscles (between the ribs) also help expand the chest cavity.
- Exhalation: When you breathe out, the diaphragm relaxes and moves upward, pushing air out of the lungs. The intercostal muscles also help by contracting to push air out more efficiently.

Oxygen is essential for every cell in our body. It's used to produce energy and keep our organs functioning properly. Carbon dioxide, on the other hand, is a waste product that must be removed to prevent it from building up in the blood.

- Oxygen Transport: Once oxygen is absorbed by the alveoli, it binds to hemoglobin in red blood cells. These oxygen-rich blood cells then travel to various tissues and organs.
- Carbon Dioxide Removal: Carbon dioxide travels from the tissues to the blood and is carried back to the lungs. From there, it's expelled when we breathe out.

Maintaining a healthy respiratory system is crucial for overall well-being. Here are some friendly tips to keep your lungs and airways in top shape:

- Avoid Smoking: Smoking can damage the airways and lungs, leading to respiratory issues and diseases. If you smoke, seek support to quit.
- Exercise Regularly: Physical activity helps strengthen the respiratory muscles and improves lung function. Aim for activities like walking, swimming, or cycling.
- Practice Deep Breathing: Incorporate deep breathing exercises into your routine. This can help expand the lungs, increase oxygen intake, and reduce stress.
- Stay Hydrated: Drinking plenty of water helps keep the mucous membranes in the respiratory system moist, which supports proper function.
- Minimize Exposure to Pollutants: Try to limit exposure to environmental pollutants and allergens. Use air purifiers if necessary and avoid areas with high pollution.

Sometimes, the respiratory system needs a little extra care. If you experience persistent symptoms such as shortness of breath, wheezing, or a chronic cough, it's important to consult a healthcare provider for proper evaluation and treatment.

Herbal Remedies for Respiratory Infections

When it comes to respiratory infections, many people turn to herbs as a natural way to support healing and soothe symptoms. Herbs have been used for centuries in various cultures to help with everything from the common cold to more serious respiratory issues. Here's a friendly guide to some of the most effective herbal remedies for respiratory infections.

Echinacea is often one of the first herbs that comes to mind when dealing with respiratory infections. Known for its immune-boosting properties, it helps your body fight off infections and can shorten the duration of colds.

- How to Use: Echinacea can be taken as a tea, tincture, or capsule. For best results, start using it at the first sign of a cold or respiratory infection.

Ginger isn't just a tasty addition to your meals—it also has powerful anti-inflammatory and antimicrobial properties. It helps to soothe a sore throat, reduce coughing, and support overall respiratory health.

- How to Use: You can make ginger tea by steeping fresh ginger slices in hot water. Adding honey and lemon can enhance its soothing effects. Ginger can also be used in cooking or taken as a supplement.

Peppermint contains menthol, which can help open up nasal passages and ease congestion. It also has antiviral and antibacterial properties, making it a great choice for respiratory infections.

- How to Use: Peppermint tea is a simple and effective way to benefit from this herb. You can also inhale peppermint steam by adding a few drops of peppermint essential oil to a bowl of hot water and breathing in the steam.

Thyme is a versatile herb with strong antimicrobial and expectorant properties. It helps to clear mucus from the respiratory tract and can soothe coughing and bronchial irritation.

- How to Use: Thyme tea is a great way to utilize this herb. Steep a teaspoon of dried thyme in a cup of hot water for 10 minutes. You can also use thyme essential oil in steam inhalation.

Marshmallow root is known for its mucilaginous properties, which help to coat and soothe the throat and respiratory tract. It's particularly useful for dry coughs and throat irritation.

- How to Use: Marshmallow root can be taken as a tea or tincture. It's also available in lozenge form, which can provide immediate relief for throat discomfort.

Licorice root has been traditionally used to ease symptoms of respiratory infections, including coughing and sore throat. It has anti-inflammatory and immune-boosting effects that can help support recovery.

- How to Use: Licorice root can be taken as a tea or tincture. However, it should be used with caution and not for extended periods, as it can affect blood pressure in some individuals.

Elderberry is well-known for its antiviral properties and can be particularly effective in reducing the severity and duration of respiratory infections like the flu.

- How to Use: Elderberry can be consumed as a syrup, tea, or capsule. It's especially beneficial when taken at the first signs of illness.

Lemon balm has calming and antiviral properties that can help ease symptoms of respiratory infections. It's great for reducing stress and promoting relaxation, which can aid the body's healing process.

- How to Use: Lemon balm can be used in tea or taken as a tincture. It's also a pleasant addition to other herbal blends.

Tips for Using Herbal Remedies

- Consult with a Healthcare Provider: If you're considering herbal remedies, especially if you have underlying health conditions or are taking other medications, it's wise to consult with a healthcare professional to ensure they're safe for you.
- Stay Hydrated: Drinking plenty of fluids helps to support your body's natural healing processes and can enhance the effectiveness of herbal remedies.
- Combine with Other Treatments: Herbal remedies can be a great complement to conventional treatments and supportive care. They work best when used as part of a comprehensive approach to health.

Managing Asthma and Allergies Naturally

Living with asthma and allergies can be challenging, but there are plenty of natural ways to help manage symptoms and support your overall respiratory health. Let's explore some friendly, natural approaches to help you breathe easier and feel more comfortable.

Understanding Asthma and Allergies

- Asthma is a chronic condition where the airways become inflamed and narrow, making it hard to breathe. Symptoms can include wheezing, shortness of breath, and coughing.
- Allergies occur when the immune system overreacts to certain substances (allergens) like pollen, dust mites, or pet dander, leading to symptoms like sneezing, itching, and congestion.

Natural Ways to Manage Asthma

- Maintain a Clean Environment: Keeping your home free of dust and allergens can help reduce asthma triggers. Use air purifiers with HEPA filters, and regularly clean bedding, carpets, and upholstery.
- Avoid Triggers: Identify and avoid common asthma triggers like smoke, strong odors, and cold air. Keeping windows closed during high pollen seasons can also help.
- Stay Hydrated: Drinking plenty of water helps keep mucus thin and easier to expel, which can help reduce asthma symptoms.
- Practice Breathing Exercises: Techniques like diaphragmatic breathing and pursed-lip breathing can improve lung function and help manage asthma symptoms. Consider adding these exercises to your daily routine.

Natural Remedies for Allergies

- Use Nasal Irrigation: Rinsing your nasal passages with a saline solution can help clear allergens and reduce congestion. You can use a neti pot or saline spray for this purpose.
- Consume Anti-Inflammatory Foods: Eating foods rich in omega-3 fatty acids (like flaxseeds and walnuts) and antioxidants (like berries and leafy greens) can help reduce inflammation and support immune health.
- Try Local Honey: Some people find relief from seasonal allergies by consuming local honey. The theory is that it may help your body build tolerance to local pollen.
- Use Essential Oils: Essential oils like lavender, eucalyptus, and peppermint can help ease allergy symptoms. You can diffuse them in your home or apply diluted oils to your skin.

Herbal Support for Asthma and Allergies

- Butterbur: This herb has been shown to reduce symptoms of allergic rhinitis (hay fever) and may help with asthma. Look for standardized extracts to ensure quality.
- Nettle Leaf: Nettle has natural anti-inflammatory properties and may help reduce allergy symptoms. It can be taken as a tea or in capsule form.
- Licorice Root: Licorice root can help soothe the respiratory tract and may support overall respiratory health. However, it should be used in moderation and not for long periods.
- Turmeric: With its potent anti-inflammatory properties, turmeric can be beneficial for managing asthma and allergies. Incorporate it into your diet or take it as a supplement.

Lifestyle Tips for Managing Symptoms

- Regular Exercise: Engaging in regular, moderate exercise can help improve lung function and reduce asthma symptoms. Just be sure to avoid exercising in cold or dry conditions, which can trigger asthma.

- Manage Stress: Stress can worsen asthma and allergy symptoms. Incorporate relaxation techniques like meditation, yoga, or deep breathing exercises into your daily routine to help manage stress.
- Maintain a Healthy Diet: A balanced diet rich in fruits, vegetables, lean proteins, and whole grains supports overall health and can help manage asthma and allergy symptoms.
- Allergy-Proof Your Home: Keep windows closed during high pollen seasons, use air purifiers, and wash bedding regularly in hot water to minimize allergens in your home.

While natural remedies can be very helpful, it's important to work closely with your healthcare provider to manage asthma and allergies effectively. If you experience severe symptoms or if natural remedies aren't providing relief, professional medical advice is essential.

Detoxifying the Lungs

Taking care of your lungs is essential for maintaining overall respiratory health and well-being. Just like the rest of our body, our lungs can benefit from a little detoxification to help them stay clear and function optimally. Let's explore some friendly and effective ways to help detoxify your lungs and keep them in tip-top shape.

Embrace Clean Air

- Avoid Pollutants: One of the best ways to support lung health is to avoid exposure to pollutants. If you live in an area with high air pollution, try to stay indoors on days with poor air quality, or use air purifiers in your home to reduce indoor pollutants.
- Go Smoke-Free: Smoking is one of the major contributors to lung damage. If you smoke, seek support to quit. Avoiding secondhand smoke is also crucial for maintaining lung health.

Stay Hydrated

- Drink Plenty of Water: Staying hydrated helps keep the mucus in your lungs thin and easier to expel. Aim to drink at least eight glasses of water a day to support your body's natural detox processes.
- Herbal Teas: Herbal teas like ginger, peppermint, and licorice root can help soothe the respiratory tract and support lung health. They also contribute to your daily fluid intake.

Incorporate Breathing Exercises

- Deep Breathing: Practice deep breathing exercises to help improve lung capacity and clear out stale air. Inhale deeply through your nose, hold for a few seconds, and exhale slowly through your mouth.
- Pursed-Lip Breathing: This technique helps improve oxygen exchange and makes it easier to expel air from the lungs. Inhale through your nose and exhale slowly through pursed lips as if you're blowing out a candle.

Use Natural Remedies

- Steam Inhalation: Inhaling steam can help loosen mucus and clear out your lungs. You can do this by taking a hot shower or placing your face over a bowl of hot water with a towel over your head. Adding a few drops of eucalyptus or peppermint oil can enhance the benefits.
- Essential Oils: Eucalyptus, peppermint, and frankincense essential oils have properties that support lung health. Diffuse these oils in your home or use them in steam inhalation to help clear your airways.

Enjoy Detoxifying Foods

- Foods Rich in Antioxidants: Include foods high in antioxidants, like berries, leafy greens, and nuts, in your diet. These foods help fight inflammation and support lung health.
- Spicy Foods: Spices like cayenne pepper and turmeric have anti-inflammatory properties and can help clear mucus from the lungs. Adding these to your meals can be both flavorful and beneficial.

Practice Regular Exercise

- Get Moving: Regular physical activity helps improve lung function and boosts overall respiratory health. Activities like walking, swimming, and cycling can help keep your lungs healthy and clear.
- Breathing Exercises in Yoga: Incorporating yoga into your routine can be particularly beneficial. Yoga encourages deep, controlled breathing and helps improve lung capacity and overall respiratory function.

Maintain a Healthy Lifestyle

- Healthy Diet: A balanced diet with plenty of fruits, vegetables, whole grains, and lean proteins supports overall health and can help keep your lungs functioning optimally.
- Avoid Environmental Toxins: Reduce exposure to chemicals and toxins in your environment, such as those found in cleaning products and personal care items. Opt for natural, non-toxic alternatives whenever possible.

Regular Health Check-Ups

- Monitor Lung Health: Regular check-ups with your healthcare provider are important for monitoring lung health and catching any potential issues early. If you have concerns or symptoms related to your lungs, don't hesitate to seek medical advice.

Breathing Techniques for Lung Health

Breathing is something we often take for granted, but it plays a crucial role in our overall health, especially when it comes to lung health. Practicing specific breathing techniques can help improve lung function, increase oxygen intake, and support respiratory well-being. Let's dive into some friendly and effective breathing techniques that can make a big difference for your lung health.

Deep Breathing

- How It Works: Deep breathing, or diaphragmatic breathing, focuses on expanding your lungs fully by engaging the diaphragm. This technique helps increase oxygen flow and promotes relaxation.
- How to Do It:

    Sit or lie down in a comfortable position.

    Place one hand on your chest and the other on your abdomen.

    Inhale deeply through your nose, allowing your abdomen to rise while keeping your chest relatively still.

    Exhale slowly and completely through your mouth.

    Repeat this process for a few minutes, focusing on deep, even breaths.

Pursed-Lip Breathing

- How It Works: Pursed-lip breathing helps improve oxygen exchange and slows down your breathing rate, which can be particularly helpful for those with respiratory conditions.
- How to Do It:
    1. Inhale slowly through your nose for a count of two.
    2. Pucker your lips as if you're going to blow out a candle.
    3. Exhale slowly and steadily through your pursed lips for a count of four.
    4. Repeat this process for a few minutes, aiming for a gentle, controlled exhale.

Box Breathing

- How It Works: Box breathing, also known as square breathing, is a technique that helps calm the mind and body while improving lung capacity and control.
- How to Do It:

    Inhale through your nose for a count of four.

    Hold your breath for a count of four.

    Exhale slowly through your mouth for a count of four.

    Hold your breath again for a count of four.

    Repeat this cycle for several minutes, focusing on maintaining a steady rhythm.

Alternate Nostril Breathing

- How It Works: Alternate nostril breathing balances the flow of air through both nostrils and can help reduce stress and anxiety while promoting lung function.

- How to Do It:

    Sit comfortably with your spine straight.

    Using your right thumb, close off your right nostril.

    Inhale deeply through your left nostril.

    Close off your left nostril with your right ring finger and release your right nostril.

    Exhale slowly through your right nostril.

    Inhale through your right nostril.

    Close off your right nostril with your thumb and release your left nostril.

    Exhale slowly through your left nostril.

    Repeat this process for several minutes.

Belly Breathing

- How It Works: Belly breathing is a variation of deep breathing that emphasizes expanding the abdomen with each breath, helping to increase lung capacity and relaxation.
- How to Do It:

    Lie on your back with your knees bent and feet flat on the floor.

    Place one hand on your chest and the other on your abdomen.

    Inhale deeply through your nose, focusing on pushing out your abdomen rather than raising your chest.

    Exhale slowly and completely through your mouth.

    Continue this pattern for several minutes, ensuring your abdomen rises and falls with each breath.

The 4-7-8 Breathing Technique

- How It Works: The 4-7-8 technique promotes relaxation and can help improve sleep and reduce anxiety.
- How to Do It:

    Inhale quietly through your nose for a count of four.

    Hold your breath for a count of seven.

Exhale completely and audibly through your mouth for a count of eight.

Complete this cycle three to four times.

Herbs and Essential Oils for Sinus Health

When it comes to managing sinus health naturally, herbs and essential oils can be incredibly effective allies. These natural remedies not only support your body's ability to fend off infections but also help ease the discomfort associated with sinus issues. Let's dive into some of the most beneficial herbs and essential oils for sinus health.

Herbs for Sinus Health

> Eucalyptus: Known for its powerful antiseptic and decongestant properties, eucalyptus can be a game-changer for sinus relief. The active compound, eucalyptol, helps clear nasal passages and reduce inflammation. You can use eucalyptus oil in a steam inhalation or apply it topically, diluted with a carrier oil, to the chest and throat.
>
> Peppermint: Peppermint is another herb with notable benefits for sinus health. Its menthol content helps relax the muscles of the respiratory tract, making it easier to breathe. Peppermint tea can soothe a sore throat and reduce sinus pressure, while peppermint oil can be used in a diffuser or applied in a diluted form to the temples.
>
> Thyme: This herb has natural antibacterial and antiviral properties that make it useful for combating sinus infections. Thyme tea can help reduce inflammation and fight off bacteria. Adding thyme to your cooking or using it as a herbal steam can offer additional relief.
>
> Ginger: Ginger is renowned for its anti-inflammatory and immune-boosting properties. It can help reduce sinus inflammation and support overall respiratory health. Drinking ginger tea or incorporating fresh ginger into your diet can help keep sinus issues at bay.
>
> Chamomile: Chamomile is known for its soothing effects, which can be beneficial for inflamed sinuses. A warm chamomile tea can ease sinus pressure and help you relax, especially before bedtime.

Essential Oils for Sinus Health

> Tea Tree Oil: With its strong antimicrobial properties, tea tree oil is excellent for clearing sinus congestion and fighting infection. It can be used in a steam inhalation or diluted with a carrier oil and applied to the chest.
>
> Lavender Oil: Lavender oil is renowned for its calming and anti-inflammatory effects. It can help soothe sinus irritation and promote relaxation. Use lavender oil in a diffuser or add a few drops to a warm bath for a comforting experience.

Frankincense Oil: This essential oil has powerful anti-inflammatory properties that can help reduce sinus congestion and support respiratory health. Diffusing frankincense oil or using it in a steam inhalation can provide relief from sinus symptoms.

Rosemary Oil: Rosemary oil is known for its ability to clear nasal congestion and improve breathing. Its expectorant properties help to expel mucus and ease sinus pressure. Use rosemary oil in a diffuser or add a few drops to a bowl of hot water for a steam inhalation.

Oregano Oil: Oregano oil has potent antimicrobial and anti-inflammatory properties that can help combat sinus infections. It can be used in a steam inhalation or diluted with a carrier oil for topical application.

Book 15: Managing Diabetes and Blood Sugar Naturally

Understanding Diabetes and Blood Sugar Imbalance

When it comes to managing diabetes and blood sugar levels, it's helpful to start with a clear understanding of what's going on in our bodies. So, let's dive into the basics in a straightforward and friendly way.

Diabetes is a condition where the body has trouble managing blood sugar (glucose) levels. Glucose is a key source of energy for our cells, but it needs insulin to get into the cells. Insulin is a hormone produced by the pancreas, and when it's not working properly, glucose can't enter the cells as it should.

There are two main types of diabetes:

> Type 1 Diabetes: This type is usually diagnosed in children and young adults. The immune system mistakenly attacks the insulin-producing cells in the pancreas, leading to little or no insulin production. People with Type 1 diabetes need to take insulin every day.

> Type 2 Diabetes: This type is more common and usually develops in adults over time. It occurs when the body becomes resistant to insulin or when the pancreas can't produce enough insulin. Lifestyle factors like diet and physical activity play a big role in managing Type 2 diabetes.

Blood sugar imbalance happens when there is too much or too little glucose in the blood. High blood sugar (hyperglycemia) can lead to symptoms like frequent urination, increased thirst, and fatigue. Low blood sugar (hypoglycemia) might cause shakiness, sweating, confusion, and irritability.

Maintaining a balanced blood sugar level is crucial for overall health. When blood sugar levels are consistently high or low, it can lead to serious complications such as heart disease, nerve damage, and kidney issues.

Several factors can contribute to blood sugar imbalances:

- Diet: Eating foods high in sugar and refined carbs can cause spikes in blood sugar. On the other hand, a diet lacking in essential nutrients can lead to blood sugar dips.
- Physical Activity: Regular exercise helps regulate blood sugar levels by improving insulin sensitivity. Lack of physical activity can contribute to higher blood sugar levels.
- Stress: Stress hormones can affect blood sugar levels by increasing insulin resistance. Managing stress is an important aspect of keeping blood sugar in check.
- Sleep: Poor sleep can impact insulin sensitivity and lead to higher blood sugar levels. Ensuring you get quality rest is key for blood sugar management.

Understanding the root causes of blood sugar imbalance is the first step toward managing it naturally. By focusing on a balanced diet, regular exercise, stress management, and proper sleep, you can help keep your blood sugar levels stable and support overall health.

Nutritional Strategies for Managing Blood Sugar

When it comes to managing blood sugar naturally, what we eat plays a big role. But don't worry; you don't have to make drastic changes overnight. By focusing on a few key nutritional strategies, you can keep your blood sugar levels more stable and support your overall well-being.

Whole foods are the backbone of a blood sugar-friendly diet. These are foods that are as close to their natural state as possible. Think fresh fruits and vegetables, whole grains, nuts, seeds, and lean proteins. They're packed with nutrients and fiber, which help keep blood sugar levels steady. Try to fill your plate with colorful veggies and fruits, whole grains like quinoa or brown rice, and lean proteins like chicken or fish.

The glycemic index (GI) measures how quickly a food raises blood sugar levels. Foods with a low GI are absorbed more slowly, helping to keep your blood sugar stable. Some great low GI options include whole grains (like barley and oats), non-starchy vegetables (like spinach and broccoli), and legumes (like lentils and chickpeas). By incorporating these foods into your meals, you'll help prevent those pesky blood sugar spikes.

Creating balanced meals is a smart way to manage your blood sugar. Try to include a mix of carbohydrates, proteins, and healthy fats in each meal. Carbohydrates provide energy, while proteins and fats help slow the absorption of sugar into the bloodstream. For example, if you're having a sandwich, opt for whole grain bread, add some lean turkey or tofu, and include a side of avocado or a handful of nuts.

Portion control is crucial for managing blood sugar. Eating large portions of even healthy foods can lead to elevated blood sugar levels. Pay attention to serving sizes and try to avoid overeating. Using smaller plates and bowls can help you manage portion sizes more effectively.

Fiber slows the digestion of carbohydrates and helps regulate blood sugar levels. Foods high in fiber include vegetables, fruits, legumes, and whole grains. Try to include a good source of fiber in each meal, such as adding a serving of beans to your salad or choosing whole grain options over refined grains.

It's no surprise that sugary foods and drinks can cause blood sugar spikes. Try to limit or avoid sugary snacks, sodas, and sweetened beverages. Instead, opt for naturally sweet options like fresh fruit or unsweetened yogurt.

Drinking enough water is important for overall health and can also help with blood sugar management. Sometimes our bodies can confuse thirst with hunger, leading us to eat more than we need. Keeping hydrated helps you stay alert and can support better blood sugar control.

Meal planning can be a game-changer for blood sugar management. By preparing healthy meals and snacks ahead of time, you can avoid the temptation of grabbing unhealthy options when you're hungry. Try to plan your meals around balanced, nutrient-dense foods and keep healthy snacks on hand.

Healthy fats, like those found in avocados, nuts, seeds, and olive oil, can help with blood sugar control. They provide essential nutrients and can make meals more satisfying. Just be mindful of portion sizes, as fats are calorie-dense.

Finally, keeping an eye on how different foods affect your blood sugar can provide valuable insights. Tracking your levels and noting any patterns can help you make informed decisions about your diet.

By incorporating these nutritional strategies into your routine, you'll be well on your way to better managing your blood sugar levels naturally. Remember, it's all about making small, sustainable changes that work for you. Enjoy experimenting with new foods and recipes that fit into your lifestyle and support your health goals!

Herbs That Support Blood Sugar Regulation

When it comes to managing blood sugar levels naturally, herbs can be a powerful ally. Many herbs have been used for centuries to support health and balance blood sugar. Let's explore some of the top herbs that can help with blood sugar regulation in a way that's easy to incorporate into your daily life.

Cinnamon is more than just a tasty spice for your oatmeal or coffee; it's also known for its blood sugar-regulating properties. Cinnamon helps improve insulin sensitivity and can lower fasting blood sugar levels. You can sprinkle cinnamon on your breakfast cereal, mix it into smoothies, or add it to your baking for a sweet and healthful boost.

Fenugreek seeds are packed with soluble fiber, which can help manage blood sugar levels. They're believed to slow the absorption of carbohydrates and improve insulin function. You can use fenugreek seeds in cooking or take fenugreek supplements after consulting with your healthcare provider.

Berberine is a compound found in several herbs, including goldenseal and barberry. It's known for its ability to support healthy blood sugar levels by improving insulin sensitivity and regulating glucose production in the liver. Berberine supplements are available, but it's best to discuss their use with your healthcare provider first.

Often referred to as the "sugar destroyer," Gymnema sylvestre is a herb that can help reduce sugar cravings and support healthy blood sugar levels. It works by blocking sugar absorption in the intestines and enhancing insulin function. You can find Gymnema sylvestre in supplement form or as a tea.

Bitter melon, a tropical fruit, has been used in traditional medicine for its blood sugar-lowering effects. It contains compounds that mimic insulin and help lower blood glucose levels. You can enjoy bitter melon as part of your meals, particularly in dishes from Asian cuisines, or take it as a supplement.

Aloe vera isn't just for soothing sunburns; it also has potential benefits for blood sugar regulation. Some studies suggest that aloe vera may help lower fasting blood glucose levels and improve overall glycemic control. You can consume aloe vera juice or supplements, but be sure to choose products without added sugars.

Turmeric, with its active compound curcumin, is renowned for its anti-inflammatory and antioxidant properties. It may also help regulate blood sugar levels by improving insulin sensitivity. You can add turmeric to your cooking, use it in smoothies, or take it as a supplement.

Clove is another spice with blood sugar-regulating benefits. It contains compounds that may help improve insulin function and reduce oxidative stress. You can use cloves in cooking or take clove supplements as directed.

Dandelion is not just a weed; it's also a herb with potential blood sugar benefits. It may help regulate blood sugar levels by improving liver function and supporting digestion. You can drink dandelion tea or use it as a salad green.

Sage is a fragrant herb that has been shown to have beneficial effects on blood sugar levels. It contains compounds that may improve glucose metabolism and support overall blood sugar balance. Sage can be used fresh or dried in cooking, or taken as a supplement.

Incorporating these herbs into your routine can be both enjoyable and beneficial. You can use them in cooking, drink them as teas, or take them in supplement form. Just remember to start with small amounts and monitor how your body responds. It's also a good idea to discuss any new herbal remedies with your healthcare provider, especially if you're on medication or have health conditions.

By adding these herbs to your diet, you're not only enhancing the flavor of your meals but also giving your body a natural boost in managing blood sugar levels. So, why not experiment with these herbal options and find the ones that work best for you?

Preventing Diabetes with a Natural Lifestyle

Preventing diabetes is all about making smart, healthful choices that support your body and keep your blood sugar levels in check. Embracing a natural lifestyle can be both enjoyable and effective. Here's how you can incorporate simple, natural strategies to help prevent diabetes and promote overall well-being.

A well-rounded diet is key to preventing diabetes. Focus on whole, nutrient-dense foods that nourish your body and help maintain stable blood sugar levels. Fill your plate with fresh fruits and vegetables, whole grains, lean proteins, and healthy fats. Try to limit processed foods, sugary snacks, and refined carbs, which can cause blood sugar spikes.

Exercise is a powerful tool for preventing diabetes. Regular physical activity helps your body use insulin more effectively and maintain a healthy weight. Aim for at least 150 minutes of moderate aerobic activity, like brisk walking, or 75 minutes of vigorous activity, like jogging, each week. Incorporate strength training exercises twice a week to build muscle and support metabolic health.

Drinking enough water is crucial for overall health and blood sugar management. Water helps your body regulate blood sugar levels and supports digestion. Aim to drink at least eight glasses of water a day. If you're active or live in a hot climate, you may need even more.

Good sleep is essential for preventing diabetes. Poor sleep can affect insulin sensitivity and lead to weight gain, both of which increase diabetes risk. Aim for 7-9 hours of quality sleep each night. Establish a regular sleep routine, create a restful environment, and avoid screens before bedtime to improve your sleep quality.

Chronic stress can impact your blood sugar levels and increase the risk of diabetes. Find healthy ways to manage stress, such as practicing mindfulness, meditation, deep breathing exercises, or engaging in hobbies you enjoy. Regular physical activity and spending time with loved ones can also help reduce stress.

Being overweight is a major risk factor for developing Type 2 diabetes. Adopting a balanced diet and regular exercise routine can help you achieve and maintain a healthy weight. Even a modest weight loss of 5-10% can significantly improve blood sugar levels and reduce diabetes risk.

Smoking and excessive alcohol consumption can increase your risk of diabetes and other health issues. If you smoke, seek support to quit, and if you drink alcohol, do so in moderation. For women, this means up to one drink per day, and for men, up to two drinks per day.

Fiber helps regulate blood sugar levels by slowing the absorption of sugar into the bloodstream. Foods high in fiber include fruits, vegetables, legumes, whole grains, and nuts. Incorporate these fiber-rich foods into your meals to support better blood sugar control.

Regular check-ups with your healthcare provider can help you monitor your risk factors for diabetes and catch any potential issues early. Discuss your lifestyle habits and get personalized advice on how to maintain your health and prevent diabetes.

Surrounding yourself with supportive friends and family can make a big difference in maintaining a healthy lifestyle. Share your goals with loved ones and encourage each other to stay on track with healthy eating, exercise, and other positive habits.

Supplements for Blood Sugar Control

When it comes to managing blood sugar levels naturally, supplements can offer valuable support. While they shouldn't replace a balanced diet and healthy lifestyle, certain supplements can help complement your efforts and keep your blood sugar in check. Here's a friendly guide to some popular supplements for blood sugar control.

Cinnamon isn't just for adding flavor to your coffee; it's also known for its potential to support blood sugar control. It can help improve insulin sensitivity and lower fasting blood glucose levels. You can take cinnamon supplements or add ground cinnamon to your meals and snacks.

Berberine is a compound found in several plants, including goldenseal and barberry. It's been shown to help regulate blood sugar levels by improving insulin sensitivity and reducing glucose production in the liver. Berberine supplements are widely available, but it's a good idea to consult with your healthcare provider before starting.

Alpha-lipoic acid is a powerful antioxidant that may help improve insulin sensitivity and reduce symptoms of nerve damage related to diabetes. It can also help lower blood sugar levels. ALA supplements can be a good addition to your routine if recommended by your healthcare provider.

Chromium is a mineral that plays a role in carbohydrate and lipid metabolism. It's thought to help improve insulin sensitivity and lower blood sugar levels. Chromium supplements are available in various forms, and incorporating them into your routine might help with blood sugar control.

Magnesium is an essential mineral that supports many bodily functions, including blood sugar regulation. Some studies suggest that magnesium supplements can help improve insulin sensitivity and reduce the risk of Type 2 diabetes. If you're not getting enough magnesium from your diet, consider discussing supplements with your healthcare provider.

Bitter melon is a fruit used in traditional medicine for its potential blood sugar-lowering effects. It contains compounds that mimic insulin and may help manage blood glucose levels. Bitter melon supplements can be found in various forms, including capsules and extracts.

Fenugreek seeds are rich in soluble fiber and may help regulate blood sugar levels by slowing carbohydrate absorption and improving insulin function. You can take fenugreek supplements or use fenugreek seeds in cooking to reap its benefits.

Gymnema sylvestre, often called the "sugar destroyer," is an herb known for its ability to reduce sugar cravings and support blood sugar regulation. It may help lower blood glucose levels and improve insulin function. Gymnema sylvestre supplements are widely available.

Turmeric contains curcumin, a compound with strong anti-inflammatory and antioxidant properties. It may help improve insulin sensitivity and support overall blood sugar management. Turmeric supplements or adding turmeric spice to your meals can be beneficial.

CoQ10 is an antioxidant that helps with energy production in cells and may support metabolic health. Some research suggests that CoQ10 supplements can help improve insulin sensitivity and reduce oxidative stress related to diabetes.

Before starting any new supplement, it's essential to consult with your healthcare provider, especially if you're on medication or have existing health conditions. They can help you determine the right dosage and ensure that the supplement won't interfere with your medications or other treatments.

Incorporating these supplements into your routine can be a helpful addition to a balanced diet and healthy lifestyle. Just remember, supplements are most effective when used in conjunction with good nutrition, regular physical activity, and other lifestyle practices that support blood sugar control. So, explore these options, and find what works best for you in your journey toward better blood sugar management.

Daily Habits to Maintain Healthy Glucose Levels

Keeping your blood sugar levels in check is all about integrating healthy habits into your daily routine. Small, consistent changes can make a big difference over time. Here's a friendly guide to daily habits that can help you maintain healthy glucose levels and support your overall well-being.

A nutritious breakfast sets the tone for the day. Aim for a meal that includes a mix of protein, healthy fats, and complex carbohydrates. For example, try Greek yogurt with berries and a sprinkle of nuts, or scrambled eggs with spinach and whole-grain toast. This balance helps stabilize blood sugar levels and keeps you energized.

Keeping an eye on portion sizes helps manage blood sugar levels and prevent overeating. Use smaller plates to help control portions and listen to your body's hunger and fullness cues. Eating moderate portions of balanced meals helps maintain steady glucose levels throughout the day.

Drinking enough water is crucial for overall health and blood sugar management. Aim for at least eight glasses of water a day. Staying hydrated helps your body process glucose more effectively and supports overall bodily functions.

Snacking smartly can help keep your blood sugar stable between meals. Opt for snacks that combine protein, fiber, and healthy fats. For instance, a handful of almonds, a piece of fruit with nut butter, or carrot sticks with hummus are great choices that provide sustained energy without causing blood sugar spikes.

Incorporate regular exercise into your routine to help regulate blood sugar levels and improve insulin sensitivity. Aim for at least 150 minutes of moderate aerobic activity per week, like brisk walking or cycling, along with strength training exercises twice a week.

Skipping meals can lead to blood sugar imbalances and cravings for unhealthy foods. Try to eat three balanced meals a day with healthy snacks if needed. Consistent meal times help maintain stable blood sugar levels and prevent overeating later on.

Chronic stress can affect blood sugar levels and overall health. Incorporate stress-reducing activities into your day, such as mindfulness meditation, deep breathing exercises, or spending time on hobbies you enjoy. Managing stress helps maintain balance in your life and supports healthy glucose levels.

Quality sleep is essential for blood sugar regulation and overall health. Aim for 7-9 hours of restful sleep each night. Establish a consistent sleep schedule, create a relaxing bedtime routine, and ensure your sleep environment is conducive to rest.

Fiber helps regulate blood sugar levels by slowing the absorption of sugar into the bloodstream. Include fiber-rich foods in your daily diet, such as whole grains, legumes, fruits, and vegetables. These foods help keep you feeling full and support stable blood sugar levels.

Regularly monitoring your blood sugar levels can provide valuable insights into how different foods and activities affect your glucose. Keeping track of your levels helps you make informed decisions and adjust your habits as needed.

Meal planning and preparation can help you make healthier choices and avoid the temptation of unhealthy options. Set aside time each week to plan your meals, prepare healthy snacks, and organize your grocery list. This helps you stay on track with your nutrition goals.

Reducing your intake of added sugars and refined carbohydrates can help prevent blood sugar spikes. Opt for whole foods and natural sweeteners instead. Check food labels to avoid hidden sugars and choose products with lower glycemic indexes.

Eating mindfully helps you pay attention to what you're eating and how it makes you feel. Take time to savor your meals, eat slowly, and listen to your body's hunger and fullness signals. Mindful eating supports better digestion and helps prevent overeating.

Book 16: Eye Health and Vision Restoration

The Importance of Nutrients for Eye Health

Your eyes are incredibly important, and taking good care of them can make a big difference in maintaining clear vision and overall eye health. One of the best ways to support your eyes is by ensuring you get the right nutrients. Let's explore why these nutrients are so vital for your eye health and how you can incorporate them into your diet.

Vitamin A is a superstar nutrient for your eyes. It helps maintain good vision, particularly in low light, and supports the health of the cornea, which is the outer layer of your eye. A deficiency in vitamin A can lead to night blindness and other vision problems. You can get vitamin A from foods like carrots, sweet potatoes, spinach, and kale. Including these foods in your diet can keep your eyes sharp and healthy.

Vitamin C is a powerful antioxidant that helps protect your eyes from oxidative damage caused by free radicals. It also plays a role in maintaining the health of the blood vessels in your eyes and can help reduce the risk of developing cataracts. Citrus fruits like oranges, strawberries, and kiwi, as well as vegetables like bell peppers and broccoli, are great sources of vitamin C.

Vitamin E is another antioxidant that helps protect your eyes from damage. It works in tandem with vitamin C to neutralize free radicals and support overall eye health. Nuts and seeds, such as almonds and sunflower seeds, as well as green leafy vegetables, are rich in vitamin E and should be part of a balanced diet.

Lutein and zeaxanthin are carotenoids found in high concentrations in the retina. They help filter harmful blue light and protect your eyes from oxidative stress. These nutrients are found in foods like spinach, kale, and corn. Adding these to your meals can help protect your eyes from age-related macular degeneration (AMD) and other vision issues.

Omega-3 fatty acids are essential for maintaining the health of the retina and preventing dry eye syndrome. They also have anti-inflammatory properties that can help protect against age-related vision problems. You can find omega-3s in fatty fish like salmon, mackerel, and sardines, as well as in flaxseeds and walnuts.

Zinc is a mineral that plays a crucial role in maintaining the health of the retina and supporting the function of enzymes involved in eye health. A deficiency in zinc can lead to night blindness and other vision problems. You can get zinc from foods like meat, shellfish, beans, and nuts.

Beta-carotene is a type of vitamin A found in colorful fruits and vegetables. It's converted into vitamin A in your body and helps support good vision and overall eye health. Foods rich in beta-carotene include carrots, sweet potatoes, butternut squash, and apricots.

Selenium is an antioxidant that helps protect your eyes from oxidative damage and supports overall eye health. You can find selenium in foods like Brazil nuts, seafood, and whole grains.

To support your eye health, aim to include a variety of these nutrients in your daily diet. Incorporate colorful fruits and vegetables, fatty fish, nuts, and seeds into your meals. A balanced diet rich in these nutrients will not only benefit your eyes but also contribute to your overall health and well-being.

By focusing on these essential nutrients, you're giving your eyes the support they need to stay healthy and vibrant. So, embrace a nutrient-rich diet, and keep your eyes in top shape for years to come!

Herbal Remedies for Eye Strain and Fatigue

If your eyes are feeling tired and strained from long hours in front of a screen or other daily activities, herbal remedies can offer some soothing relief. Many herbs have properties that help ease eye strain and reduce fatigue, making them a great addition to your wellness routine. Here's a friendly guide to herbal remedies that can help you relax your eyes and restore their vitality.

Chamomile is well-known for its calming and anti-inflammatory properties. It can be particularly soothing for tired eyes. You can use chamomile tea bags as a warm compress by placing them over your closed eyes for about 10-15 minutes. This can help reduce puffiness and relieve eye strain. Drinking chamomile tea can also help promote overall relaxation.

As its name suggests, eyebright is an herb traditionally used to support eye health. It has anti-inflammatory and astringent properties that can help soothe irritated eyes. You can use eyebright as an herbal tea or a wash to help reduce eye strain and fatigue. Be sure to consult with a healthcare provider before using it, especially if you have any underlying health conditions.

Calendula, or marigold, is another herb with soothing properties. It's often used in eye washes and compresses to help relieve irritation and inflammation. You can make a gentle calendula eye wash by steeping dried calendula flowers in hot water, allowing it to cool, and then using it to rinse your eyes.

Green tea is rich in antioxidants and has anti-inflammatory properties that can benefit your eyes. You can use cooled green tea bags as a compress to help reduce puffiness and soothe tired eyes. Drinking green tea also provides systemic benefits that support overall health and well-being.

Rose water is known for its soothing and anti-inflammatory effects. It can help refresh tired eyes and reduce redness. You can use rose water as a gentle eye rinse or apply it to a cotton pad and place it over your closed eyes for a few minutes.

Fennel seeds have antioxidant and anti-inflammatory properties that can help ease eye strain. You can make a fennel seed infusion by steeping the seeds in hot water, straining the mixture, and using it as an eye rinse. This can help reduce discomfort and promote relaxation.

Ginkgo biloba is an herb that supports blood circulation, including to the eyes. Improved circulation can help reduce symptoms of eye fatigue and strain. You can take ginkgo biloba supplements as directed or consult with a healthcare provider to determine the best form and dosage for your needs.

Licorice root has anti-inflammatory properties that can help reduce eye strain and support overall eye health. You can use it as an herbal tea or as part of a topical eye compress.

As with other herbs, it's important to use licorice root under the guidance of a healthcare provider, especially if you have any existing health conditions.

While herbal remedies can be very effective, it's important to use them safely. Always follow the recommended dosages and consult with a healthcare provider before starting any new herbal treatments, especially if you have allergies, are pregnant, or are taking other medications.

Incorporating these herbal remedies into your routine can offer soothing relief from eye strain and fatigue. Whether you're using them as a compress, a tea, or a rinse, these herbs can help refresh and rejuvenate your tired eyes, allowing you to feel more comfortable and relaxed. So, give these natural remedies a try and enjoy the soothing benefits they bring to your eye health!

Protecting Your Eyes from Environmental Damage

Your eyes are delicate and deserve a little extra care, especially when it comes to environmental factors that can cause damage. Whether it's harsh sunlight, pollution, or dry air, there are simple and effective ways to shield your eyes from environmental harm. Here's a friendly guide to help you protect your precious vision and keep your eyes healthy.

Sunglasses aren't just a stylish accessory—they're essential for protecting your eyes from harmful UV rays. Prolonged exposure to UV radiation can increase the risk of cataracts and macular degeneration. Choose sunglasses that offer 100% UV protection and cover your eyes completely. Polarized lenses can also reduce glare and improve visibility.

In addition to sunglasses, wearing a wide-brimmed hat or visor can provide extra protection from the sun's rays. A hat can help shield your eyes and the delicate skin around them from direct sunlight, reducing your risk of sun-related eye issues.

Wind and dust can irritate your eyes and cause discomfort. If you're outdoors in windy conditions or in dusty environments, consider wearing protective eyewear, such as goggles or wraparound glasses. This can help keep foreign particles out and protect your eyes from dryness.

Proper hydration is crucial for maintaining the moisture balance of your eyes. Drinking plenty of water throughout the day helps keep your eyes lubricated and can prevent dryness and irritation. If you're in a dry or air-conditioned environment, consider using a humidifier to add moisture to the air.

If you're working with hazardous materials or engaging in activities that pose a risk to your eyes (like DIY projects or sports), wearing appropriate protective eyewear is a must. Safety goggles or glasses can shield your eyes from debris, chemicals, and other potential dangers.

Extended screen time can lead to digital eye strain, causing symptoms like dryness, blurred vision, and headaches. Follow the 20-20-20 rule to reduce strain: every 20 minutes, take a 20-second break and look at something 20 feet away. Adjusting your screen's brightness and using blue light filters can also help reduce eye strain.

Protect your eyes from infection and irritation by practicing good hygiene. Wash your hands regularly, especially before touching your face or eyes. Avoid sharing eye makeup or using expired products, and clean your contact lenses according to the recommended guidelines.

Regular eye exams are crucial for detecting and addressing any potential issues before they become serious. An eye care professional can help monitor your eye health and provide personalized advice on how to protect your eyes from environmental damage.

A diet rich in vitamins and antioxidants supports overall eye health and can help protect your eyes from environmental damage. Foods high in vitamins A, C, and E, as well as omega-3 fatty acids, contribute to maintaining healthy vision and reducing oxidative stress.

Some medications can cause dry eyes or increase sensitivity to sunlight. If you're taking any medications, discuss potential side effects with your healthcare provider and take necessary precautions to protect your eyes.

Natural Approaches to Improving Vision

Taking care of your eyes doesn't always mean resorting to glasses or contacts. There are plenty of natural approaches you can use to help improve your vision and support overall eye health. Here's a friendly guide to some effective and natural ways to give your eyes a little extra TLC.

Just like your body needs exercise, so do your eyes! Simple eye exercises can help reduce strain and improve focus. Try this one: hold your finger a few inches away from your eyes, focus on it, and then slowly move it away while keeping your gaze fixed. Do this a few times, and it helps strengthen your eye muscles and improve flexibility.

Your diet plays a big role in eye health. Incorporate foods rich in vitamins and antioxidants that support vision. Leafy greens like spinach and kale, orange vegetables like carrots and sweet potatoes, and fatty fish like salmon are excellent choices. These foods are packed with nutrients like vitamin A, lutein, and omega-3 fatty acids, all of which are great for your eyes.

Keeping your body hydrated helps maintain moisture in your eyes. Drink plenty of water throughout the day to keep your eyes lubricated and reduce the risk of dryness and irritation. If you're in a dry environment, consider using a humidifier to add moisture to the air.

Adequate sleep is crucial for your eye health. During sleep, your eyes get a chance to rest and repair. Aim for 7-9 hours of quality sleep each night to keep your eyes feeling refreshed and to maintain optimal vision.

Sunlight can damage your eyes over time, increasing the risk of cataracts and macular degeneration. Wear sunglasses that offer 100% UV protection when you're outdoors to shield your eyes from harmful UV rays. A wide-brimmed hat can also provide additional protection.

If you spend a lot of time in front of screens, it's important to give your eyes regular breaks. Follow the 20-20-20 rule: every 20 minutes, take a 20-second break and look at something 20 feet away. This helps reduce digital eye strain and keeps your vision sharp.

Certain herbs can support eye health and improve vision. Bilberry is known for its potential benefits in improving night vision, while ginkgo biloba may help with circulation to the eyes. Always consult with a healthcare provider before starting any new supplements to ensure they're right for you.

Keeping your eyes clean and free from irritation is important for maintaining good vision. Wash your hands regularly and avoid touching your eyes with dirty hands. If you wear contact lenses, follow the cleaning and replacement instructions carefully to prevent infections and discomfort.

Nutrients like lutein and zeaxanthin, found in foods such as leafy greens and egg yolks, can help protect your eyes from oxidative damage and support overall vision. Including these nutrients in your diet can contribute to better eye health.

Excessive exposure to blue light from screens can contribute to eye strain. Consider using blue light filters on your devices, and practice good screen habits, such as taking regular breaks and adjusting the brightness to a comfortable level.

Preventing Eye Diseases with Nutrition and Herbs

Your eyes are one of your most precious assets, and keeping them healthy is crucial for maintaining clear vision throughout your life. One of the best ways to protect your eyes from diseases is through a balanced diet and the use of supportive herbs. Here's a friendly guide to how you can prevent eye diseases with the right nutrition and herbal remedies.

What you eat can have a big impact on your eye health. Here's how to make your diet work for you:

- Vitamin A: Essential for maintaining good vision, especially in low light, vitamin A helps keep your eyes' surface tissues healthy. Foods rich in vitamin A include carrots, sweet potatoes, spinach, and kale. Aim to include these in your diet regularly to support your eye health.
- Vitamin C: This powerful antioxidant helps protect your eyes from oxidative damage and supports the health of blood vessels in the eyes. Citrus fruits like oranges and grapefruits, strawberries, and bell peppers are great sources of vitamin C.
- Vitamin E: Another antioxidant, vitamin E helps protect eye cells from damage and supports overall eye health. Nuts, seeds, and green leafy vegetables are rich in vitamin E and should be part of your diet.
- Lutein and Zeaxanthin: These carotenoids are found in high concentrations in the retina and help protect your eyes from harmful light and oxidative stress. Incorporate foods like spinach, kale, and corn into your meals to get these important nutrients.
- Omega-3 Fatty Acids: Omega-3s support the health of the retina and may help prevent dry eyes and age-related macular degeneration (AMD). Fatty fish like salmon, mackerel, and sardines are excellent sources of omega-3 fatty acids.

Certain herbs have been traditionally used to support eye health and prevent diseases. Here's a look at some helpful herbs:

- Bilberry: Known for its potential to improve night vision and support overall eye health, bilberry is rich in antioxidants called anthocyanins. You can take bilberry supplements or drink bilberry tea to benefit from its eye-supportive properties.

- Ginkgo Biloba: This herb is thought to improve circulation, including to the eyes, which can help reduce the risk of certain eye conditions. Ginkgo biloba supplements may help enhance visual function and reduce symptoms of eye fatigue.
- Eyebright: Traditionally used to relieve eye irritation and strain, eyebright has anti-inflammatory properties that can benefit eye health. It can be taken as a tea or used as an eye wash (consult with a healthcare provider for proper use).
- Calendula: Known for its soothing and anti-inflammatory effects, calendula can be used in eye washes or as a topical remedy to help reduce irritation and support eye health.

Hydration is key to maintaining the health of the eye's surface and preventing dry eyes. Drinking plenty of water throughout the day helps keep your eyes moist and comfortable. Consider incorporating hydrating foods like cucumbers and watermelon into your diet as well.

Limiting your exposure to harmful substances like smoking and excessive alcohol can also support eye health. Smoking, in particular, is a significant risk factor for age-related macular degeneration and cataracts, so avoiding it is a proactive step for eye care.

No matter how well you eat or how many herbs you take, regular eye exams are essential for catching any potential issues early. Schedule regular check-ups with your eye care provider to monitor your eye health and address any concerns promptly.

By focusing on these nutritional strategies and herbal remedies, you can take proactive steps to prevent eye diseases and support your overall eye health. With a little care and attention, you can keep your vision sharp and your eyes feeling great. So, embrace these natural approaches and give your eyes the nourishment and support they deserve!

Exercises for Eye Strength and Focus

Just like your body benefits from exercise, your eyes can also get stronger and more focused with a little workout. Regular eye exercises can help reduce strain, improve focus, and enhance overall eye health. Here's a friendly guide to some simple and effective eye exercises you can incorporate into your daily routine.

If you spend long hours in front of screens, this exercise is a game-changer. Every 20 minutes, take a 20-second break and look at something 20 feet away. This helps relax your eye muscles and reduce digital eye strain. It's a quick and easy way to give your eyes a much-needed rest!

This exercise helps improve your eye flexibility and focus. Start by holding your thumb a few inches from your eyes. Focus on your thumb for about 5 seconds, then slowly move it away while keeping your gaze fixed. Focus on something further away for another 5 seconds. Return to your thumb and repeat this process 10 times. It's a great way to strengthen your eye muscles and improve your ability to shift focus.

Eye rolling is a simple exercise that helps relieve tension and improve circulation around your eyes. Sit comfortably and close your eyes. Gently roll your eyes in a circular motion, first clockwise and then counterclockwise. Do this for 10-15 seconds in each direction. It's a relaxing way to refresh your eyes and ease any strain.

Palming is a soothing exercise that helps reduce eye fatigue. Rub your hands together to generate warmth, then gently cup your palms over your closed eyes without applying pressure. Breathe deeply and relax for about 30 seconds. This technique helps reduce stress on your eyes and gives them a chance to rest.

This exercise improves your ability to focus on objects at different distances. Hold a pen or another small object about 6 inches from your eyes and focus on it for 10-15 seconds. Then, shift your focus to something in the distance, like a picture on the wall, for another 10-15 seconds. Repeat this process 5 times. It helps train your eyes to switch focus more efficiently.

Tracing a figure eight with your eyes helps enhance eye muscle control and flexibility. Imagine a large figure eight lying on its side (or the infinity symbol) about 10 feet in front of you. Trace the shape with your eyes slowly, without moving your head. Do this for about 1-2 minutes, and then switch directions. This exercise helps improve your eye coordination and strength.

Frequent blinking helps keep your eyes moist and reduces strain. Make a habit of blinking more often, especially if you're staring at a screen. Set a timer to remind yourself to blink every few minutes, or try blinking rapidly for 10 seconds to refresh your eyes.

This exercise helps with eye coordination and focusing skills. Hold your thumb up and focus on it. Slowly bring your thumb closer to your nose, maintaining your focus. When it gets too close to focus clearly, move it back to arm's length. Repeat this process 10 times. It's a great way to strengthen your eye muscles and improve your focus.

A gentle eye massage can help relax your eye muscles and reduce tension. Using your fingertips, lightly massage the area around your eyes in a circular motion. Be gentle and avoid applying too much pressure. This can help relieve eye strain and improve circulation.

Book 17: Detoxification and Heavy Metal Cleansing

Understanding the Impact of Heavy Metals on Health

Heavy metals are elements like lead, mercury, arsenic, and cadmium that can be harmful when they accumulate in the body. They're often found in the environment due to pollution, industrial processes, and certain foods. While we might not always think about them, heavy metals can have a significant impact on our health. Here's a friendly guide to understanding how these metals affect us and what you can do to minimize their impact.

Heavy metals are naturally occurring elements that can be toxic in large amounts. They include:

- Lead: Found in old paint, plumbing pipes, and contaminated soil.
- Mercury: Present in some fish, dental fillings, and industrial waste.
- Arsenic: Found in contaminated water and certain pesticides.
- Cadmium: Present in batteries, some fertilizers, and cigarette smoke.

Heavy metals can affect various systems in the body and lead to a range of health issues:

- Neurological Issues: Lead and mercury can impact brain function and development. Symptoms may include memory problems, difficulty concentrating, and mood swings.
- Kidney Damage: Cadmium and lead can harm the kidneys, potentially leading to chronic kidney disease or impairing kidney function over time.
- Cardiovascular Problems: Exposure to heavy metals like lead can contribute to high blood pressure and heart disease.
- Digestive Issues: Arsenic exposure has been linked to gastrointestinal problems and an increased risk of certain cancers.
- Immune System Suppression: Heavy metals can weaken the immune system, making you more susceptible to infections and diseases.

Understanding where heavy metals come from can help you reduce your exposure:

- Food: Some fish, like tuna and swordfish, can contain high levels of mercury. Certain crops may have absorbed heavy metals from contaminated soil or water.
- Water: Contaminated water sources can contain harmful levels of arsenic and other heavy metals.
- Household Items: Items like old paint, batteries, and certain industrial products can be sources of lead and cadmium.
- Environmental Pollution: Heavy metals can be released into the air and soil from industrial processes and waste.

Be aware of symptoms that might suggest heavy metal exposure:

- Fatigue and Weakness
- Headaches
- Digestive Problems
- Memory Loss
- Unexplained Joint or Muscle Pain

You can take steps to limit your exposure to heavy metals:

- Eat a Balanced Diet: Focus on a varied diet with plenty of fruits, vegetables, and whole grains. This helps reduce your risk of exposure to contaminated foods.
- Choose Safe Seafood: Opt for fish low in mercury, such as salmon, sardines, and trout. Limit your intake of high-mercury fish.
- Use Filtered Water: If you're concerned about contaminants, consider using a water filter that removes heavy metals.
- Be Mindful of Household Products: Avoid using products that contain heavy metals, like old paint, and properly dispose of items like batteries.
- Support Detoxification: Foods rich in antioxidants, like garlic and cilantro, may help support your body's natural detoxification processes.

If you suspect heavy metal exposure, consider gentle detoxification methods to help your body eliminate these toxins. Eating a diet high in fiber, staying well-hydrated, and incorporating foods known for their detoxifying properties can support your body's natural cleansing processes.

If you have concerns about heavy metal exposure or symptoms of toxicity, it's a good idea to consult with a healthcare professional. They can provide testing, personalized advice, and guidance on safe detoxification methods.

Chelation Therapy and Natural Detoxification

Detoxifying your body from heavy metals is a key step toward maintaining overall health, and there are two main approaches to consider: chelation therapy and natural detoxification. Both methods aim to remove harmful toxins, but they work in different ways. Here's a friendly guide to understanding each approach and how they can help you achieve a healthier, cleaner body.

Chelation therapy is a medical treatment used to remove heavy metals from the body. It involves using specific agents called chelators that bind to heavy metals and help eliminate them through urine. Here's how it works:

- How It Works: Chelators, such as EDTA (ethylenediaminetetraacetic acid), are administered either orally or through intravenous (IV) infusions. These chelators bind to heavy metals in the bloodstream, allowing them to be excreted more easily by the kidneys.
- Benefits: Chelation therapy can be effective for individuals with high levels of heavy metals and specific health conditions related to heavy metal toxicity. It's used under medical supervision and can help alleviate symptoms associated with metal poisoning.

- Considerations: While chelation therapy can be beneficial, it's important to undergo this treatment under the guidance of a healthcare professional. They will monitor for any potential side effects and ensure the therapy is appropriate for your situation.

Natural detoxification involves supporting your body's own detox processes through lifestyle and dietary changes. It's a gentler approach compared to chelation therapy and can be incorporated into your daily routine. Here's how you can support your body's natural detoxification:

- Hydration: Drinking plenty of water helps flush out toxins through your kidneys and urine. Aim for at least 8 glasses of water a day to support overall detoxification.
- Fiber-Rich Foods: Foods high in fiber, like fruits, vegetables, and whole grains, help support digestion and regular bowel movements, which are essential for toxin elimination.
- Antioxidant-Rich Foods: Incorporate foods rich in antioxidants, such as berries, nuts, and green leafy vegetables. Antioxidants help neutralize free radicals and reduce oxidative stress on your body.
- Herbs and Spices: Certain herbs and spices, like cilantro, garlic, and turmeric, are known for their detoxifying properties. Adding these to your meals can help support your body's natural cleansing processes.
- Regular Exercise: Physical activity promotes circulation and sweating, which aids in the elimination of toxins through the skin. Aim for at least 30 minutes of exercise most days of the week.
- Saunas and Steam Rooms: Using saunas or steam rooms can help promote sweating, which is another way your body can release toxins. Just make sure to stay hydrated during these sessions.

Some people may benefit from combining chelation therapy with natural detoxification methods. If you're considering chelation therapy, supporting it with a natural detox plan can enhance overall results and promote better health. Always consult with your healthcare provider before starting any new treatment or detox plan to ensure it's safe and appropriate for you.

Regardless of the method you choose, it's important to listen to your body and make adjustments as needed. Pay attention to how you feel during the detox process and communicate with your healthcare provider if you experience any concerns or symptoms.

Beyond detoxification, maintaining a healthy lifestyle is crucial for long-term well-being. Focus on eating a balanced diet, staying hydrated, exercising regularly, and avoiding exposure to environmental toxins. These habits will support your body's natural ability to stay clean and healthy.

Herbal and Nutritional Support for Heavy Metal Detox

Detoxifying your body from heavy metals is an important step for maintaining good health, and incorporating the right herbs and nutrients can play a big role in this process. If you're looking for natural ways to support your body's detox efforts, here's a friendly guide to some helpful herbs and nutrients that can assist with heavy metal cleansing.

Herbs are powerful allies in detoxification. They can help your body eliminate toxins, including heavy metals, and support overall health. Here are a few herbs known for their detoxifying properties:

- Cilantro: This herb is famous for its ability to help remove heavy metals from the body. It works by binding to metals like mercury and lead, helping to flush them out through urine.
- Chlorella: A type of green algae, chlorella is known for its detoxifying properties. It can help remove heavy metals from the body and also supports liver function.
- Milk Thistle: Milk thistle contains silymarin, which supports liver health and helps in detoxification processes. A healthy liver is crucial for processing and eliminating toxins.
- Dandelion Root: Often used in traditional medicine, dandelion root supports liver and kidney function, aiding in the removal of toxins and heavy metals.
- Garlic: Garlic is well-known for its detoxifying effects. It contains sulfur compounds that help the liver process toxins and supports overall detoxification.

Along with herbs, specific nutrients can support your body's detoxification processes. Here's a look at some key nutrients that can help:

- Vitamin C: This antioxidant vitamin helps neutralize free radicals and supports the immune system. It also plays a role in the detoxification process by helping to excrete toxins from the body.
- Vitamin E: Another powerful antioxidant, vitamin E helps protect cells from oxidative stress and supports overall detoxification.
- Zinc: Zinc is important for immune function and helps the body process and eliminate toxins. It also supports the liver's detoxification abilities.
- Selenium: Selenium is a trace mineral that works as an antioxidant and supports the detoxification process. It helps protect the body from oxidative damage caused by heavy metals.
- B Vitamins: B vitamins, particularly B6, B12, and folate, play a role in detoxification and support liver function. They also help in the metabolism of heavy metals.

Adding these herbs and nutrients to your daily routine can be simple and enjoyable:

- Herbal Teas: Enjoy teas made from cilantro, dandelion root, or milk thistle. These can be a soothing way to incorporate detoxifying herbs into your diet.
- Smoothies: Add chlorella or spinach (which contains high levels of vitamin C) to your smoothies for a detoxifying boost.
- Supplements: If you find it challenging to get enough herbs and nutrients from food alone, consider supplements. Choose high-quality products and consult with a healthcare provider to determine the right dosage for you.
- Cooking: Incorporate garlic and other herbs into your cooking. Not only will they add flavor, but they'll also provide detoxifying benefits.

Along with specific herbs and nutrients, maintaining a balanced diet rich in fruits, vegetables, whole grains, and lean proteins is crucial for overall health and effective detoxification. Eating a variety of nutrient-dense foods supports your body's natural detox processes and helps ensure you're getting the vitamins and minerals you need.

As you incorporate these herbs and nutrients into your routine, pay attention to how you feel. Everyone's body responds differently, so it's important to monitor any changes and consult with a healthcare provider if you have any concerns or experience any unusual symptoms.

How to Avoid Heavy Metal Exposure

Avoiding heavy metal exposure is a key step in protecting your health and ensuring that your body stays as toxin-free as possible. Heavy metals like lead, mercury, arsenic, and cadmium can accumulate in your body and cause various health issues, so it's wise to be proactive in reducing your exposure. Here's a friendly guide to help you avoid heavy metals in your daily life.

Be Mindful of Your Food Choices

- Opt for Low-Mercury Fish: Fish can be a great source of nutrients, but some types have higher mercury levels. Choose fish like salmon, sardines, and trout, which are lower in mercury, and limit consumption of high-mercury fish like tuna, swordfish, and shark.
- Wash Your Fruits and Vegetables: Thoroughly wash and peel fruits and vegetables to reduce the risk of ingesting pesticides and other contaminants. Organic produce can also be a good option as it is less likely to be treated with harmful chemicals.
- Avoid Contaminated Water: If you're concerned about heavy metals in your water supply, consider using a water filter designed to remove contaminants or drink bottled water that is tested for purity.

Be Cautious with Household Products

- Check for Lead in Paint: If you live in an older home, it's a good idea to have the paint checked for lead. Lead-based paint was commonly used before it was banned, and lead dust can be a source of exposure.
- Handle Batteries Safely: Batteries can contain heavy metals like cadmium and mercury. Dispose of old batteries properly at designated recycling centers, and avoid using disposable batteries when possible.
- Avoid Certain Traditional Remedies: Some traditional or herbal remedies, especially those from international sources, might contain heavy metals. Ensure you source supplements and remedies from reputable suppliers and check for certifications.

Minimize Exposure to Environmental Pollution

- Stay Informed About Air Quality: Pay attention to air quality reports in your area, especially if you live in an industrial or heavily polluted area. Avoid outdoor activities on days with poor air quality to reduce inhalation of airborne pollutants.
- Reduce Soil Exposure: If you have a garden, be aware of potential contamination in the soil. Use clean soil and avoid planting in areas where heavy metal contamination is a concern. Consider using raised beds or container gardening if soil quality is a worry.

Choose Safe Personal Care Products

- Check Labels for Harmful Ingredients: Personal care products, such as cosmetics and lotions, can sometimes contain heavy metals. Opt for products labeled as free from heavy metals and choose natural or organic options when possible.
- Avoid Certain Types of Jewelry: Some inexpensive jewelry, especially from sources that don't adhere to strict safety standards, might contain metals like lead. Choose jewelry from reputable brands that comply with safety regulations.

Practice Safe Work Habits

- Follow Safety Protocols: If you work in an industry where heavy metal exposure is a risk, make sure to follow all safety guidelines and use personal protective equipment (PPE) as required.
- Proper Ventilation: Ensure good ventilation in workspaces where chemicals or metals are handled to reduce inhalation and absorption of toxic substances.

Regular Health Checkups

- Monitor Your Health: Regular health checkups can help detect any issues related to heavy metal exposure early on. If you have symptoms or concerns, discussing them with your healthcare provider can lead to timely interventions.

Support Natural Detoxification

- Stay Hydrated and Eat Well: Drinking plenty of water and eating a balanced diet rich in antioxidants and fiber can support your body's natural detoxification processes, helping to eliminate any minor exposures to heavy metals.

Daily Detox Habits for a Clean Body

Incorporating daily detox habits into your routine can help keep your body clean and functioning at its best. These habits support your body's natural detoxification processes, helping you feel energized and vibrant. Here's a friendly guide to some easy and effective daily habits that can make a big difference in your overall health.

- Drink Plenty of Water: Water is essential for flushing out toxins and keeping your organs functioning properly. Aim for at least 8 glasses a day, and consider adding a splash of lemon for an extra detox boost. Lemon water can help stimulate digestion and support liver function.
- Herbal Teas: Incorporate herbal teas like dandelion, ginger, or green tea into your daily routine. These teas have natural detoxifying properties and can help support digestion and liver health.

Eat a Balanced, Nutrient-Rich Diet

- Focus on Whole Foods: Base your meals around fresh fruits, vegetables, whole grains, and lean proteins. These foods are rich in nutrients and antioxidants that support your body's detox processes.
- Include Detoxifying Foods: Foods like beets, carrots, garlic, and leafy greens are known for their detoxifying properties. Incorporate these into your meals to help support liver and kidney function.
- Limit Processed Foods: Reduce your intake of processed and sugary foods, as they can contribute to toxin buildup and inflammation in the body.

Exercise Regularly

- Get Moving: Regular physical activity promotes circulation and sweating, both of which help your body eliminate toxins. Aim for at least 30 minutes of exercise most days of the week, whether it's a brisk walk, a workout class, or yoga.
- Try Sweating It Out: Consider incorporating activities that make you sweat, such as saunas or hot baths. Sweating helps your body release toxins through the skin.

Support Digestive Health

- Eat Fiber-Rich Foods: Fiber supports healthy digestion and regular bowel movements, which are crucial for eliminating toxins. Include foods like chia seeds, beans, and whole grains in your diet.
- Stay Consistent: Maintain a regular eating schedule to support your digestive system. Avoid skipping meals and try to eat at regular intervals throughout the day.

Get Quality Sleep

- Prioritize Rest: Good quality sleep is vital for detoxification and overall health. Aim for 7-9 hours of sleep each night to allow your body to repair and regenerate.
- Create a Sleep-Friendly Environment: Make your bedroom a restful space by keeping it cool, dark, and quiet. Establish a relaxing bedtime routine to help you wind down.

Practice Mindful Stress Management

- Manage Stress: Chronic stress can impact your body's ability to detoxify and recover. Incorporate stress-reducing practices like meditation, deep breathing exercises, or journaling into your daily routine.
- Take Breaks: Ensure you're taking regular breaks throughout the day to relax and recharge, especially if you have a demanding or sedentary job.

Support Skin Health

- Dry Brushing: Consider dry brushing your skin before a shower to stimulate circulation and help remove dead skin cells. This can support your body's natural detox processes.
- Use Gentle Skincare Products: Choose natural or organic skincare products to avoid exposing your skin to potentially harmful chemicals.

Limit Toxin Exposure

- Be Mindful of Your Environment: Reduce exposure to environmental toxins by using natural cleaning products, avoiding smoking, and ensuring good ventilation in your home.
- Choose Safe Personal Care Products: Opt for personal care items that are free from harmful chemicals and heavy metals. Look for products with natural or organic ingredients.

Listen to Your Body

- Pay Attention to How You Feel: Regularly check in with yourself to see how your body is responding to your detox habits. Adjust your routine as needed to ensure you're feeling your best.

Rebuilding Health After Heavy Metal Exposure

If you've been exposed to heavy metals, it's important to focus on rebuilding your health and restoring balance in your body. Heavy metal exposure can take a toll, but with the right steps, you can support your body's recovery and help restore your well-being. Here's a friendly guide to help you get back on track after exposure to heavy metals.

- Avoid Further Exposure: The first step in rebuilding health is to eliminate or reduce any ongoing sources of heavy metal exposure. This might mean making changes in your diet, environment, or work practices to minimize contact with harmful metals.
- Consult a Healthcare Professional: If you suspect heavy metal toxicity, it's a good idea to consult with a healthcare provider. They can provide personalized advice and may recommend tests to assess your levels and overall health.

Support Detoxification

- Hydrate Well: Drinking plenty of water helps flush out toxins and supports your body's natural detox processes. Aim for at least 8 glasses of water a day, and consider adding a splash of lemon for added benefits.
- Incorporate Detoxifying Foods: Eating foods that support detoxification can aid in your recovery. Include fruits and vegetables high in antioxidants, such as berries, leafy greens, and cruciferous vegetables. These foods help combat oxidative stress and support liver function.
- Consider Detox Herbs: Herbal supplements like cilantro, chlorella, and milk thistle can assist in detoxification. These herbs help bind and eliminate heavy metals from the body. Always consult a healthcare provider before starting any new supplement.

Support Your Digestive System

- Eat Fiber-Rich Foods: Fiber helps with digestion and elimination, which is crucial for removing toxins from your body. Include foods like whole grains, legumes, and vegetables in your diet to promote healthy bowel movements.
- Maintain Regular Digestion: Establishing a regular eating schedule and avoiding overeating or undereating can help keep your digestive system in balance. A well-functioning digestive system is key for effective detoxification.

Focus on Nutritional Support

- Boost Your Nutrient Intake: Certain nutrients are particularly helpful for recovery. Vitamin C, vitamin E, zinc, and selenium are known for their antioxidant properties and support detoxification. Incorporate foods rich in these nutrients, like citrus fruits, nuts, seeds, and whole grains.

- Consider a Multivitamin: If your diet may be lacking in certain nutrients, a high-quality multivitamin can help fill in the gaps. Choose one that is free from heavy metals and contaminants.

Prioritize Rest and Recovery

- Get Adequate Sleep: Quality sleep is essential for your body to repair and regenerate. Aim for 7-9 hours of sleep per night to support your overall health and recovery.
- Manage Stress: Chronic stress can impact your body's ability to detoxify and recover. Practice stress-reducing techniques like meditation, deep breathing, or gentle exercise to support your well-being.

Exercise Regularly

- Stay Active: Regular physical activity helps improve circulation, supports your body's detoxification systems, and promotes overall health. Aim for at least 30 minutes of moderate exercise most days of the week.
- Sweat It Out: Activities that induce sweating, like exercise or saunas, can help your body eliminate toxins through the skin.

Support Your Liver and Kidneys

- Focus on Liver Health: The liver is a key player in detoxification. Support liver health by eating liver-friendly foods like beets, artichokes, and green tea. Avoid excessive alcohol and processed foods that can strain the liver.
- Keep Kidneys Healthy: Your kidneys also play a crucial role in detoxification. Stay hydrated and eat foods that support kidney function, such as cranberries and watermelon.

Monitor Your Progress

- Track Your Health: Keep an eye on your overall health and well-being as you implement these changes. Note any improvements or issues and discuss them with your healthcare provider.
- Adjust as Needed: Recovery is a gradual process, and it's important to be patient. Adjust your habits and strategies based on how your body responds and any guidance from your healthcare provider.

Liver Support for Efficient Detoxification

Your liver is like your body's natural detox powerhouse, working tirelessly to filter out toxins and keep everything running smoothly. Supporting your liver is key to efficient detoxification and overall health. Here's a friendly guide to help you keep your liver in tip-top shape and make the most of its detoxifying abilities.

- Load Up on Vegetables: Vegetables like beets, carrots, and Brussels sprouts are fantastic for liver health. They contain nutrients and antioxidants that support liver function and help it process toxins more effectively.

- Include Leafy Greens: Spinach, kale, and arugula are rich in chlorophyll, which can help remove toxins from your bloodstream and support liver health.
- Opt for Healthy Fats: Incorporate sources of healthy fats like avocados, nuts, and olive oil. These fats support liver cell health and help with the absorption of fat-soluble vitamins that aid detoxification.

Stay Hydrated

- Drink Plenty of Water: Water is essential for liver function. It helps flush out toxins and supports all your body's natural processes. Aim to drink at least 8 glasses of water a day, and consider adding a splash of lemon for an extra detox boost.
- Herbal Teas: Teas like dandelion, milk thistle, and green tea are known for their liver-supportive properties. They can help stimulate liver function and provide antioxidants that protect liver cells.

Support Your Liver with Herbs

- Milk Thistle: This herb is renowned for its liver-protective qualities. It contains silymarin, a powerful antioxidant that helps protect liver cells from damage and supports overall liver function.
- Dandelion Root: Dandelion root acts as a gentle diuretic, promoting bile production and helping to cleanse the liver. It's great for supporting digestion and liver health.
- Turmeric: Turmeric contains curcumin, which has anti-inflammatory and antioxidant properties that can help support liver health and detoxification.

Avoid Excessive Alcohol and Processed Foods

- Limit Alcohol Intake: Excessive alcohol can overwhelm the liver and lead to inflammation and damage. If you drink, do so in moderation and ensure you give your liver plenty of time to recover between drinks.
- Cut Back on Processed Foods: Processed and sugary foods can burden your liver and contribute to inflammation. Focus on whole, natural foods to support liver health and overall well-being.

Maintain a Healthy Weight

- Watch Your Weight: Being overweight can lead to fatty liver disease, which impairs liver function. Maintaining a healthy weight through balanced eating and regular exercise supports liver health.
- Exercise Regularly: Physical activity helps improve circulation and supports liver function. Aim for at least 30 minutes of moderate exercise most days of the week.

Practice Safe Medication Use

- Be Cautious with Medications: Some medications and over-the-counter drugs can put a strain on your liver. Use medications as directed and consult with your healthcare provider about any potential liver impacts.
- Avoid Unnecessary Supplements: Not all supplements are liver-friendly. Choose supplements from reputable sources and avoid those that may contain contaminants or unnecessary additives.

Get Regular Checkups

- Monitor Liver Health: Regular checkups with your healthcare provider can help monitor liver function and catch any potential issues early. If you have any concerns about your liver health, discuss them with your doctor.
- Get Liver Enzyme Tests: If you're at risk for liver issues, your doctor may recommend liver enzyme tests to check for any signs of dysfunction or damage.

Practice Stress Management

- Manage Stress: Chronic stress can affect liver health and overall well-being. Incorporate stress-reducing practices into your daily routine, such as meditation, yoga, or deep breathing exercises.
- Take Time for Yourself: Make sure to schedule regular relaxation and self-care activities to keep stress levels in check.

Book 18: Healing Inflammation Naturally

The Root Causes of Inflammation

Inflammation is a fundamental aspect of the body's defense mechanism, serving as an alert system to identify and address injury or infection. However, when inflammation becomes chronic, it shifts from being a protective response to a potential threat to overall health. Understanding the root causes of inflammation is crucial for managing and mitigating its impacts.

One of the primary contributors to chronic inflammation is poor diet. Modern diets often include a high intake of processed foods, refined sugars, and unhealthy fats, all of which can promote inflammatory processes within the body. These types of foods can lead to an imbalance in the body's natural inflammatory responses. Conversely, a diet rich in anti-inflammatory foods—such as fruits, vegetables, whole grains, and healthy fats—can help combat inflammation and support overall health. Emphasizing a diet that incorporates these wholesome ingredients can play a significant role in managing inflammation.

Another significant factor is a lack of physical activity. A sedentary lifestyle, characterized by prolonged periods of inactivity and insufficient exercise, has been linked to increased levels of inflammation. Physical activity helps regulate the body's inflammatory responses and promotes overall well-being. Regular exercise, even in moderate amounts, can help keep inflammation in check and improve overall health.

Chronic stress is also a notable contributor to inflammation. Stress is not merely a mental or emotional burden; it has tangible effects on the body. Persistent stress keeps the body in a constant state of alert, leading to the release of inflammatory markers and contributing to chronic inflammation. Managing stress through techniques such as mindfulness, relaxation exercises, and adequate rest can help mitigate its inflammatory effects.

Environmental toxins present another significant challenge. Exposure to pollutants, chemicals, and other environmental toxins can irritate the body and lead to inflammatory responses. Reducing exposure to these harmful substances, when possible, is an essential step in controlling inflammation. Adopting lifestyle choices that minimize contact with environmental pollutants can contribute to a reduction in inflammation levels.

Sleep plays a crucial role in inflammation as well. Inadequate or poor-quality sleep disrupts the body's natural processes, including those related to inflammation. Ensuring sufficient and restful sleep is vital for maintaining balanced inflammatory responses. Good sleep hygiene practices, such as maintaining a consistent sleep schedule and creating a restful sleep environment, can significantly impact inflammation levels.

Allergies and sensitivities are also relevant factors. When the body reacts to certain substances—whether they are environmental allergens or food sensitivities—it can trigger an inflammatory response. Identifying and managing these triggers is essential for controlling inflammation. For those with known allergies or sensitivities, avoiding these triggers can help reduce inflammation and improve overall health.

Lastly, chronic infections and diseases, such as autoimmune conditions, contribute to persistent inflammation. These conditions can lead to ongoing inflammatory responses, affecting various aspects of health. Effective management of chronic infections and diseases, often in consultation with healthcare professionals, is crucial for controlling inflammation and maintaining overall well-being.

Anti-Inflammatory Foods for Everyday Health

In the pursuit of maintaining optimal health and managing inflammation, the foods we choose to include in our diet play a pivotal role. Inflammation, while a natural and necessary part of the body's healing process, can become problematic when it becomes chronic. Incorporating anti-inflammatory foods into our daily routine offers a proactive approach to reducing inflammation and promoting overall well-being. Understanding which foods have anti-inflammatory properties can empower us to make dietary choices that support a healthier, more balanced body.

Berries are a prime example of foods that can combat inflammation effectively. Blueberries, strawberries, raspberries, and blackberries are not only delicious but also rich in antioxidants known as anthocyanins. These compounds are responsible for the vibrant colors of berries and play a crucial role in reducing inflammatory markers in the body. Regular consumption of berries can help lower inflammation levels, making them a valuable addition to breakfast smoothies, yogurt, or enjoyed as a simple snack.

Leafy greens such as spinach, kale, and Swiss chard are another important category of anti-inflammatory foods. These vegetables are abundant in vitamins, minerals, and antioxidants that contribute to the body's natural anti-inflammatory processes. Leafy greens are versatile and can be incorporated into a variety of meals, from fresh salads to blended smoothies or sautéed as a nutritious side dish.

Nuts and seeds offer a wealth of anti-inflammatory benefits. Almonds, walnuts, chia seeds, and flaxseeds are rich in healthy fats, fiber, and antioxidants that help regulate inflammation. These small but powerful foods can be easily added to a daily diet by sprinkling them on salads, blending them into oatmeal, or simply enjoying a handful as a snack.

Fatty fish such as salmon, mackerel, and sardines are renowned for their high omega-3 fatty acid content, which has been shown to have potent anti-inflammatory effects. Omega-3s help reduce the production of inflammatory chemicals in the body. Incorporating fatty fish into the diet, whether grilled, baked, or added to salads, provides a significant boost to managing inflammation.

Turmeric is a spice celebrated for its anti-inflammatory properties, primarily due to its active compound, curcumin. Curcumin has been widely studied for its ability to reduce inflammation and improve overall health. Adding turmeric to various dishes, such as curries, soups, or even golden milk, can enhance flavor while providing an anti-inflammatory benefit.

Ginger has a long history of use for its medicinal properties, including its role in reducing inflammation. Fresh ginger can be added to smoothies, teas, or used as a flavorful ingredient in cooking. Its natural compounds help mitigate inflammatory responses, making it a valuable addition to a health-conscious diet.

Olive oil, particularly extra virgin olive oil, is a staple in the Mediterranean diet known for its anti-inflammatory benefits. It contains oleocanthal, a compound with properties similar to non-steroidal anti-inflammatory drugs. Using olive oil in cooking, as a salad dressing, or as a dip for whole-grain bread can provide an easy way to incorporate anti-inflammatory benefits into daily meals.

Tomatoes are rich in lycopene, an antioxidant that helps combat inflammation. Lycopene is particularly available in cooked tomatoes, such as in sauces and soups. Including tomatoes in your diet can help support your body's ability to manage inflammation, making them a valuable component of a balanced diet.

Avocados are another powerful anti-inflammatory food. Packed with healthy fats, fiber, and antioxidants, avocados also contain magnesium, which aids in reducing inflammatory responses. They can be enjoyed in a variety of ways, such as in salads, on toast, or blended into smoothies, making them a versatile addition to any meal.

Whole grains like brown rice, quinoa, and oats provide significant fiber content, which is beneficial for reducing inflammation. Fiber supports overall health by promoting healthy digestion and reducing inflammatory responses. Incorporating whole grains into meals as side dishes, bases for salads, or part of breakfast can contribute to a balanced and anti-inflammatory diet.

Herbal Remedies for Reducing Inflammation

Herbs have been used for ages to help soothe inflammation and support overall health. If you're interested in exploring natural ways to manage inflammation, here are some herbal remedies that might be just what you need.

Turmeric is a standout herb in the world of inflammation relief. Its key component, curcumin, is renowned for its powerful anti-inflammatory effects. You can easily incorporate turmeric into your diet by adding it to dishes like curries, soups, or even smoothies. For a comforting drink, try turmeric tea, often called "golden milk," which can be both soothing and beneficial.

Ginger is another fantastic option for tackling inflammation. Known for its warming and digestive-soothing properties, fresh ginger can be added to your teas, smoothies, or meals. If you prefer a more concentrated form, ginger supplements are also available.

Green tea is not just a relaxing beverage; it's packed with antioxidants called catechins, which help fight inflammation. A daily cup of green tea can be a simple yet effective way to support your body's inflammatory response. For a bit of variety, try adding a slice of lemon or a touch of honey.

Boswellia, also known as frankincense, is an herb that has been used in traditional medicine for its anti-inflammatory benefits. It can be taken in supplement form and is known for its potential to help reduce inflammation and support joint health.

Incorporating these herbs into your daily routine can offer a natural and soothing approach to managing inflammation. Whether you enjoy them in teas, meals, or supplements, they provide a gentle yet effective way to support your body's health and well-being.

The Role of the Gut in Inflammation

The connection between gut health and inflammation is a fascinating and crucial aspect of overall wellness. Your gut, often referred to as your digestive system, is not just responsible for processing food; it also plays a significant role in regulating inflammation throughout your body. Understanding this relationship can provide valuable insights into how to manage and reduce inflammation naturally.

At the heart of this connection is the gut microbiome, a diverse community of trillions of microorganisms—including bacteria, viruses, fungi, and other microbes—living in your digestive tract. These microorganisms are not only essential for breaking down food and absorbing nutrients but also play a critical role in maintaining a balanced immune response. A healthy gut microbiome helps regulate inflammation by producing beneficial compounds and supporting the gut lining, which acts as a barrier against harmful substances.

When the balance of the gut microbiome is disrupted, a condition known as dysbiosis can occur. This imbalance can be triggered by various factors, such as a diet high in processed foods and sugars, chronic stress, antibiotics, or other medications. Dysbiosis can lead to increased inflammation as the gut loses its ability to manage harmful substances effectively. This imbalance can contribute to chronic inflammatory conditions and impact overall health.

Another key concept related to gut health and inflammation is leaky gut syndrome. The lining of your gut is made up of a single layer of cells that act as a barrier between your digestive tract and the bloodstream. When this barrier becomes damaged or compromised, it can lead to a condition known as leaky gut. In leaky gut syndrome, gaps between the gut lining cells widen, allowing partially digested food particles, toxins, and microbes to leak into the bloodstream. This can trigger an immune response, leading to systemic inflammation and potentially contributing to various health issues, including autoimmune conditions and chronic diseases.

The good news is that you can support gut health and manage inflammation through dietary and lifestyle choices. A diet rich in fiber, prebiotics, and probiotics can help nourish and maintain a healthy gut microbiome. Fiber, found in fruits, vegetables, whole grains, and legumes, acts as a food source for beneficial gut bacteria. Prebiotics, which are a type of fiber, specifically encourage the growth of healthy gut bacteria. Probiotics, found in fermented foods like yogurt, kefir, sauerkraut, and kimchi, provide live beneficial bacteria that can help restore balance to the gut microbiome.

In addition to dietary choices, other lifestyle factors can impact gut health and inflammation. Managing stress through practices like mindfulness, meditation, or regular physical activity can help support a balanced gut microbiome. Adequate sleep is also essential, as poor sleep can affect gut health and contribute to inflammation. Avoiding overuse of antibiotics and other medications, when possible, is another way to protect gut health.

Managing Chronic Inflammatory Conditions

Managing chronic inflammatory conditions can indeed feel overwhelming, but with a thoughtful approach and consistent effort, you can significantly improve your health and quality of life. Chronic inflammation is a persistent state of inflammation that can contribute to various health issues, including arthritis, cardiovascular diseases, and autoimmune disorders. Here's a comprehensive guide to help you manage these conditions effectively and improve your overall well-being.

Embrace an Anti-Inflammatory Diet: One of the most impactful ways to manage chronic inflammation is through diet. An anti-inflammatory diet focuses on foods that help reduce inflammation and supports overall health. Incorporate a variety of fruits and vegetables, particularly those high in antioxidants, such as berries, leafy greens, and bell peppers. Fatty fish, like salmon and mackerel, are excellent sources of omega-3 fatty acids, which are known for their anti-inflammatory properties.

Nuts, seeds, and whole grains also play a crucial role in an anti-inflammatory diet. On the flip side, limit your intake of processed foods, sugary snacks, and refined carbohydrates, as these can exacerbate inflammation. Reducing your consumption of red and processed meats can also be beneficial.

Stay Active: Regular physical activity is another key component in managing inflammation. Exercise helps to lower inflammatory markers in the body, improves cardiovascular health, and boosts your mood. It doesn't have to be intense; even moderate exercise like brisk walking, cycling, or swimming can be effective. Find activities that you enjoy, as you're more likely to stick with a routine that you find pleasant. Incorporating strength training and flexibility exercises, such as yoga or pilates, can also be beneficial for maintaining overall health and managing inflammation.

Manage Stress: Chronic stress is known to have a significant impact on inflammation and overall health. Finding effective ways to manage stress is crucial. Techniques such as mindfulness, meditation, and deep breathing exercises can help reduce stress and support a balanced immune response. Engaging in activities that you find relaxing or fulfilling, such as reading, gardening, or spending time with friends and family, can also help manage stress levels. Regular practice of relaxation techniques can help calm the mind and body, reducing the impact of stress on inflammation.

Prioritize Quality Sleep: Sleep plays a critical role in managing inflammation. During sleep, your body repairs and restores itself, and insufficient or poor-quality sleep can increase inflammatory markers. Aim for 7 to 9 hours of quality sleep each night. Establishing a consistent sleep schedule, creating a calming bedtime routine, and maintaining a comfortable sleep environment can all contribute to better sleep. Avoiding screens and stimulating activities before bed can help improve your sleep quality.

Stay Hydrated: Proper hydration is essential for maintaining overall health and can support your body's ability to manage inflammation. Water helps with nutrient transport, digestion, and detoxification processes. Aim to drink plenty of water throughout the day and limit your intake of sugary beverages and excessive caffeine, which can contribute to inflammation and disrupt hydration balance.

Avoid Smoking and Limit Alcohol Consumption: Smoking and excessive alcohol consumption can both exacerbate inflammation and negatively affect your health. If you smoke, seek support to quit, as smoking is a significant risk factor for chronic inflammation and various health issues. Additionally, try to limit alcohol intake to moderate levels, as excessive alcohol consumption can lead to increased inflammation and a range of other health problems.

Consider Supplements: Certain supplements can offer additional support in managing inflammation. Omega-3 fatty acids, found in fish oil supplements, are known for their anti-inflammatory effects. Turmeric, particularly its active compound curcumin, is also recognized for its potential to reduce inflammation. However, it's important to consult with a healthcare provider before starting any new supplements to ensure they are appropriate for your specific health needs.

Work Closely with Your Healthcare Team: Managing chronic inflammatory conditions often requires a collaborative approach. Regular consultations with your healthcare provider can help you develop a personalized management plan that addresses your unique needs. Your healthcare team can offer guidance on dietary changes, physical activity, and other lifestyle modifications, and they can help monitor your progress and make adjustments as needed.

Educate Yourself and Stay Informed: Understanding your condition and staying informed about the latest research and treatments can empower you to take an active role in your health. Educate yourself about your specific inflammatory condition and explore reliable sources of information. This knowledge can help you make informed decisions and advocate for your health effectively.

Exercise and Lifestyle Changes for Inflammation

Managing inflammation isn't just about what you eat; it's also about how you live your life. Incorporating regular exercise and making thoughtful lifestyle changes can have a significant impact on reducing inflammation and enhancing your overall health. Here's a friendly guide to help you incorporate exercise and lifestyle changes to keep inflammation in check.

Exercise Regularly: Engaging in regular physical activity is one of the most effective ways to combat inflammation. Exercise helps reduce the production of inflammatory markers and improves your body's ability to manage stress. You don't need to commit to intense workouts to see benefits—consistent moderate exercise, like walking, swimming, or cycling, can make a big difference. Aim for at least 150 minutes of moderate aerobic activity or 75 minutes of vigorous activity per week, combined with strength training exercises on two or more days. Finding activities you enjoy can make it easier to stick with an exercise routine, so explore different options and see what feels best for you.

Prioritize Sleep: Quality sleep is essential for managing inflammation. During sleep, your body undergoes important repair processes and regulates inflammatory responses. Aim for 7 to 9 hours of restful sleep each night. To improve your sleep quality, establish a regular sleep schedule, create a relaxing bedtime routine, and make your sleep environment as comfortable as possible. Avoid screens and stimulating activities before bed, and consider practices like reading or gentle stretching to help wind down.

Manage Stress Effectively: Chronic stress can significantly contribute to inflammation, so finding ways to manage stress is crucial. Incorporate stress-reducing practices into your daily routine, such as mindfulness, meditation, deep breathing exercises, or yoga. Engaging in activities you find relaxing or enjoyable, such as hobbies, spending time with loved ones, or immersing yourself in nature, can also help lower stress levels. Regular physical activity is another great way to manage stress, as exercise releases endorphins that improve mood and promote relaxation.

Stay Hydrated: Proper hydration supports your body's ability to manage inflammation. Drinking plenty of water throughout the day helps with digestion, nutrient absorption, and the removal of toxins from your system. Aim to drink at least eight glasses of water daily, and adjust based on your activity level and climate. Try to limit your intake of sugary drinks and excessive caffeine, which can contribute to inflammation.

Avoid Smoking and Limit Alcohol: Smoking and excessive alcohol consumption can both increase inflammation and negatively affect your health. If you smoke, seek support to quit, as smoking is a major contributor to chronic inflammation and various health issues. Additionally, try to limit alcohol intake to moderate levels, as excessive alcohol can lead to inflammation and other health problems.

Incorporate Relaxation Techniques: Incorporating relaxation techniques into your daily routine can also help manage inflammation. Practices like tai chi, qigong, or gentle stretching can promote relaxation and reduce stress. Regularly taking time for yourself to relax and unwind is essential for maintaining balance and supporting your body's ability to manage inflammation.

Create a Supportive Environment: Your environment can influence your stress levels and overall well-being. Surround yourself with supportive people, and create a home environment that promotes relaxation and comfort. Consider organizing your space in a way that reduces stress and fosters a sense of calm.

Listen to Your Body: Pay attention to how your body responds to different activities and lifestyle changes. If you notice that certain exercises or practices are causing discomfort or exacerbating inflammation, make adjustments as needed. It's important to find a balance that works for you and supports your health goals.

Understanding the Link Between Inflammation and Disease

Inflammation is a natural response by your body's immune system to protect itself from harm. It's like your body's built-in alarm system, kicking into gear to fight off infections, heal injuries, and deal with harmful stimuli. However, when inflammation becomes chronic, it can be a different story, potentially contributing to a range of diseases. Let's dive into how inflammation is linked to various health conditions and why understanding this connection is important.

Acute vs. Chronic Inflammation: To get a clear picture, it's helpful to distinguish between acute and chronic inflammation. Acute inflammation is short-term and often a direct response to an injury or infection. For example, if you cut yourself, the area becomes red, swollen, and warm—that's acute inflammation in action, working to heal the wound. This type of inflammation is typically beneficial and resolves once the body has addressed the issue.
Chronic inflammation, on the other hand, is long-term and can persist even after the initial cause has been resolved. This ongoing inflammation can be less obvious but can still cause damage over time. It's like having your body's alarm system stuck on "high alert," which can lead to various health problems.

Inflammation and Chronic Diseases: Chronic inflammation has been linked to a range of serious health conditions. One major area is cardiovascular disease. Inflammation can contribute to the buildup of plaque in the arteries, which increases the risk of heart attacks and strokes. It's like having a persistent, low-grade irritation that gradually wears down the arteries, making them less efficient and more prone to damage.
Another significant link is with autoimmune diseases, where the immune system mistakenly attacks the body's own tissues. Conditions like rheumatoid arthritis, lupus, and multiple sclerosis involve chronic inflammation as the immune system targets healthy cells, leading to pain, swelling, and tissue damage.
Diabetes is another condition where inflammation plays a role. In type 2 diabetes, chronic inflammation can affect how your body processes insulin, the hormone that helps regulate blood sugar levels. This disruption can lead to insulin resistance, where the body's cells don't respond properly to insulin, contributing to elevated blood sugar levels and the development of diabetes.

Cancer and Inflammation: There is also evidence suggesting that chronic inflammation can increase the risk of certain types of cancer. Inflammatory processes can cause changes in the cells of tissues, potentially leading to cancerous growths. For instance, persistent inflammation in the digestive tract, such as in inflammatory bowel disease, can increase the risk of colorectal cancer.

The Role of Lifestyle: Understanding the link between inflammation and disease underscores the importance of lifestyle choices in managing inflammation. Diet, exercise, stress management, and avoiding harmful habits like smoking can all impact inflammation levels. For instance, an anti-inflammatory diet rich in fruits, vegetables, and healthy fats can help reduce chronic inflammation, while regular physical activity helps regulate inflammation and supports overall health.

Monitoring and Prevention: Keeping an eye on inflammation levels, especially if you have a condition that is known to be associated with chronic inflammation, is crucial. Regular check-ups with your healthcare provider can help monitor inflammation markers and assess your risk for related diseases. Additionally, adopting a proactive approach to your health by maintaining a balanced diet, staying active, managing stress, and avoiding harmful substances can make a big difference in reducing inflammation and preventing disease.

Book 19: Bone and Joint Health with Natural Remedies

Understanding Bone Health and Aging

As we age, maintaining strong and healthy bones becomes increasingly important, yet it's something many people don't think about until they face issues like osteoporosis or frequent fractures. Understanding bone health and how it changes with age can help you take proactive steps to keep your bones in good shape throughout your life.

Bone Health Basics: Our bones are living tissues that constantly undergo a process of remodeling. This involves the breakdown of old bone tissue by cells called osteoclasts and the formation of new bone tissue by cells called osteoblasts. In our youth, this process is balanced, and bones are continuously strengthened. However, as we age, the balance can shift. The rate of bone breakdown may surpass the rate of bone formation, leading to a gradual loss of bone density.

The Impact of Aging: Aging affects bone health in several ways. One of the key factors is hormonal changes. For women, menopause leads to a significant drop in estrogen levels, a hormone that helps protect bone density. This decrease can accelerate bone loss, increasing the risk of osteoporosis. For men, a gradual decline in testosterone levels can also contribute to bone density loss, although the effect is generally less abrupt than in women.
Bone density naturally decreases with age, starting in our mid-30s. After this peak, bones can become more porous and brittle. This loss of bone density can make bones more susceptible to fractures and breaks, even from minor falls or injuries.

Nutrition and Bone Health: What you eat plays a crucial role in maintaining bone health as you age. Calcium and vitamin D are particularly important. Calcium is a major component of bone tissue, and getting enough of it helps maintain bone strength. Vitamin D is essential for calcium absorption and bone metabolism. You can get calcium from dairy products, leafy greens, and fortified foods, while vitamin D can be obtained from sunlight exposure and foods like fatty fish and fortified dairy products.

Physical Activity: Regular weight-bearing and muscle-strengthening exercises are beneficial for bone health. Activities like walking, jogging, and resistance training help stimulate bone formation and improve bone density. Exercise also enhances muscle strength and balance, reducing the risk of falls and fractures. Incorporating activities like yoga or tai chi can improve flexibility and stability, further supporting bone health.

Bone Health and Lifestyle Choices: Several lifestyle choices can impact bone health. Smoking and excessive alcohol consumption can weaken bones and increase the risk of fractures. Smoking impairs bone healing and decreases bone density, while heavy drinking can interfere with calcium absorption and hormone levels related to bone health.

Preventive Measures: It's never too early to start caring for your bones. Adopting a bone-healthy lifestyle, including a balanced diet rich in calcium and vitamin D, regular exercise, and avoiding harmful habits, can make a big difference. For those already experiencing age-related bone loss, medications and supplements may be recommended by a healthcare provider to help manage bone density.

Regular Check-ups: Regular bone density screenings can help assess bone health and detect any early signs of bone loss. Your healthcare provider can offer personalized recommendations based on your bone density and overall health.

Natural Remedies for Arthritis and Joint Pain

Managing arthritis and joint pain naturally can be a powerful way to enhance your quality of life and reduce discomfort. By incorporating various natural remedies into your routine, you can alleviate symptoms and support overall joint health. Here's an in-depth look at some effective natural approaches that may help you find relief.

Embrace Anti-Inflammatory Foods: Diet plays a crucial role in managing inflammation and supporting joint health. Certain foods are known for their anti-inflammatory properties and can help reduce joint pain. Fruits and vegetables rich in antioxidants, such as berries, cherries, oranges, and leafy greens, help combat oxidative stress and inflammation. Omega-3 fatty acids, found in fatty fish like salmon, mackerel, and sardines, are also beneficial. These healthy fats can help reduce inflammation and improve joint function. Nuts, seeds, and olive oil are other great additions to your diet, as they contain monounsaturated fats that support overall joint health. Additionally, whole grains like quinoa and brown rice can provide fiber and nutrients that help manage inflammation.

Incorporate Turmeric and Ginger: Turmeric and ginger are two herbs with a long history of use in traditional medicine for their anti-inflammatory and pain-relieving properties. Turmeric contains curcumin, a compound that has been shown in studies to reduce inflammation and pain associated with arthritis. You can add turmeric to your cooking, blend it into smoothies, or drink it as a tea. Ginger, another potent anti-inflammatory herb, can be used fresh, dried, or as a tea. Incorporating these herbs into your diet regularly can help manage symptoms and provide relief from joint pain.

Utilize Heat and Cold Therapy: Heat and cold therapy are simple yet effective methods for managing joint pain and inflammation. Applying heat, such as through warm baths, heating pads, or hot packs, can help relax tight muscles, improve blood flow, and reduce stiffness in the joints. Cold therapy, on the other hand, can reduce inflammation and numb pain. Ice packs or cold compresses applied to the affected area can help alleviate acute pain and swelling. Alternating between heat and cold therapy can be particularly beneficial, offering combined effects of muscle relaxation and inflammation reduction.

Engage in Gentle Exercise: Regular physical activity is essential for maintaining joint health and managing pain. Gentle exercises like swimming, walking, and cycling are low-impact and can help keep your joints flexible while reducing stiffness. Strengthening exercises that target the muscles around your joints can also provide support and improve stability, reducing the risk of further injury. Yoga and stretching routines can enhance flexibility, balance, and overall joint function. It's important to choose activities that you enjoy and that feel comfortable, as overexertion or high-impact exercises can sometimes aggravate symptoms.

Explore Herbal Supplements: Several herbal supplements are known for their potential to support joint health and reduce inflammation. Boswellia, also known as Indian frankincense, has been used in traditional medicine for centuries for its anti-inflammatory effects. Studies suggest that it can help reduce symptoms of arthritis and improve joint function. Devil's Claw is another herb with pain-relieving properties that has been researched for its effectiveness in managing arthritis pain. Before starting any herbal supplements, it's essential to consult with a healthcare provider to ensure they are safe for you and won't interact with any other medications you may be taking.

Maintain a Healthy Weight: Extra weight can place additional stress on your joints, especially those in the lower body. Managing your weight through a balanced diet and regular exercise can help reduce this stress and alleviate joint pain. Even a small amount of weight loss can have a positive impact on joint health and reduce symptoms. Focus on a diet rich in whole foods, lean proteins, healthy fats, and plenty of fruits and vegetables to support a healthy weight and overall well-being.

Practice Stress Management: Chronic stress can exacerbate arthritis symptoms and contribute to pain perception. Incorporating stress-reducing practices into your daily routine can help manage inflammation and improve your overall quality of life. Techniques such as mindfulness, meditation, and deep breathing exercises can promote relaxation and reduce stress levels. Engaging in activities you enjoy, such as hobbies, spending time with loved ones, or taking leisurely walks, can also help manage stress and support emotional well-being.

Ensure Proper Sleep: Quality sleep is vital for managing arthritis and joint pain. During sleep, your body has the opportunity to repair and regenerate tissues, including those in your joints. Aim for 7 to 9 hours of restful sleep each night to support overall health and reduce pain. Create a comfortable sleep environment by maintaining a consistent sleep schedule, keeping your bedroom cool and dark, and avoiding stimulating activities before bed.

Consider Epsom Salt Baths: Epsom salt baths are a popular remedy for joint pain due to the magnesium content in Epsom salt. Magnesium helps relax muscles and reduce inflammation, which can provide temporary relief from joint discomfort. Add a cup or two of Epsom salt to a warm bath and soak for 15-20 minutes to experience the soothing effects. This can be a relaxing and effective way to ease joint pain and promote relaxation.

Stay Hydrated: Proper hydration is essential for maintaining joint health. Water helps keep the joints lubricated and supports the body's ability to flush out toxins. Aim to drink plenty of water throughout the day to stay hydrated and support overall joint function. Limiting your intake of sugary drinks and excessive caffeine can also contribute to better hydration and overall health.

Nutritional Support for Strong Bones

Strong, healthy bones are crucial for overall well-being, and what you eat plays a vital role in maintaining bone strength and density. By focusing on the right nutrients, you can support your bone health and help prevent conditions like osteoporosis. Here's a friendly guide to nutritional support for keeping your bones strong and resilient.

Calcium is one of the most essential nutrients for bone health. It's a key component of bone tissue and helps maintain bone density. To ensure you're getting enough calcium, include dairy products like milk, cheese, and yogurt in your diet. If you prefer non-dairy options, many plant-based milks, such as almond or soy milk, are fortified with calcium.

Leafy green vegetables like kale and bok choy, as well as fortified cereals and juices, are also great sources of calcium. For those who need a little extra boost, calcium supplements can be considered, but it's always best to consult with a healthcare provider before starting any new supplements.

Vitamin D is crucial because it helps your body absorb calcium more effectively. Without adequate vitamin D, your bones may not get the full benefit of the calcium you consume. Sunlight is a natural source of vitamin D, so spending time outdoors can help boost your levels. You can also find vitamin D in foods like fatty fish (salmon, mackerel, and sardines), egg yolks, and fortified foods. If you live in a region with limited sunlight, especially during the winter months, you might need to consider vitamin D supplements. Again, consulting with a healthcare provider can help determine the right dosage for you.

Magnesium plays a supportive role in bone health by aiding in the regulation of calcium levels and contributing to bone formation. Good sources of magnesium include nuts (especially almonds and cashews), seeds (like pumpkin and flaxseeds), whole grains, and legumes. Incorporating these foods into your diet can help ensure you're getting enough magnesium to support your bones.

Vitamin K is another important nutrient for bone health, as it helps in the regulation of calcium in your bones and blood. It plays a role in bone mineralization and helps prevent bone loss. Leafy green vegetables, such as spinach, kale, and broccoli, are excellent sources of vitamin K. Including these greens in your meals can contribute to strong and healthy bones.

Protein is essential for maintaining bone strength and structure. It provides the building blocks needed for bone repair and growth. Incorporate a variety of protein sources into your diet, including lean meats, poultry, fish, eggs, and plant-based options like beans, lentils, and tofu. Balancing your protein intake with other nutrients can help support overall bone health.

Omega-3 fatty acids, found in fatty fish like salmon and mackerel, as well as in flaxseeds and walnuts, can help reduce inflammation in the body. Chronic inflammation can negatively impact bone health, so including omega-3-rich foods in your diet may help support your bones and overall well-being.

Vitamin C is vital for the production of collagen, a protein that provides structure to your bones. A diet rich in vitamin C can help maintain bone integrity. Citrus fruits, strawberries, bell peppers, and tomatoes are all great sources of vitamin C. Adding these colorful fruits and vegetables to your diet can support collagen production and bone health.

A well-balanced diet that includes a variety of nutrients is essential for bone health. Aim for a mix of calcium, vitamin D, magnesium, vitamin K, protein, and other key nutrients to support strong bones. Eating a variety of foods from different food groups ensures that you're getting all the nutrients your body needs to maintain bone strength and overall health.

Herbal Approaches to Bone Healing

When it comes to healing bones and supporting bone health, nature has provided us with a wealth of herbal remedies that can complement conventional treatments. Herbal approaches can help improve bone strength, accelerate healing, and reduce inflammation. Here's a friendly guide to some effective herbs that are known for their beneficial effects on bone health.

Turmeric: Turmeric, with its active compound curcumin, is renowned for its powerful anti-inflammatory and antioxidant properties. Inflammation can slow down the healing process of bones, so reducing inflammation can aid in faster recovery. Turmeric can be incorporated into your diet as a spice in curries, soups, and stews, or taken as a supplement. Its benefits extend beyond just bone health, making it a versatile addition to your herbal toolkit.

Ginger: Ginger is another herb with strong anti-inflammatory properties that can support bone healing. It helps in reducing swelling and pain associated with bone injuries. You can enjoy ginger in various forms, such as fresh ginger root in teas, dried ginger in cooking, or ginger supplements. Including ginger in your diet can aid in alleviating discomfort and promoting a quicker recovery.

Boswellia: Often referred to as Indian frankincense, boswellia has been used traditionally to support joint and bone health. It contains compounds that help reduce inflammation and improve joint function. Boswellia supplements are available and can be particularly useful for managing chronic bone inflammation or supporting recovery after bone injuries.

Nettle: Nettle is a powerhouse of nutrients that are beneficial for bone health, including calcium, magnesium, and vitamins A and C. These nutrients support bone strength and healing. Nettle can be used as a tea, tincture, or in capsule form. It's also a great addition to soups and stews for a nutritional boost.

Horsetail: Horsetail is rich in silica, a mineral that is essential for bone health and the formation of collagen. Silica helps improve bone density and supports the healing process of bones. Horsetail can be consumed as a tea or taken in supplement form. It's a valuable herb for strengthening bones and promoting overall bone health.

Red Clover: Red clover contains isoflavones, which are plant compounds that have been shown to support bone health and reduce the risk of osteoporosis. It can be used in teas or taken as a supplement. Red clover's bone-supporting properties make it a helpful herb for maintaining bone density and strength.

Alfalfa: Alfalfa is rich in vitamins and minerals that support bone health, including calcium, magnesium, and vitamin K. It helps in maintaining bone density and strength. Alfalfa can be consumed as a tea, in capsule form, or as a green powder added to smoothies. Its nutrient-rich profile makes it a great addition to any bone-health regimen.

Gotu Kola: Gotu kola is known for its ability to promote wound healing and strengthen connective tissues. It supports the repair of bone tissues and enhances overall bone health. Gotu kola can be taken as a tea, tincture, or supplement. Its benefits extend to improving circulation, which can also aid in the healing process.

Comfrey: Comfrey has been used traditionally for its ability to promote bone healing and reduce inflammation. It contains allantoin, which helps in the repair of tissues and bones. Comfrey is typically used in topical applications, such as poultices or ointments, to support healing of bone injuries. However, it's important to use comfrey topically and not internally, as it can be toxic if ingested.

Dandelion: Dandelion is rich in calcium, magnesium, and potassium, all of which support bone health. Its leaves and roots can be used to make teas or tinctures that help in strengthening bones and supporting overall health. Dandelion is a gentle herb that can be a valuable part of your bone-health regimen.

Preventing Osteoporosis Naturally

Osteoporosis is a condition characterized by weakened bones that are more prone to fractures and breaks. While it's commonly associated with aging, the good news is that there are many natural ways to help prevent osteoporosis and support bone health throughout life. By adopting a holistic approach that includes dietary choices, physical activity, and lifestyle changes, you can strengthen your bones and reduce your risk of osteoporosis.

A nutritious diet is fundamental to maintaining bone density and preventing osteoporosis. One of the most crucial nutrients for bone health is calcium, which forms the structure of your bones. To ensure you're getting enough calcium, include dairy products such as milk, cheese, and yogurt in your diet. If you're lactose intolerant or prefer plant-based options, consider fortified plant-based milks like almond, soy, or oat milk, which often contain added calcium. Leafy green vegetables, such as kale, collard greens, and bok choy, are also excellent sources of calcium. For those who have difficulty meeting their calcium needs through diet alone, calcium supplements can be an option, but it's always wise to consult with a healthcare provider before starting any new supplement.

Vitamin D is equally important as it enhances the absorption of calcium in the body. Your skin produces vitamin D when exposed to sunlight, so spending some time outdoors can boost your levels. Foods like fatty fish (salmon, mackerel, and sardines), egg yolks, and fortified cereals and orange juice also provide vitamin D. In regions with limited sunlight, especially during winter months, a vitamin D supplement may be necessary. Again, checking with a healthcare provider can help determine the right dosage for you.

In addition to calcium and vitamin D, a diet rich in other essential nutrients can support bone health. Magnesium is a key mineral involved in bone formation and maintenance. Good sources of magnesium include nuts (such as almonds and cashews), seeds (like pumpkin and flaxseeds), whole grains, and legumes. Vitamin K, found in green leafy vegetables such as spinach, kale, and broccoli, is important for bone mineralization and helps to maintain bone density. Protein also plays a role in bone health, as it provides the building blocks for bone tissue. Incorporate a variety of protein sources, including lean meats, poultry, fish, eggs, and plant-based options like beans and tofu, to support bone strength.

Exercise is a powerful tool in preventing osteoporosis and maintaining bone health. Engaging in weight-bearing and resistance exercises helps to stimulate bone formation and increase bone density. Weight-bearing exercises include activities that force you to work against gravity, such as walking, jogging, dancing, and hiking. These activities help to build and maintain bone strength. Resistance exercises, such as lifting weights or using resistance bands, also contribute to bone health by stimulating bone-forming cells and improving muscle strength.

Aim for at least 30 minutes of weight-bearing exercise most days of the week. Incorporating strength-training exercises two to three times a week can further enhance bone density and support overall musculoskeletal health. If you're new to exercise or have any health concerns, consider starting with lower-impact activities and gradually increasing intensity.

Consulting with a fitness professional or physical therapist can help create a personalized exercise plan that suits your needs and fitness level.

Maintaining a healthy lifestyle is integral to preventing osteoporosis. One significant factor is avoiding smoking, which can weaken bones and decrease bone density. Smoking impairs the function of bone-forming cells and reduces the absorption of essential nutrients. Quitting smoking is one of the best things you can do for your bone health and overall well-being.
Excessive alcohol consumption can also negatively impact bone health by interfering with calcium absorption and bone-forming cells. Limit alcohol intake to moderate levels—generally defined as up to one drink per day for women and up to two drinks per day for men. Reducing alcohol consumption can help support bone density and reduce the risk of fractures.

Maintaining a healthy weight is important for bone health. Being underweight can increase the risk of bone loss and fractures, while being overweight can put additional stress on your bones. Achieving and maintaining a healthy weight through a balanced diet and regular physical activity supports bone strength and overall health. If you have concerns about your weight, consider seeking guidance from a healthcare provider or registered dietitian for personalized recommendations.

Chronic stress can negatively impact bone health by influencing hormone levels that affect bone density. Incorporate stress-reducing practices into your routine, such as mindfulness, meditation, or yoga, to support emotional and physical well-being. Engaging in activities that promote relaxation and balance can contribute to overall health, including bone health.
Quality sleep is also crucial for bone health, as the body repairs and regenerates tissues during sleep. Aim for 7 to 9 hours of restful sleep each night to support bone repair and maintenance. Creating a consistent sleep schedule, practicing good sleep hygiene, and managing stress can help improve sleep quality.

For individuals at higher risk of osteoporosis, regular bone density screenings can be beneficial in monitoring bone health and detecting potential issues early. Your healthcare provider can recommend when to start screenings based on factors such as age, family history, and lifestyle. Early detection allows for timely interventions and adjustments to your prevention strategy.

Certain herbs have been traditionally used to support bone health and prevent osteoporosis. Herbs like horsetail, which is rich in silica, and red clover, which contains isoflavones, can help support bone density. Nettle, with its high calcium and magnesium content, and turmeric, known for its anti-inflammatory properties, are also beneficial. Always consult with a healthcare provider before incorporating new herbal supplements to ensure they are appropriate for your needs.

Maintaining Joint Mobility and Flexibility

Maintaining joint mobility and flexibility is crucial for a vibrant, active life. As we age or face various health challenges, our joints can become less flexible and more prone to stiffness and discomfort. Thankfully, there are numerous natural strategies to help keep your joints moving smoothly and comfortably. Here's an in-depth look at how you can support joint mobility and flexibility through a combination of exercise, lifestyle choices, and mindful practices.

Engaging in regular exercise is one of the most effective ways to support joint health. Exercise helps keep your joints flexible by strengthening the muscles that surround them, which provides better support and stability.

Aim for a balanced routine that includes aerobic exercises, strength training, and flexibility work. Activities such as walking, swimming, and cycling are excellent for maintaining overall joint function. Swimming, in particular, is low-impact and provides a full-body workout without stressing the joints.

Strength training is also vital. Incorporating resistance exercises, such as using weights or resistance bands, helps build muscle mass, which can support and protect your joints. Strengthening the muscles around key joints like the knees, hips, and shoulders can reduce the strain on these areas and improve mobility.

In addition to aerobic and strength exercises, flexibility exercises play a critical role. Yoga and Pilates are great choices for enhancing flexibility and joint range of motion. These practices involve gentle stretching and controlled movements that help maintain and increase joint flexibility. Regularly participating in these activities can also improve balance, coordination, and overall body awareness, which contributes to joint health.

Incorporating stretching into your daily routine is essential for maintaining joint flexibility. Stretching helps keep the muscles and tendons around your joints flexible and can alleviate stiffness. Focus on stretches that target major joints, including your shoulders, hips, knees, and ankles. Gentle, consistent stretching can enhance blood flow to the muscles and improve overall mobility.

Dynamic stretching, which involves moving parts of your body through their full range of motion, is particularly beneficial before exercising. This type of stretching warms up the muscles and prepares them for activity. On the other hand, static stretching, where you hold a stretch for a period of time, is best done after exercising to help relax and lengthen the muscles.

Consider incorporating stretching exercises that target specific problem areas. For instance, if you experience stiffness in your lower back, perform stretches that focus on the lower back and hips. For tight hamstrings, include hamstring stretches in your routine. Tailoring your stretches to your specific needs can provide targeted relief and enhance overall flexibility.

Good posture has a significant impact on joint health. Poor posture can place extra strain on your joints, leading to stiffness and discomfort. Being mindful of how you sit, stand, and move throughout the day can help maintain proper alignment and reduce joint stress.

When sitting, ensure that your chair provides adequate support for your lower back and that your feet are flat on the floor. Use a chair with adjustable height and lumbar support if possible. When standing, distribute your weight evenly on both feet and avoid locking your knees. Incorporate ergonomic adjustments into your workspace to promote proper posture while working at a desk.

Engaging in exercises that strengthen your core muscles can also support better posture. A strong core helps stabilize your spine and pelvis, reducing strain on your joints. Consider incorporating core-strengthening exercises such as planks, bridges, and abdominal crunches into your fitness routine.

Maintaining a healthy weight is crucial for joint health. Excess weight places additional stress on weight-bearing joints like the knees, hips, and lower back. This added stress can contribute to joint pain and increase the risk of developing conditions such as osteoarthritis.

Achieving and maintaining a healthy weight through a balanced diet and regular exercise can reduce the burden on your joints. Focus on eating a variety of nutrient-dense foods, including fruits, vegetables, lean proteins, and whole grains. These foods provide essential vitamins and minerals that support overall health and help manage weight effectively.

If you're concerned about your weight, consider seeking guidance from a registered dietitian or healthcare provider. They can provide personalized recommendations and help you develop a sustainable plan to achieve and maintain a healthy weight.

When performing daily activities, using techniques that minimize joint stress can help maintain joint health. For example, when lifting objects, use your legs to lift rather than your back, and avoid twisting your body. Proper lifting techniques can reduce strain on your spine and joints.

For tasks that involve repetitive motions, take regular breaks to avoid overloading your joints. Incorporate ergonomic tools and supports, such as cushioned mats or specialized grips, to reduce joint strain. If you spend long hours at a desk, use an ergonomic chair and desk setup to promote proper posture and minimize joint discomfort.

Hydration is important for joint health. Water helps keep the cartilage in your joints lubricated, which can reduce stiffness and improve movement. Proper hydration also supports overall bodily functions and helps maintain healthy tissues.

Aim to drink plenty of water throughout the day. If you find plain water unappealing, consider infusing it with slices of fruits or herbs for added flavor. Eating hydrating foods like fruits and vegetables can also contribute to your daily fluid intake.

Hot and cold therapies can provide relief from joint stiffness and pain. Applying a warm compress or heating pad to stiff joints can help relax muscles and improve blood flow. Warmth can also soothe discomfort and increase flexibility.
Conversely, cold packs can reduce inflammation and numb pain. Applying a cold pack to swollen or painful joints can help manage acute inflammation. Alternating between hot and cold treatments can offer relief and support joint mobility.

Certain supplements may support joint health and flexibility. Omega-3 fatty acids, found in fish oil and flaxseed oil, have anti-inflammatory properties that can benefit joint function. Glucosamine and chondroitin are often used to support cartilage health and reduce joint pain. Additionally, turmeric, known for its anti-inflammatory properties, can be included in your diet or taken as a supplement.
Always consult with a healthcare provider before starting any new supplements. They can help determine the appropriate dosage and ensure that the supplements are safe and beneficial for your individual needs.

Gentle activities that promote joint mobility without putting excessive strain on your body can be very beneficial. Swimming, for example, provides a low-impact way to exercise and improve joint flexibility. The buoyancy of the water supports your body and reduces joint stress while still allowing for effective movement and stretching.
Water aerobics is another excellent option. These classes offer a low-impact workout that can help improve joint flexibility, strengthen muscles, and enhance cardiovascular fitness.

It's important to listen to your body and be mindful of any signs of joint pain or discomfort. If you experience pain or stiffness, take a break and allow your body to rest. Overdoing it can lead to injury or exacerbate existing issues. Gradually increase the intensity of your exercises and ensure you're using proper techniques to prevent strain.

If you have specific concerns or conditions affecting your joints, consider consulting with a healthcare provider or physical therapist. They can provide personalized advice and support tailored to your needs and help you develop a plan to maintain joint mobility and flexibility.

Exercises and Habits for Long-Term Bone Health

Maintaining strong, healthy bones is essential for overall well-being and quality of life, especially as we age. Incorporating regular exercise and adopting healthy habits can significantly impact bone health and help prevent conditions like osteoporosis. Here's a comprehensive look at how to support long-term bone health through a combination of exercise, lifestyle choices, and mindful practices.

Weight-bearing exercises are vital for bone health. These activities require you to work against gravity, stimulating bone formation and strengthening the bones. Simple activities such as walking can be incredibly beneficial; aim for brisk walks of at least 30 minutes a day to promote bone health. Jogging or running also supports bone strength through higher-impact activities, while dancing adds a fun element and strengthens bones in your legs, hips, and spine. Hiking, with its varied terrain, adds an extra challenge and supports bone health through weight-bearing and balance.

Strength training complements weight-bearing exercises by building muscle, which supports and protects the bones. Engaging in weight lifting, whether with free weights or weight machines, helps strengthen the arms, legs, and core. Resistance bands are another excellent tool for adding resistance without heavy weights, and bodyweight exercises like squats, lunges, push-ups, and planks can build muscle strength effectively.

Balance and flexibility exercises are also essential for maintaining bone health and preventing falls. Yoga, with its focus on flexibility, balance, and strength, is beneficial for enhancing bone strength and mobility. Poses such as the tree pose, warrior pose, and downward dog are particularly effective. Tai Chi, a gentle martial art involving slow, controlled movements, is excellent for improving balance and coordination, further supporting bone health.

Nutrition plays a crucial role in bone health. A diet rich in essential nutrients like calcium and vitamin D is vital. Calcium, which strengthens bones, is found in dairy products such as milk, yogurt, and cheese, as well as in leafy greens like kale and spinach, and fortified plant-based milks. Vitamin D aids in calcium absorption and can be obtained through sunlight exposure, fatty fish such as salmon, and fortified foods. Protein also supports bone health and muscle strength, so include lean meats, beans, nuts, and seeds in your diet.

Proper hydration is important for maintaining bone health. Water helps maintain the balance of minerals in the body and supports bone and muscle functions. Aim to drink plenty of water throughout the day, and include hydrating foods like fruits and vegetables in your diet.

Certain habits can negatively impact bone health, so it's important to be mindful of them. Smoking weakens bones and reduces bone density, so if you smoke, seek support to quit. Excessive alcohol consumption can interfere with bone formation and lead to bone loss, so it's advisable to limit alcohol intake to moderate levels.

Regular health check-ups are essential for monitoring bone health and identifying potential issues early. Discuss your bone health with your healthcare provider, especially if you have risk factors for bone loss. They can recommend appropriate screenings, such as bone density tests, and offer personalized advice. Allowing your body adequate time to rest and recover is crucial. Overtraining can lead to injuries and strain on your bones, so incorporate rest days into your exercise routine and listen to your body's signals. Proper rest supports muscle recovery and overall bone health.

Functional exercises that mimic everyday activities can also support bone health. For instance, standing on one leg improves balance and strengthens the muscles around your hips and knees. Step-ups using a platform or step strengthen the legs and support bone health, while chair squats help build leg strength and improve stability.

Lastly, maintaining a positive mindset and consistent habits is important for overall well-being. Set realistic goals, celebrate your progress, and stay motivated by engaging in activities you enjoy. Finding joy in your exercise routine and daily habits can make maintaining bone health a rewarding part of your lifestyle.

Book 20: Gut-Brain Connection and Mental Health

Understanding the Gut-Brain Axis

The gut-brain axis is an incredible and intricate connection between your digestive system and your brain, and it plays a crucial role in your overall health and well-being. This fascinating link helps explain how what happens in your gut can affect your mood, mental health, and even your cognitive functions. Let's dive into how this connection works and why it's so important.

At its core, the gut-brain axis is a bidirectional communication network that links your gut and brain through various pathways. This connection allows signals to travel back and forth between the two, influencing how you feel mentally and physically. Imagine your gut as a complex ecosystem filled with trillions of microorganisms, including bacteria, viruses, and fungi, known collectively as the gut microbiota. This microbial community plays a crucial role in maintaining gut health, digesting food, and even producing neurotransmitters—the chemical messengers that help regulate mood and mental functions.

One of the primary ways the gut and brain communicate is through the vagus nerve, a major nerve that runs from the brainstem down to the abdomen. It acts like a communication superhighway, transmitting signals between the gut and the brain. When your gut bacteria break down food, they produce various metabolites and compounds, some of which can influence brain function. For example, certain gut bacteria can produce neurotransmitters like serotonin, which is often referred to as the "feel-good" chemical because of its role in regulating mood. In fact, about 90% of your body's serotonin is produced in the gut, highlighting just how intertwined your gut and mental health are.

The gut-brain axis also involves the immune system. Your gut houses a large portion of your body's immune cells, which can release inflammatory cytokines in response to an imbalance in gut bacteria or infections. These cytokines can travel through the bloodstream and affect brain function, potentially influencing mood and cognitive processes. For instance, chronic inflammation in the gut has been linked to mental health conditions like depression and anxiety.

Stress is another factor that impacts the gut-brain axis. When you're stressed, your body releases stress hormones like cortisol, which can affect gut function and alter the composition of your gut microbiota. This can lead to gastrointestinal issues and exacerbate mental health problems. On the flip side, an imbalance in gut bacteria can increase susceptibility to stress and anxiety, creating a feedback loop that can be challenging to break.

Understanding the gut-brain axis highlights the importance of maintaining a healthy gut to support mental well-being. Eating a balanced diet rich in fiber, prebiotics, and probiotics can help nourish your gut microbiota and promote a healthy gut-brain connection. Fiber helps feed beneficial gut bacteria, while probiotics are live microorganisms that can support a healthy microbial balance. Additionally, managing stress through practices like mindfulness, exercise, and adequate sleep can positively impact both your gut and brain health.

Healing the Gut to Improve Mental Clarity

Your gut and brain are intricately linked, and taking care of one can significantly benefit the other. If you've ever felt foggy-headed or mentally sluggish, it might be worth looking into how your gut health is affecting your mental clarity. By focusing on healing and nourishing your gut, you can enhance your cognitive function and enjoy sharper, clearer thinking.

To begin with, understanding the connection between your gut and brain is crucial. Your gut, often called the "second brain," houses a vast network of neurons and beneficial bacteria that play a significant role in your overall mental function. When your gut is out of balance, it can impact your mood, focus, and cognitive performance. This is because the gut-brain axis, the communication network between your gut and brain, influences how well your brain functions.

One of the first steps in healing your gut is improving your diet. Eating a diet rich in fiber from fruits, vegetables, and whole grains helps promote a healthy balance of gut bacteria. Fiber acts as food for beneficial bacteria, which can enhance their growth and activity. In turn, these good bacteria produce compounds that support brain health and mental clarity. Including fermented foods like yogurt, kefir, and sauerkraut in your diet can also be beneficial, as they provide probiotics that support a healthy gut microbiota.

Additionally, reducing your intake of processed foods and sugars can make a significant difference. Processed foods and high sugar consumption can lead to an imbalance in gut bacteria and increase inflammation, which can negatively affect mental clarity. Opt for whole, unprocessed foods that nourish your body and your gut.

Hydration is another essential aspect of gut health. Drinking plenty of water supports digestion and helps maintain a healthy gut lining. Proper hydration can also help clear brain fog and improve focus. Aim to drink enough water throughout the day and consider incorporating herbal teas like ginger or peppermint, which can also aid digestion.

Managing stress is a key factor in healing your gut and improving mental clarity. Chronic stress can disrupt the balance of gut bacteria and lead to digestive issues. Engaging in stress-reducing activities such as mindfulness, meditation, and regular exercise can help maintain a healthy gut and support clear thinking. Exercise, in particular, boosts blood flow to the brain and promotes the release of endorphins, which can enhance mood and cognitive function.

Paying attention to your gut's health can also involve identifying and addressing food sensitivities or intolerances. Common culprits like gluten, dairy, and certain additives can cause gut inflammation and affect mental clarity. Keeping a food diary and noting any symptoms can help you identify any problematic foods and make necessary adjustments.

Incorporating gut-healing supplements can also be beneficial. Probiotics, which are live bacteria that support a healthy gut microbiota, can help restore balance in the gut. Prebiotics, which are dietary fibers that feed beneficial bacteria, can also support gut health. Consult with a healthcare professional before starting any new supplements to ensure they're appropriate for you.

Finally, getting enough sleep is essential for both gut and brain health. Quality sleep allows your body to repair and regenerate, including your gut lining. Aim for 7-9 hours of restful sleep each night to support overall health and mental clarity.

Probiotics for Mental Health

When it comes to nurturing your mental health, the concept of "good bacteria" might seem a bit unconventional, but it's a concept that's gaining increasing attention in the world of wellness. Probiotics, often referred to as beneficial bacteria, play a fascinating role in supporting not just your digestive system but also your mental well-being. Let's explore how these tiny microbes can have a big impact on your mental health.

Probiotics are live microorganisms that, when consumed in adequate amounts, can provide health benefits. They're commonly found in fermented foods like yogurt, kefir, sauerkraut, and kombucha. These good bacteria help maintain a balanced gut microbiota, which is crucial for optimal gut function. But their influence doesn't stop there—recent research suggests that probiotics also play a significant role in mental health, thanks to the gut-brain axis.

The gut-brain axis is a communication network linking your gut and brain. This connection means that what happens in your gut can affect your brain and vice versa. Probiotics contribute to a healthy gut microbiota, which can positively influence this gut-brain communication. By supporting the balance of good bacteria in your gut, probiotics can help manage inflammation and produce neurotransmitters that affect mood and cognitive functions.

One of the key ways probiotics support mental health is by reducing inflammation. An imbalance in gut bacteria can lead to chronic inflammation, which has been linked to mood disorders like depression and anxiety. Probiotics can help restore balance in the gut microbiota, thereby reducing inflammation and potentially alleviating symptoms of these conditions.

Probiotics also play a role in the production of neurotransmitters, the chemicals that transmit signals in the brain. For example, certain probiotics can enhance the production of serotonin, a neurotransmitter often referred to as the "feel-good" hormone. Since a significant portion of serotonin is produced in the gut, having a healthy balance of gut bacteria can support the production and regulation of serotonin, which can improve mood and emotional well-being.

Moreover, probiotics may help improve the gut's barrier function. A healthy gut lining is crucial for preventing harmful substances from entering the bloodstream, which can contribute to inflammation and impact mental health. By supporting a strong gut barrier, probiotics help maintain a healthy environment for both the gut and the brain.

Choosing the right probiotics is important for reaping these benefits. Look for probiotic supplements or foods with strains that have been shown to support mental health, such as Lactobacillus and Bifidobacterium species. These strains have been researched for their potential to improve mood and reduce symptoms of anxiety and depression.

Incorporating probiotics into your diet can be simple and enjoyable. Enjoy a serving of yogurt with live cultures, sip on some kombucha, or add fermented vegetables like kimchi to your meals. If you prefer supplements, choose high-quality products with well-researched strains and follow the recommended dosage.

While probiotics can be a valuable part of a mental health regimen, they are not a cure-all.

They work best when combined with other healthy habits such as a balanced diet, regular exercise, adequate sleep, and stress management. If you have specific mental health concerns or conditions, it's always a good idea to consult with a healthcare provider before starting any new supplement regimen.

How Nutrition Affects Mood and Emotions

You might be surprised to learn just how closely linked your diet is to your mood and emotions. The foods you eat have a powerful impact on your mental well-being, influencing everything from your energy levels to your overall mood. Understanding this connection can help you make dietary choices that support not just your physical health, but also your emotional and mental balance.

Nutrition plays a crucial role in brain function. Your brain needs a steady supply of nutrients to function optimally, and deficiencies in certain vitamins and minerals can affect your mood and emotional health. For instance, omega-3 fatty acids, found in fatty fish like salmon, walnuts, and flaxseeds, are essential for brain health and have been shown to reduce symptoms of depression. These healthy fats help maintain the structure of brain cells and support neurotransmitter function, which is vital for mood regulation.

B vitamins, particularly B6, B12, and folate, are also crucial for mental health. They help produce neurotransmitters like serotonin and dopamine, which play key roles in mood regulation. A deficiency in these vitamins can lead to feelings of fatigue, irritability, and even depression. Foods rich in B vitamins, such as leafy greens, whole grains, and lean meats, can help keep your mood stable and support overall emotional health.

Another important player in mood regulation is magnesium. This mineral helps manage stress and can improve symptoms of anxiety and depression. Magnesium is found in foods like almonds, spinach, and black beans. Ensuring you get enough magnesium can help your body handle stress more effectively and promote a sense of calm.

Additionally, the gut-brain connection plays a significant role in how nutrition affects your mood. Your gut, often referred to as your "second brain," is home to trillions of bacteria that can influence your brain function. A diet high in fiber from fruits, vegetables, and whole grains supports a healthy gut microbiota, which in turn supports better mental health. Probiotic-rich foods like yogurt and fermented vegetables can help maintain a balanced gut microbiota, potentially improving mood and reducing symptoms of anxiety and depression.

On the flip side, certain foods can negatively impact your mood. Highly processed foods and those high in refined sugars can lead to fluctuations in blood sugar levels, which can cause mood swings and irritability. These foods can also contribute to inflammation, which has been linked to mood disorders. Reducing your intake of sugary snacks and processed foods and focusing on whole, nutrient-dense options can help stabilize your mood and support emotional health.

Hydration is another key factor. Dehydration can lead to fatigue and irritability, impacting your mood. Drinking plenty of water throughout the day ensures that your body and brain are well-hydrated, which can help you stay focused and maintain a positive outlook.

Finally, adopting a balanced diet with regular meals can prevent energy crashes and support steady mood levels. Skipping meals or eating irregularly can lead to low blood sugar levels, which can make you feel cranky and affect your overall emotional well-being.

Herbal Remedies for Anxiety and Depression

When it comes to managing anxiety and depression, many people are turning to herbal remedies as a natural way to support their mental health. Herbal remedies can be a gentle and effective addition to your wellness routine, helping to soothe the mind and lift your spirits. Let's explore some of the most popular herbs known for their calming and mood-boosting properties.

One of the most well-known herbs for easing anxiety is chamomile. Chamomile tea has been a go-to for centuries due to its gentle, calming effects. It contains antioxidants and compounds that may help relax the nervous system and promote better sleep. Drinking a warm cup of chamomile tea before bedtime can be a soothing way to unwind and ease anxiety.

Lavender is another herb with a reputation for reducing anxiety and improving mood. Lavender essential oil is often used in aromatherapy for its calming effects. Simply diffusing lavender oil in your home or adding a few drops to a warm bath can help create a peaceful environment and ease stress. Lavender tea is also an option, offering a gentle way to calm your nerves and enhance relaxation.

For those struggling with depression, St. John's Wort is a well-regarded herb. This herb has been used for centuries as a natural remedy for improving mood. It's believed to work by increasing the levels of neurotransmitters like serotonin in the brain, which can help lift your mood. However, it's important to consult with a healthcare professional before starting St. John's Wort, as it can interact with certain medications and isn't suitable for everyone.

Ashwagandha is another powerful herb known for its adaptogenic properties, which help the body cope with stress. Ashwagandha can support overall emotional balance and reduce symptoms of anxiety and depression. It works by helping to regulate stress hormones and support a healthy response to stress. Taking ashwagandha in supplement form can be an effective way to enhance your resilience to stress and support mental well-being.

Valerian root is often used as a natural remedy for anxiety and insomnia. This herb has sedative properties that can help relax the mind and body, making it easier to fall asleep and stay asleep. Valerian root can be taken as a supplement or brewed into a tea. Its calming effects can help reduce anxiety and improve overall sleep quality.

Passionflower is another herb known for its calming effects. It's often used to ease symptoms of anxiety and promote relaxation. Passionflower can be consumed as a tea or taken in supplement form. Its calming properties can help soothe the nervous system and improve sleep quality.

Lastly, lemon balm is a gentle herb that can help reduce anxiety and promote a sense of calm. It's often used in teas or tinctures to ease stress and improve mood. Lemon balm has a soothing effect on the nervous system, making it a great choice for those looking for a natural way to support emotional balance.

Incorporating these herbs into your routine can provide additional support for managing anxiety and depression. However, it's essential to remember that herbal remedies are best used in conjunction with other strategies for mental health, such as a balanced diet, regular exercise, and stress management techniques. Always consult with a healthcare professional before starting any new herbal remedies, especially if you're taking medications or have underlying health conditions.

The Role of Detoxification in Mental Wellness

Detoxification often brings to mind images of juice cleanses or elaborate fasting regimens, but it's much more than just a trend. At its core, detoxification is about supporting your body's natural ability to remove toxins and maintain balance, which can have a profound impact on your mental wellness. Understanding how detoxification works can help you appreciate its role in keeping both your body and mind in harmony.

Our bodies are constantly exposed to various toxins from the environment, food, and even stress. These toxins can accumulate over time and potentially disrupt our physical and mental health. Detoxification is the process by which your body eliminates these harmful substances, primarily through the liver, kidneys, lungs, and skin. When these organs are functioning optimally, they help clear out toxins, which can lead to improved mood, mental clarity, and overall well-being.

One of the primary benefits of detoxification is its impact on reducing inflammation. Chronic inflammation is often linked to mood disorders such as depression and anxiety. By supporting your body's detoxification processes, you can help reduce inflammation and potentially alleviate symptoms of these conditions. For example, drinking plenty of water, eating a diet rich in fruits and vegetables, and getting regular exercise can enhance your body's ability to flush out toxins and reduce inflammation.

Another important aspect of detoxification is its role in gut health. The gut plays a crucial role in mental wellness, as it is home to a large portion of your body's serotonin, the neurotransmitter that regulates mood. A healthy gut is better equipped to handle toxins and maintain a balanced microbiome, which can positively influence your mood and mental clarity. Incorporating detoxifying foods like fiber-rich vegetables and probiotic-rich foods into your diet can support gut health and enhance your mental well-being.

Detoxification also supports liver function, which is essential for breaking down and eliminating toxins from your body. A healthy liver can help improve your mood and energy levels. Foods such as beets, cruciferous vegetables (like broccoli and cauliflower), and herbal teas (such as dandelion root) are known to support liver health and promote efficient detoxification. By including these foods in your diet, you can help your liver perform its vital functions more effectively.

Moreover, reducing your exposure to environmental toxins is another important aspect of detoxification. Simple changes like using natural cleaning products, avoiding excessive use of plastics, and choosing organic foods can minimize your toxin load and support overall mental wellness. A cleaner environment can help reduce the stress on your body's detoxification systems and contribute to a more balanced mood.

It's worth noting that detoxification should be approached with a balanced mindset. Extreme detox diets or overly restrictive practices can sometimes lead to stress or nutritional deficiencies, which can negatively affect your mental health. Instead,

Focus on incorporating healthy habits that support your body's natural detoxification processes, such as staying hydrated, eating a balanced diet, and engaging in regular physical activity.

Mindfulness and Mental Well-Being

Mindfulness might seem like just another buzzword, but it's actually a powerful practice with deep roots in improving mental well-being. At its core, mindfulness is about being fully present in the moment, observing your thoughts and feelings without judgment. This simple yet profound practice can have a remarkable impact on your mental health, helping you manage stress, enhance emotional resilience, and improve overall well-being.

The essence of mindfulness lies in paying attention to the present moment. Often, our minds are cluttered with worries about the past or anxieties about the future. Mindfulness teaches us to focus on the here and now, which can help break the cycle of negative thinking and reduce feelings of stress and anxiety. By learning to stay grounded in the present, you can gain a better perspective on your thoughts and emotions, making them easier to manage.

One of the key benefits of mindfulness is its ability to reduce stress. When you practice mindfulness, you activate the body's relaxation response, which counteracts the stress response. This can lower levels of cortisol, the stress hormone, and help you feel more calm and centered. Simple mindfulness techniques, like deep breathing exercises or mindful meditation, can be incredibly effective in managing stress and creating a sense of inner peace.

Mindfulness also enhances emotional resilience. It helps you become more aware of your emotional patterns and reactions, allowing you to respond to challenging situations with greater clarity and balance. Instead of reacting impulsively, mindfulness encourages a pause, giving you the space to choose how you want to respond. This can lead to more thoughtful and constructive ways of dealing with difficult emotions and situations.

Moreover, mindfulness can improve your overall mental well-being by fostering a greater sense of self-awareness and self-compassion. By observing your thoughts and feelings without judgment, you can develop a kinder, more accepting relationship with yourself. This self-compassion can help reduce feelings of self-criticism and enhance your overall mood and sense of well-being.

Incorporating mindfulness into your daily life doesn't have to be complicated. You can start with just a few minutes each day. Try setting aside a short period for mindful breathing or meditation. Focus on your breath, observe your thoughts, and gently bring your attention back to the present moment whenever your mind starts to wander. Even simple practices like mindful eating—where you pay full attention to the taste, texture, and experience of your food—can be a great way to cultivate mindfulness throughout your day.

Another way to integrate mindfulness is by practicing mindful movement, such as yoga or tai chi. These activities combine physical movement with mindful awareness, helping you connect with your body and breath while also reducing stress and improving mental clarity.

Remember, mindfulness is a skill that develops over time. It's normal for your mind to wander or for you to encounter challenges along the way. The key is to approach your mindfulness practice with patience and curiosity. Over time, you'll likely find that mindfulness becomes a natural and valuable part of your daily routine, contributing to a more balanced, calm, and joyful life

Book 21: Natural Remedies for Children's Health

Strengthening Children's Immune System Naturally

Keeping children healthy is a top priority for any parent, and a strong immune system plays a crucial role in safeguarding their well-being. While traditional medicine has its place, there are many natural ways to bolster your child's immune system and help them stay vibrant and resilient. Let's explore some simple, effective strategies for enhancing your child's immunity naturally.

One of the best ways to support your child's immune system is through a balanced diet. Nutrition is the cornerstone of a strong immune system, and including a variety of nutrient-rich foods can make a big difference. Encourage your child to eat a colorful array of fruits and vegetables. Foods like oranges, strawberries, and bell peppers are packed with vitamin C, which is known to boost immune function. Leafy greens, such as spinach and kale, provide essential vitamins and antioxidants that help protect the body from illness.

Incorporating whole grains and lean proteins into their meals also supports immune health. Foods like brown rice, quinoa, and chicken provide the body with necessary nutrients and amino acids. Don't forget the power of healthy fats, which are found in foods like avocados, nuts, and seeds. These fats are important for maintaining healthy cell membranes and overall immune function.

Probiotics are another great addition to your child's diet. These beneficial bacteria support gut health, which is closely linked to immune function. Yogurt, kefir, and fermented foods like sauerkraut are excellent sources of probiotics. A healthy gut helps ensure that your child's immune system is functioning optimally and can better fend off infections.

Hydration is also key to a healthy immune system. Ensure your child drinks plenty of water throughout the day. Proper hydration supports overall bodily functions and helps flush out toxins. If your child is reluctant to drink water, try offering it with a splash of fresh fruit juice for added flavor.

Getting enough sleep is vital for maintaining a robust immune system. Children need more sleep than adults, and adequate rest helps their bodies repair and regenerate. Establishing a consistent bedtime routine and ensuring your child gets sufficient sleep each night can significantly impact their immune health.

Physical activity is another important factor in boosting immunity. Encourage your child to engage in regular physical exercise, whether it's playing outside, participating in sports, or simply being active. Exercise promotes good circulation, which helps immune cells move efficiently throughout the body and improves overall health.

In addition to these lifestyle habits, consider incorporating some natural supplements if needed. For example, echinacea and elderberry are herbs that have been traditionally used to support the immune system. Always consult with a healthcare provider before introducing new supplements, especially for children.

Finally, managing stress is crucial for maintaining a healthy immune system. Although children may not experience stress in the same way adults do, they can still be affected by changes in their environment or routine. Providing a stable, nurturing environment and helping your child learn coping strategies can help keep their stress levels in check and support their overall immune health.

Herbal Remedies for Common Childhood Illnesses

When it comes to caring for children, natural remedies can be a gentle and effective way to support their health, especially for common childhood ailments. Herbal remedies have been used for centuries to treat a variety of conditions, and many are safe and beneficial for children when used appropriately. Here's a look at some of the herbal options that can help address common childhood issues.

For colds and respiratory infections, herbs like chamomile and peppermint can be very soothing. Chamomile is well-known for its calming properties and can be used as a gentle tea to help ease a sore throat or cough. It also has mild anti-inflammatory effects that can reduce irritation in the throat. Peppermint, on the other hand, has menthol, which acts as a natural decongestant. A warm peppermint tea or a steam inhalation can help clear nasal congestion and make it easier for your child to breathe.

When dealing with digestive issues like tummy aches or indigestion, ginger and fennel are excellent choices. Ginger has been traditionally used to soothe nausea and aid digestion. You can make a mild ginger tea by steeping fresh ginger slices in hot water. Fennel seeds are another great remedy for digestive discomfort and can help relieve gas and bloating. Fennel tea is easy to prepare and has a pleasant flavor that children usually find enjoyable.

For minor skin irritations and rashes, calendula and aloe vera are gentle and effective. Calendula has anti-inflammatory and healing properties, making it ideal for soothing skin irritations and promoting healing. You can use calendula cream or ointment on affected areas. Aloe vera is also soothing and can help relieve itching and inflammation. Applying pure aloe vera gel directly to the skin can provide immediate relief.

If your child is experiencing difficulty sleeping or anxiety, valerian root and lavender can be very calming. Valerian root is known for its sedative properties and can be used in small amounts to help your child relax and improve sleep. Lavender, with its soothing aroma, can be used in a calming bath or as a few drops of lavender essential oil on a pillow to promote relaxation and better sleep.

For immune support, echinacea is a popular choice. It's believed to stimulate the immune system and can be helpful in preventing or shortening the duration of colds. Echinacea is available in various forms, including teas and tinctures, but it's best to consult with a healthcare provider to determine the appropriate dosage for your child.

It's important to remember that while herbal remedies can be beneficial, they should be used with caution and in moderation. Always start with a small amount and observe how your child responds. Additionally, it's wise to consult with a healthcare provider before introducing new herbs, especially if your child has existing health conditions or is taking other medications.

Natural Approaches to Managing ADHD

Managing ADHD (Attention-Deficit/Hyperactivity Disorder) in children can be challenging, but natural approaches offer valuable tools to help support your child's well-being and improve their quality of life. While medication is often prescribed for ADHD, many families find that incorporating natural strategies can complement conventional treatments and enhance overall management of the condition.

One of the most impactful natural approaches is dietary adjustment. A balanced diet rich in whole, unprocessed foods can have a positive effect on ADHD symptoms. Focus on incorporating plenty of fruits, vegetables, lean proteins, and whole grains. Foods rich in omega-3 fatty acids, such as salmon, walnuts, and flaxseeds, are particularly beneficial. Omega-3s are known to support brain health and cognitive function, and some studies suggest they may help improve attention and behavior in children with ADHD.

In addition to omega-3s, consider reducing your child's intake of artificial additives and sugars. Some studies have found that certain food colorings and preservatives may exacerbate ADHD symptoms. By opting for natural, unprocessed foods and minimizing sugar and artificial ingredients, you can help reduce potential triggers for hyperactivity and impulsiveness.

Another important aspect of managing ADHD naturally is ensuring your child gets regular physical activity. Exercise helps improve focus, mood, and energy levels. Activities like biking, swimming, or even a daily walk can be beneficial. Physical exercise not only supports overall health but also helps children with ADHD channel their energy in a positive way.

Incorporating mindfulness and relaxation techniques into your child's routine can also be helpful. Techniques such as deep breathing exercises, meditation, and yoga can assist in managing stress and improving focus. These practices teach children how to calm their minds and enhance their ability to concentrate, which can be particularly beneficial for those with ADHD.

Establishing a structured routine and a consistent environment is crucial for children with ADHD. A predictable schedule helps them understand what to expect and can reduce feelings of chaos or frustration. Create a daily routine that includes time for schoolwork, play, and relaxation. Use visual schedules and reminders to help your child stay on track and manage their time effectively.

Sleep is another vital factor in managing ADHD. Ensure that your child gets adequate and consistent sleep each night. A regular bedtime routine and a sleep-friendly environment can significantly improve their rest and overall behavior. Lack of sleep can exacerbate ADHD symptoms, so fostering good sleep habits is essential.

Herbal remedies can also play a supportive role. For instance, herbs like chamomile and valerian root are known for their calming properties and may help with relaxation and focus. However, it's important to consult with a healthcare provider before introducing any new supplements or herbs to ensure they are safe and appropriate for your child.

Finally, consider behavioral therapy as part of a comprehensive approach to managing ADHD. While not a natural remedy per se, behavioral therapy can complement natural strategies by helping children develop coping skills, improve organizational abilities, and manage their behavior more effectively.

Nutrition for Healthy Growth and Development

Ensuring that children receive proper nutrition is crucial for supporting their healthy growth and development. Proper nutrition lays the groundwork for robust physical health, cognitive development, and emotional well-being. A well-balanced diet tailored to their needs helps children grow up strong, focused, and energetic. Here's a comprehensive guide to understanding how different nutrients contribute to your child's development and how to incorporate them into their diet effectively.

Balanced Diet: A balanced diet is the cornerstone of healthy growth. This means incorporating a variety of foods from all the major food groups to ensure that your child gets a broad spectrum of nutrients. Aim for a plate that includes fruits, vegetables, whole grains, lean proteins, and healthy fats. Each of these groups provides essential nutrients that support different aspects of development and health.

Fruits and Vegetables: Fruits and vegetables are rich sources of essential vitamins, minerals, and antioxidants that play a crucial role in a child's development. For instance, vitamin C from citrus fruits and berries supports immune function and helps the body absorb iron from plant-based foods. Vegetables like spinach and broccoli are packed with vitamins A and K, which are important for vision and bone health, respectively. Incorporate a rainbow of fruits and vegetables into your child's diet to ensure they receive a wide range of nutrients.

Whole Grains: Whole grains, such as brown rice, whole wheat, quinoa, and oats, provide vital fiber that supports digestive health and prevents constipation. Fiber also helps to regulate blood sugar levels and can contribute to maintaining a healthy weight. Additionally, whole grains are a good source of B vitamins, which are necessary for energy production and brain function. Encourage your child to choose whole grain options over refined grains to maximize their nutrient intake.

Lean Proteins: Protein is essential for growth, muscle development, and repair. Lean meats like chicken, turkey, and fish provide high-quality protein and important nutrients such as iron and zinc. For plant-based options, beans, lentils, tofu, and tempeh are excellent sources of protein. Protein is also crucial for the production of enzymes and hormones, making it a key player in overall health. Include a variety of protein sources in your child's diet to meet their growing needs.

Healthy Fats: Fats are an important part of a child's diet, supporting brain development and energy levels. Focus on incorporating healthy fats from sources like avocados, nuts, seeds, and olive oil. Omega-3 fatty acids, which are found in fatty fish like salmon and in plant sources such as flaxseeds and chia seeds, are particularly beneficial for brain health and cognitive function. These healthy fats help to maintain cell structure and support the absorption of fat-soluble vitamins.

Dairy or Alternatives: Dairy products such as milk, cheese, and yogurt are rich in calcium and vitamin D, both of which are essential for building strong bones and teeth. If your child is lactose intolerant or follows a vegan diet, fortified plant-based milk alternatives like almond milk or soy milk can be used. These alternatives often come with added calcium and vitamin D to ensure your child still gets these critical nutrients.

Hydration: Adequate hydration is fundamental to maintaining energy levels and supporting various bodily functions. Encourage your child to drink plenty of water throughout the day. Proper hydration helps maintain focus, supports digestion, and keeps skin healthy. Limit sugary drinks like sodas and fruit juices, which can contribute to weight gain and dental issues.

Portion Sizes and Meal Timing: Managing portion sizes and maintaining regular meal times are key to promoting healthy eating habits. Offer balanced meals and snacks at consistent times to help regulate your child's appetite and energy levels. Smaller, frequent meals can also prevent overeating and help maintain steady blood sugar levels. Pay attention to hunger cues and avoid pressuring your child to eat more than they need.

Avoiding Excess Sugar and Processed Foods: Reducing the intake of sugary snacks and heavily processed foods is crucial for maintaining optimal health. These foods can lead to weight gain, energy crashes, and nutritional deficiencies. Instead, opt for whole, natural foods and encourage healthy snacks like fresh fruit, nuts, and yogurt.

Encouraging Healthy Eating Habits: Foster positive eating habits by setting a good example. Children often mimic the behaviors of adults, so showing them your own healthy eating practices can have a significant impact. Involve your child in meal planning and preparation to make them more interested in trying new, nutritious foods. Creating a pleasant mealtime environment where family members sit together and enjoy their meals can also make eating a positive experience.

Remedies for Skin Conditions in Children

Children's skin is sensitive and prone to various conditions, from mild irritations to more persistent issues. Fortunately, natural remedies can offer effective relief and help soothe and heal their delicate skin. Here's a guide to some gentle and natural remedies that can help address common skin conditions in children.

Eczema: Eczema, or atopic dermatitis, is a common skin condition characterized by itchy, inflamed patches. To soothe eczema flare-ups, try applying coconut oil or almond oil to the affected areas. These oils have moisturizing and anti-inflammatory properties that can help relieve dryness and irritation. Another soothing option is colloidal oatmeal baths, which can calm itching and reduce inflammation. Simply add finely ground oatmeal to a warm bath and let your child soak for 15-20 minutes.

Diaper Rash: Diaper rash is a frequent issue for babies and toddlers. To prevent and treat diaper rash naturally, keep the area clean and dry. After each diaper change, gently clean the area with warm water and a soft cloth, avoiding harsh wipes. Allow the skin to air dry before putting on a fresh diaper. Applying a natural barrier cream, such as one made with zinc oxide or shea butter, can help protect the skin and promote healing.

Acne: While acne is more common in teenagers, younger children can also experience pimples and breakouts. For gentle acne treatment, consider using tea tree oil, known for its antibacterial properties. Dilute a few drops of tea tree oil with a carrier oil, like coconut oil, and apply it to the affected areas. Additionally, a honey mask can help; honey has natural antibacterial and moisturizing properties that can reduce inflammation and clear blemishes.

Bug Bites: Bug bites can be itchy and uncomfortable. To relieve the itching and reduce swelling, try applying a paste made from baking soda and water to the bite area. Baking soda has soothing properties that can help calm the skin. Alternatively, aloe vera gel is a great natural remedy with anti-inflammatory and healing benefits. Simply apply a thin layer of aloe vera gel to the bite and allow it to dry.

Rashes: Skin rashes can arise from various causes, including allergies or irritants. For general rash relief, try using chamomile tea compresses. Chamomile has anti-inflammatory properties that can soothe irritated skin. Brew chamomile tea, let it cool, and then soak a clean cloth in the tea. Apply the cloth to the rash for 10-15 minutes. Additionally, calendula ointment can be applied to the rash to help promote healing and reduce redness.

Sunburn: If your child gets a sunburn, soothe the skin with cool, damp cloths and ensure they stay hydrated. Aloe vera gel is a fantastic remedy for sunburn, as it provides cooling relief and helps the skin heal. Apply the gel generously to the affected areas. You can also mix aloe vera gel with a bit of coconut oil for added moisturizing benefits.

Dry Skin: Dry, flaky skin can be uncomfortable. To combat dryness, regularly apply a natural moisturizer, such as shea butter or jojoba oil, to your child's skin. These natural oils help lock in moisture and prevent dryness. Additionally, adding a few drops of essential oils like lavender or chamomile to a bath can help soothe and moisturize the skin.

Itchy Skin: Itching can be caused by various conditions, including dry skin or allergies. To relieve itching, consider an oatmeal bath, as mentioned earlier. Another option is to use a natural anti-itch cream made with ingredients like aloe vera, calendula, and chamomile. Applying a cool, damp cloth to the itchy areas can also provide temporary relief.
When using natural remedies, always do a patch test first to ensure your child doesn't have a sensitivity or allergy to the ingredients. Also, remember that while natural remedies can be effective, it's essential to consult with a healthcare professional if the skin condition persists or worsens. They can provide guidance and ensure that there are no underlying health issues that need addressing.

Managing Allergies and Asthma in Children

Managing allergies and asthma in children involves a multifaceted approach that combines lifestyle changes, natural remedies, and medical care. By understanding the nature of these conditions and implementing effective strategies, you can help your child lead a more comfortable and healthy life. Here's an in-depth guide to managing allergies and asthma in children with a focus on natural and supportive approaches.

Allergies occur when the immune system overreacts to normally harmless substances known as allergens. Common allergens include pollen, pet dander, dust mites, and certain foods. This overreaction can lead to symptoms such as sneezing, itching, runny nose, and watery eyes. Asthma, on the other hand, is a chronic condition characterized by inflammation and narrowing of the airways, leading to difficulty breathing, wheezing, coughing, and shortness of breath. Allergies can often trigger asthma symptoms, making the management of both conditions particularly important.

The environment where your child spends most of their time plays a crucial role in managing allergies and asthma. Regular cleaning is essential to minimize dust and allergens. Use a vacuum cleaner equipped with a HEPA filter to trap small particles and prevent them from being released back into the air. Dust surfaces with a damp cloth rather than dry dusting, which can stir up allergens. Consider using an air purifier with a HEPA filter to improve indoor air quality. Keeping pets out of bedrooms and minimizing their access to other parts of the home can help reduce exposure to pet dander.

Pollen is a major trigger for seasonal allergies, and managing exposure is key to minimizing symptoms. Check pollen counts regularly to determine when levels are high and try to keep your child indoors during these times, particularly on windy days. If your child spends time outdoors, encourage them to change clothes and shower immediately upon coming inside to remove pollen from their skin and hair. Using air conditioning with clean filters can help reduce the amount of pollen that enters your home. Additionally, planting low-pollen or hypoallergenic plants in your garden can reduce pollen levels around your home.

Nutrition plays a significant role in managing allergies and asthma. A well-balanced diet can help support a healthy immune system and reduce inflammation. Encourage a diet rich in fruits, vegetables, whole grains, and lean proteins. Foods high in antioxidants, such as berries, spinach, and kale, can help combat oxidative stress and inflammation. Omega-3 fatty acids, found in fish like salmon, flaxseeds, and walnuts, have anti-inflammatory properties that can benefit asthma and allergy management. Ensure your child avoids known food allergens and maintains a balanced intake of essential nutrients to support overall health.

Herbs can provide natural relief from allergy and asthma symptoms. Butterbur and nettle are known for their antihistamine properties, which can help reduce the severity of allergic reactions. Butterbur has been shown to be as effective as some antihistamine medications in clinical studies. Nettle, often used as a tea or supplement, can also help alleviate allergy symptoms. For asthma relief, herbs like licorice root and mullein can support lung health and reduce inflammation. Licorice root has been used traditionally to soothe respiratory inflammation, while mullein is known for its ability to clear mucus from the lungs. Always consult with a healthcare provider before introducing new herbal remedies, especially for children.

Breathing exercises are beneficial for managing asthma and improving lung function. Techniques such as diaphragmatic breathing, where your child breathes deeply from their diaphragm rather than shallowly from their chest, can help control asthma symptoms and increase lung capacity. Pursed-lip breathing, which involves inhaling slowly through the nose and exhaling through pursed lips, can help your child control their breath during an asthma attack. Regular practice of these exercises can improve respiratory efficiency and reduce the frequency of asthma symptoms.

Stress can exacerbate both allergies and asthma, so it's important to help your child manage stress effectively. Encourage relaxation techniques such as deep breathing, progressive muscle relaxation, and mindfulness. Activities like yoga and tai chi, which incorporate gentle movement and focused breathing, can also be beneficial. Creating a supportive and calm environment at home can help reduce stress levels and contribute to overall well-being. Engage in regular physical activities that your child enjoys, as exercise can be a great stress reliever.

Regular visits to a healthcare provider are essential for monitoring and managing allergies and asthma. Ensure that your child's condition is well-managed with appropriate medications and treatment plans. If your child's symptoms change or worsen, consult with your healthcare provider to adjust their treatment plan accordingly. Keeping track of any triggers and symptom patterns can provide valuable information for your healthcare provider.

For severe allergies, immunotherapy, also known as allergy shots, may be recommended by an allergist. This treatment involves gradually exposing the immune system to small amounts of allergens to build tolerance over time.

Immunotherapy can be an effective long-term solution for reducing the severity of allergic reactions and improving quality of life. This treatment is usually considered when other management strategies are insufficient.

Educating your child about their allergies and asthma can empower them to take an active role in managing their health. Teach them to recognize their symptoms and understand what steps to take during an allergic reaction or asthma attack. Encourage them to communicate openly about their condition and involve them in their own care routine. This sense of responsibility can lead to better adherence to treatment and overall better management of their condition.

Building Emotional Resilience in Kids

Building emotional resilience in children is like giving them a sturdy toolbox to handle life's ups and downs. Emotional resilience helps kids bounce back from challenges, manage stress, and maintain a positive outlook, even when things get tough. By nurturing resilience, you empower your child to cope with difficulties more effectively and develop a strong sense of self. Here's a friendly guide to fostering emotional resilience in kids.

One of the most important aspects of building emotional resilience is fostering open and honest communication. Create a safe space where your child feels comfortable expressing their feelings and thoughts without fear of judgment. Listen actively and validate their emotions, whether they're happy, sad, or frustrated. Encourage them to talk about their experiences and offer support and understanding. By validating their feelings, you help them understand and manage their emotions better.

Resilient children are good problem-solvers who can think critically and find solutions to challenges. Teach your child problem-solving skills by involving them in decision-making and encouraging them to think through problems and potential solutions. Ask questions like, "What do you think we can do to solve this?" or "How can we approach this challenge differently?" This helps them develop a proactive mindset and confidence in their ability to overcome obstacles.

Positive thinking can significantly impact emotional resilience. Help your child recognize and challenge negative thoughts by encouraging them to focus on positive aspects of situations. Teach them to reframe setbacks as opportunities for growth and learning. For example, if they didn't do well on a test, remind them that it's a chance to learn and improve for next time. Celebrate their efforts and progress, not just the outcomes.

Strong relationships with family, friends, and mentors provide a solid support network for children. Encourage your child to build and maintain positive relationships with others. Spend quality time together, engage in meaningful conversations, and show affection and support. Building a network of caring relationships helps children feel secure and valued, which is crucial for developing resilience.

Teaching your child healthy ways to cope with stress and challenges is vital for emotional resilience. Encourage activities that help them relax and unwind, such as reading, drawing, or engaging in hobbies they enjoy. Introduce them to mindfulness practices like deep breathing or meditation, which can help them manage stress and stay grounded. By providing them with effective coping tools, you help them handle difficult situations with greater ease.

Building resilience involves helping children become more independent and self-reliant. Allow them to take on age-appropriate responsibilities and make decisions for themselves.

Encourage them to tackle tasks and challenges on their own, while offering guidance and support as needed. This fosters a sense of accomplishment and confidence in their abilities, reinforcing their resilience.

Children learn a great deal by observing the adults in their lives. Model resilient behavior by demonstrating how you handle challenges and setbacks. Share your experiences with them, including how you cope with stress and find solutions to problems. Show them that it's okay to experience difficulties and that perseverance and a positive attitude can lead to overcoming challenges.

Helping your child become more aware of their emotions is an important step in building resilience. Teach them to identify and label their feelings, and discuss how different emotions can affect their behavior and reactions. This emotional awareness helps them understand their responses to various situations and develop better strategies for managing their emotions.

Fostering a growth mindset—the belief that abilities and intelligence can be developed through effort and learning—can enhance resilience. Encourage your child to view challenges and failures as opportunities for growth rather than as fixed limitations. Praise their effort and perseverance, and emphasize that learning and improvement come through practice and persistence.

Consistent support and encouragement from parents and caregivers play a crucial role in building resilience. Offer reassurance and praise for their efforts and achievements, and provide a stable and supportive environment. Knowing that they have a reliable support system helps children feel more confident in their ability to face challenges and build resilience over time.

Book 22: Healing the Liver and Gallbladder Naturally

The Role of the Liver and Gallbladder in Detoxification

Think of your liver and gallbladder as the dynamic duo responsible for keeping your body's internal environment clean and balanced. These organs work closely together to process and eliminate toxins, ensuring that you stay healthy and energetic.

The liver, situated in the upper right side of your abdomen, is often referred to as the body's primary detoxifier. It handles a vast array of responsibilities, with detoxification being one of its most critical roles. The liver processes nutrients and substances that enter your body, including drugs, alcohol, and environmental pollutants. It breaks these substances down into less harmful forms, which are then prepared for elimination. One of the liver's essential functions is producing bile, a digestive fluid that helps in the breakdown and absorption of fats and fat-soluble vitamins. Bile also acts as a vehicle for carrying waste products out of the liver and into the intestines, where they are eventually excreted from the body.

Just below the liver is the gallbladder, a small, pear-shaped organ that plays a vital role in the digestive process. The gallbladder's main job is to store and concentrate bile produced by the liver. When you eat a meal, especially one that contains fats, the gallbladder releases concentrated bile into the small intestine. This bile is crucial for breaking down dietary fats and aiding in the absorption of fat-soluble vitamins like A, D, E, and K. In addition to its digestive functions, the gallbladder helps in the elimination of waste products, including cholesterol and bilirubin, by expelling them through the bile.

Supporting the health of your liver and gallbladder is essential for maintaining their efficiency in detoxification. A balanced diet rich in fruits, vegetables, and whole grains provides the nutrients your liver needs to function optimally. Foods high in antioxidants, such as berries and leafy greens, help protect the liver from oxidative stress. Staying hydrated by drinking plenty of water supports liver function by aiding in toxin elimination and maintaining bile production.

Limiting processed foods and alcohol can significantly reduce the burden on these organs. Processed foods often contain additives and unhealthy fats that can stress the liver, while excessive alcohol consumption can lead to liver damage. Incorporating liver-friendly herbs, like milk thistle and dandelion root, into your diet can also support liver health. Milk thistle is known for its protective properties, while dandelion root helps promote bile production and liver detoxification.

Signs of Liver Overload and How to Address Them

Your liver is an incredible multitasker, handling everything from detoxifying harmful substances to aiding in digestion. However, just like any hardworking organ, it can sometimes become overwhelmed. Understanding the signs of liver overload and knowing how to address them can help you keep this vital organ in top shape.

When your liver is overloaded, it might not be able to process toxins as effectively as it normally does. This can lead to a range of symptoms that signal it's time to give your liver a little extra care. Common signs of liver overload include persistent fatigue, which can make even simple tasks feel exhausting. If you're feeling unusually tired despite getting enough rest, your liver might be struggling to keep up with its workload.

Another sign to watch for is unexplained digestive issues. This could manifest as frequent bloating, gas, or discomfort after eating. Your liver plays a key role in digesting fats and producing bile, so if it's overwhelmed, these processes can be disrupted. Skin issues, such as unexplained rashes or jaundice (a yellowing of the skin and eyes), are also potential indicators. When the liver is under stress, toxins can build up and affect your skin's appearance.

You might also notice mood swings or irritability, which can be linked to the liver's role in regulating hormones and detoxifying substances. A compromised liver can affect your overall mood and mental clarity. Additionally, if you find yourself experiencing frequent headaches or brain fog, this could be a result of the liver's reduced ability to detoxify and eliminate waste effectively.

To address these signs of liver overload, consider making some lifestyle adjustments to support your liver's natural detoxification processes. Start by improving your diet. Focus on consuming whole foods rich in antioxidants, such as fruits, vegetables, and whole grains. These foods help protect your liver from oxidative stress and support its detoxification functions.

Hydration is also key. Drinking plenty of water aids in flushing out toxins and maintaining healthy liver function. Reducing your intake of processed foods and alcohol can further alleviate the strain on your liver. Processed foods often contain additives and unhealthy fats, while alcohol can exacerbate liver stress and lead to damage over time.

Incorporating liver-friendly herbs into your diet can also be beneficial. Milk thistle, for instance, is known for its protective effects on liver cells and can help support liver regeneration. Dandelion root is another excellent herb that promotes bile production and helps with detoxification.

Regular exercise and sufficient sleep play important roles in liver health as well. Exercise boosts circulation and helps the liver process and eliminate toxins more efficiently. Quality sleep allows your body to repair and regenerate, including your liver.

Herbal Remedies for Liver Support

Your liver is your body's powerhouse for detoxification, and keeping it in top shape is crucial for overall health. Herbal remedies have been used for centuries to support liver health, offering natural ways to enhance its function and help it handle its many responsibilities. Let's explore some effective herbal remedies that can give your liver the support it needs to stay strong and healthy.

Milk Thistle is one of the most renowned herbs for liver support. Its active compound, silymarin, is known for its powerful antioxidant and anti-inflammatory properties. Silymarin helps protect liver cells from damage caused by toxins and supports liver regeneration. It's often used to aid in liver detoxification and to promote overall liver health. You can find milk thistle in various forms, including capsules, teas, and tinctures.

Dandelion Root is another fantastic herb for liver health. It's a natural diuretic, which means it helps the body eliminate excess fluids and toxins. Dandelion root also stimulates bile production, which aids in digestion and helps the liver process fats more efficiently. You can enjoy dandelion root as a tea or take it in supplement form.

Turmeric is well-known for its bright yellow color and its role in curries, but it's also a powerful liver supporter. The active ingredient in turmeric, curcumin, has strong anti-inflammatory and antioxidant effects. It helps reduce inflammation in the liver and supports its detoxification processes. Turmeric can be added to your diet in various forms, including fresh, powdered, or as a supplement.

Artichoke Leaf is another herb that benefits the liver. It contains compounds that help increase bile flow, which supports digestion and helps the liver detoxify. Artichoke leaf is also known for its antioxidant properties, which can help protect the liver from damage. You can find it in supplement form or enjoy artichoke as a delicious vegetable in your meals.

Ginger isn't just a tasty addition to your dishes—it's also great for your liver. Ginger has anti-inflammatory properties and can help reduce nausea, which may be beneficial if you're experiencing digestive discomfort. It supports overall digestion and can aid in the liver's detoxification processes. Fresh ginger can be added to teas, smoothies, or meals, while ginger supplements are also available.

Schisandra is a lesser-known but powerful herb for liver support. It's often used in traditional Chinese medicine for its detoxifying properties. Schisandra helps protect the liver from oxidative stress and supports its ability to process toxins. It can be taken as a tincture, tea, or supplement.

The Gallbladder Cleanse and Its Benefits

The gallbladder might be a small organ, but it plays a big role in your digestive health. Located just beneath the liver, the gallbladder stores and concentrates bile, a fluid essential for digesting fats. Sometimes, however, the gallbladder can get a bit sluggish or develop issues like gallstones. That's where a gallbladder cleanse comes into play—a natural method designed to help refresh and rejuvenate this vital organ.

A gallbladder cleanse involves a series of steps aimed at flushing out accumulated bile, waste products, and, in some cases, even small gallstones. The idea is to stimulate the gallbladder and liver to work more efficiently, promoting better digestion and overall digestive health. While it may sound a bit like a detox, it's more about supporting the body's natural processes rather than a complete overhaul.
One of the main benefits of a gallbladder cleanse is improved digestion. When the gallbladder is functioning optimally, it releases bile more effectively, which helps break down fats and absorb essential nutrients. This can lead to a reduction in symptoms like bloating, gas, and discomfort after meals. If you've been experiencing digestive issues, a cleanse might provide the support your gallbladder needs to get back on track.

Another benefit is the potential for reducing the risk of gallstones. Gallstones can form when there's an imbalance in the substances that make up bile, such as cholesterol and bilirubin. By promoting a healthy flow of bile and helping to clear out any built-up waste, a gallbladder cleanse can potentially help prevent the formation of new gallstones or help manage existing ones. While it's not a guaranteed solution, many people find it a helpful complementary approach.

There are several ways to approach a gallbladder cleanse. A common method involves drinking a mixture of olive oil and lemon juice. Olive oil is thought to help stimulate the gallbladder to release bile, while lemon juice adds a bit of acidity that can further aid in digestion. Another approach is to incorporate foods and herbs known for their gallbladder-supporting properties, such as beets, artichokes, and dandelion root. These can help encourage bile production and support overall liver and gallbladder health.

It's important to remember that while a gallbladder cleanse can offer benefits, it should be approached with caution. If you have existing gallbladder issues or any other health conditions, it's wise to consult with a healthcare professional before starting a cleanse. They can help ensure that it's a safe and appropriate option for your specific needs.

Nutrition for Liver Health

Your liver is like your body's personal detox center, working tirelessly to process nutrients, filter out toxins, and keep everything running smoothly. To keep this vital organ in top shape, what you eat plays a crucial role. Let's dive into the best nutritional choices for supporting liver health and ensuring it continues to function at its best.

Start with a colorful plate. Incorporating a variety of fruits and vegetables into your diet provides your liver with essential vitamins, minerals, and antioxidants. Vegetables like leafy greens (spinach, kale), cruciferous veggies (broccoli, Brussels sprouts), and root vegetables (beets, carrots) are particularly beneficial. These foods are rich in antioxidants and nutrients that help combat oxidative stress and support the liver's detoxification processes.

Whole grains are another important component of a liver-friendly diet. Foods like brown rice, quinoa, and oats are high in fiber, which helps your digestive system run smoothly and supports liver health by reducing the workload on this critical organ. Fiber helps in the elimination of waste and toxins from the body, preventing them from accumulating and potentially causing harm.

Healthy fats are also essential for liver health. Opt for sources of unsaturated fats like avocados, nuts, seeds, and olive oil. These fats provide the liver with the necessary nutrients to produce bile, which is vital for digesting fats and absorbing fat-soluble vitamins. They also help reduce inflammation, which is beneficial for maintaining liver health.

Lean proteins such as chicken, fish, and legumes provide your liver with the building blocks it needs to repair and regenerate. Proteins are essential for the production of enzymes and other substances that support liver function. Fish like salmon and sardines are particularly beneficial due to their high content of omega-3 fatty acids, which have anti-inflammatory properties and help maintain a healthy liver.

Hydration is another key aspect of liver health. Drinking plenty of water helps the liver flush out toxins more effectively. Aim for at least 8 glasses of water a day, and consider incorporating herbal teas like dandelion or milk thistle, which are known for their liver-supportive properties.

Limit or avoid alcohol and excessive consumption of processed foods. Alcohol can put a strain on the liver, leading to inflammation and potential damage over time. Processed foods, often high in sugar and unhealthy fats, can contribute to liver fat buildup and other health issues. Instead, focus on whole, unprocessed foods to give your liver the best chance to thrive.

Green tea is another great addition to your diet. It's packed with antioxidants called catechins that help improve liver function and reduce fat accumulation. Drinking a cup or two of green tea daily can provide a gentle boost to your liver's natural detoxification abilities.

Managing Gallstones Naturally

Gallstones can be a painful and troublesome condition, but managing them naturally can help alleviate symptoms and support overall gallbladder health. Gallstones form when there's an imbalance in the substances that make up bile, like cholesterol and bilirubin. They can range in size from tiny grains to larger stones and may cause issues if they block the bile ducts. While medical intervention is sometimes necessary, there are several natural approaches you can explore to help manage and potentially reduce gallstones.

Start with your diet. A balanced diet plays a crucial role in managing gallstones. Incorporate foods that promote healthy bile flow and reduce the risk of stone formation. High-fiber foods like fruits, vegetables, and whole grains can help keep bile flowing smoothly and reduce cholesterol levels, which may help prevent the formation of new gallstones. Additionally, healthy fats from sources like avocados, nuts, and olive oil can support bile production and help your gallbladder function more effectively.

Stay hydrated. Drinking plenty of water is essential for maintaining good gallbladder health. Proper hydration helps keep bile diluted and prevents it from becoming too concentrated, which can reduce the risk of stone formation. Aim for at least 8 glasses of water a day, and consider herbal teas such as dandelion or milk thistle, which are known to support liver and gallbladder health.

Consider natural supplements. Certain supplements may help support gallbladder health and reduce the risk of gallstones. Milk thistle is known for its liver-supportive properties and may help improve bile production and flow. Artichoke extract can stimulate bile production and help with fat digestion. Turmeric contains curcumin, which has anti-inflammatory properties and may help keep the bile ducts healthy. Always consult with a healthcare professional before starting any new supplements to ensure they are appropriate for your situation.

Maintain a healthy weight. Being overweight or rapidly losing weight can increase the risk of gallstones. Gradual weight loss through a balanced diet and regular exercise can help reduce the risk of gallstone formation. Aim for a steady and sustainable weight loss of 1-2 pounds per week to avoid putting additional stress on your gallbladder.

Exercise regularly. Physical activity helps keep your digestive system functioning smoothly and supports overall gallbladder health. Aim for at least 30 minutes of moderate exercise most days of the week. Activities like walking, swimming, and cycling can help maintain a healthy weight and promote good bile flow.

Be mindful of meal timing. Eating smaller, more frequent meals can help keep bile flowing regularly and prevent it from becoming too concentrated. Try to avoid large, heavy meals that can overload your digestive system and strain your gallbladder.

Incorporate foods with gallbladder-friendly properties. Foods like beets, which support liver function, and ginger, which aids digestion, can be beneficial for managing gallstones. Additionally, foods rich in antioxidants, such as berries and leafy greens, can help reduce inflammation and support overall gallbladder health.

Daily Practices for Liver and Gallbladder Maintenance

Taking care of your liver and gallbladder is crucial for maintaining overall health and well-being. These two organs work together to process nutrients, detoxify the body, and aid in digestion. Incorporating some daily practices into your routine can help keep them functioning optimally and prevent potential issues. Here's a friendly guide to keeping your liver and gallbladder in tip-top shape every day.

Start your day with a glass of water. Hydration is essential for liver and gallbladder health. Drinking a glass of water first thing in the morning helps kickstart your metabolism and aids in the detoxification process. You might also consider adding a splash of lemon juice, which can stimulate bile production and support liver function.

Eat a balanced breakfast. A nutritious breakfast sets the tone for the day and provides your body with the energy and nutrients it needs. Opt for a meal rich in fiber, healthy fats, and lean protein. Think oatmeal topped with berries and a sprinkle of nuts or a smoothie with spinach, banana, and a scoop of chia seeds. This helps keep bile flowing smoothly and supports overall digestion.

Incorporate liver-friendly foods into your diet. Throughout the day, focus on eating foods that support liver and gallbladder health. Include plenty of fruits and vegetables, especially those high in antioxidants like leafy greens, beets, and citrus fruits. Whole grains, such as brown rice and quinoa, and healthy fats from sources like avocados and nuts also support liver function.

Practice mindful eating. Eating smaller, more frequent meals can help keep your digestive system working efficiently and prevent bile from becoming too concentrated. Avoid overeating or consuming large meals, as this can put extra strain on your liver and gallbladder.

Get regular physical activity. Exercise is not just good for your body; it also benefits your liver and gallbladder. Aim for at least 30 minutes of moderate exercise most days of the week. Activities like walking, cycling, or yoga can help improve digestion, support healthy weight management, and enhance bile flow.

Limit alcohol consumption. Alcohol can put significant strain on your liver, so it's best to consume it in moderation. If possible, consider reducing or eliminating alcohol from your diet to give your liver a break and support its natural detoxification processes.

Stay hydrated throughout the day. In addition to your morning glass of water, continue to drink water throughout the day. Proper hydration supports liver function and helps keep bile from becoming too concentrated, which can reduce the risk of gallstone formation.

Incorporate herbal teas. Herbal teas like dandelion root, milk thistle, and ginger can provide additional support for liver and gallbladder health. Drinking a cup of these teas daily can help stimulate bile production, support liver detoxification, and improve digestion.

Prioritize sleep. A good night's sleep is essential for overall health, including liver and gallbladder function. Aim for 7-9 hours of quality sleep each night to give your body time to repair and regenerate. Establish a relaxing bedtime routine and maintain a consistent sleep schedule to support restorative rest.

Manage stress. Chronic stress can impact your digestive system and liver health. Practice stress-reducing techniques such as deep breathing, meditation, or gentle exercise to help keep stress levels in check and support overall well-being.

Book 23: Weight Loss and Metabolic Health with Natural Approaches

Understanding the Metabolism and Weight Management

Metabolism is one of those terms we often hear but don't always fully understand. Yet, it plays a crucial role in how our bodies function, particularly when it comes to weight management. In the simplest terms, metabolism refers to all the chemical processes that occur in your body to maintain life. These processes include everything from breathing and blood circulation to digesting food and repairing cells. When we talk about metabolism in relation to weight management, we are specifically referring to how efficiently your body converts the food you eat into energy and how that energy is used or stored.

At the core of your metabolic function is something called your basal metabolic rate (BMR). This is the number of calories your body needs just to carry out its most basic functions, like breathing, pumping blood, and regulating body temperature. Even when you're completely at rest—sitting on the couch or sleeping—your body is still burning calories to keep you alive and functioning. This baseline rate varies from person to person and is influenced by several factors such as age, muscle mass, hormone levels, and genetics.

As you get older, your BMR tends to decrease. This is partly because you naturally lose muscle mass with age, and muscle burns more calories than fat. So, even if you're eating the same amount and doing the same activities as you did when you were younger, you might find it harder to maintain or lose weight as you age. Hormones also play a significant role in metabolism. For instance, thyroid hormones help regulate how quickly your body burns calories. If you have an underactive thyroid (hypothyroidism), your metabolism may slow down, making it harder to lose weight. Similarly, certain hormonal changes that occur during menopause can also slow metabolism, leading to weight gain.

Genetics, too, plays a role in how efficiently your body burns calories. Some people are naturally predisposed to having a faster or slower metabolism. You might know someone who seems to eat whatever they want without gaining weight, while others struggle with their weight despite eating relatively little. This variability is largely due to genetic factors that influence your metabolic rate. However, just because you may have a slower metabolism doesn't mean you're stuck with it. There are ways to naturally boost your metabolism and support weight management.

One of the most effective ways to increase your metabolic rate is through physical activity. When you exercise, especially when you engage in strength training, you build muscle. And the more muscle you have, the more calories your body burns throughout the day, even when you're not working out. Think of muscle as a calorie-burning engine that keeps running, even when you're resting. This is why strength training is particularly effective for boosting metabolism and aiding in weight loss. It helps you build and maintain muscle, which in turn keeps your metabolic fire burning brightly.

In addition to exercise, how you eat can also affect your metabolism. Skipping meals or drastically cutting calories may seem like a good idea for losing weight, but it can actually slow your metabolism.

When your body senses that it's not getting enough energy, it goes into "starvation mode," slowing down the rate at which it burns calories in an effort to conserve energy. On the other hand, eating smaller, balanced meals and snacks throughout the day can keep your metabolism steady. Foods rich in protein are particularly helpful for boosting metabolism, as your body burns more calories digesting protein compared to fats or carbohydrates.

Staying hydrated is another simple yet effective way to support your metabolism. Water is essential for all of your body's processes, including those that involve burning calories. When you're dehydrated, your metabolism can slow down because your body isn't able to function as efficiently. Drinking enough water throughout the day helps keep your metabolism working at its best. Some studies even suggest that drinking cold water can temporarily boost your metabolism, as your body uses energy to heat the water to body temperature.

Sleep also plays a significant role in metabolism and weight management. When you don't get enough sleep, it can throw off your body's hunger-regulating hormones, making you more likely to overeat and less likely to make healthy food choices. Lack of sleep also slows down your metabolism and makes it harder for your body to process carbohydrates, which can lead to weight gain over time. Prioritizing good quality sleep is crucial for maintaining a healthy metabolism and supporting your weight loss goals.

Stress is another factor that can negatively affect your metabolism. When you're stressed, your body produces higher levels of cortisol, a hormone that can cause your body to store more fat, particularly in the abdominal area. Chronic stress can also lead to overeating and cravings for high-calorie, comfort foods, making it even more difficult to manage your weight. Finding healthy ways to cope with stress, such as through exercise, meditation, or relaxation techniques, can help keep your cortisol levels in check and support a healthy metabolism.

Weight management isn't just about counting calories or following strict diets; it's about understanding how your body works and making lifestyle changes that support your natural metabolism. By focusing on building muscle through exercise, eating balanced meals, staying hydrated, prioritizing sleep, and managing stress, you can give your metabolism the boost it needs to work more efficiently. These small but sustainable changes can have a big impact on your overall health and help you manage your weight in a healthy, natural way.

Natural Appetite Suppressants and Fat Burners

When it comes to weight loss, many people struggle with managing hunger and cravings. It's completely normal to feel hungry, especially when you're making changes to your eating habits. But did you know there are natural ways to help curb your appetite and boost fat burning? These approaches can help you stay on track without feeling deprived or overwhelmed by constant hunger.

Natural appetite suppressants work by helping you feel full for longer or reducing the intensity of cravings. They aren't meant to eliminate hunger altogether (which wouldn't be healthy!), but instead, they can help you control portions and prevent overeating. The best part? These natural options are safe and can easily be incorporated into your daily routine.

One of the simplest ways to curb your appetite is by eating foods high in fiber. Fiber-rich foods like vegetables, fruits, whole grains, and legumes take longer to digest, which means they keep you feeling full for a longer period.

When you feel satisfied, you're less likely to snack or overeat at your next meal. Additionally, fiber helps regulate blood sugar levels, which can prevent the spikes and crashes that often lead to cravings.

Another great appetite suppressant is water. Sometimes, we confuse thirst with hunger, so drinking a glass of water before meals can help reduce overeating. Water can also fill your stomach temporarily, making you feel fuller. Similarly, foods with high water content, such as cucumbers, watermelon, and leafy greens, not only hydrate you but also help you feel satisfied without many calories.

Herbal teas are another gentle way to suppress your appetite. Green tea, for instance, contains compounds like catechins and caffeine that can increase metabolism and help reduce hunger. Ginger tea is known for helping to regulate blood sugar levels and reduce cravings, while peppermint tea can naturally reduce feelings of hunger by calming the digestive system.

Proteins are another key element in natural appetite suppression. Foods high in protein, such as eggs, chicken, fish, tofu, and legumes, take longer to break down, which helps you feel full longer. Including a good amount of protein in your meals can help control your appetite throughout the day. Plus, protein-rich foods are essential for building muscle, which boosts your metabolism and helps burn more calories.

When it comes to fat burning, it's not just about cutting calories but also about giving your metabolism a little help. Natural fat burners can give your body that extra boost it needs to efficiently burn fat and support weight loss.

One of the most popular natural fat burners is green tea. Not only does it help suppress your appetite, but the caffeine and antioxidants in green tea also help speed up your metabolism. Studies have shown that green tea can increase fat oxidation, meaning your body uses fat as fuel more efficiently. Drinking a few cups of green tea throughout the day can support your weight loss goals.

Another excellent fat-burning ingredient is cayenne pepper. The spicy compound in cayenne, called capsaicin, has been shown to increase the rate at which your body burns fat. Adding a pinch of cayenne to your meals can raise your body temperature slightly, boosting your metabolism and encouraging your body to burn more calories, even at rest.

Coconut oil is another surprising natural fat burner. It contains medium-chain triglycerides (MCTs), which are types of fat that your body uses quickly for energy instead of storing. Adding a small amount of coconut oil to your diet can help your body burn fat more efficiently, especially belly fat.

Coffee, when consumed in moderation, can also act as a natural fat burner. The caffeine in coffee stimulates the nervous system, signaling your body to break down stored fat and use it as energy. Just be mindful of what you add to your coffee, as sugar and cream can add extra calories.

Apple cider vinegar is a popular natural remedy for weight loss. It works by reducing appetite and increasing feelings of fullness. Some studies suggest that it can help reduce body fat by improving digestion and regulating blood sugar levels. Simply diluting a tablespoon of apple cider vinegar in water and drinking it before meals can have a subtle but helpful effect on your weight loss efforts.

Protein, once again, plays a big role here. Eating more protein not only keeps you full but also has a higher thermic effect than fats or carbs, meaning your body burns more calories digesting protein. This makes protein not just an appetite suppressant but also a great fat burner. Foods like lean meats, fish, eggs, and plant-based proteins can help rev up your metabolism and support fat loss.

While appetite suppressants and fat burners can help on their own, they work even better when combined with healthy eating habits and regular physical activity. Incorporating more natural, whole foods into your diet, staying active, and focusing on hydration and sleep are key components to achieving lasting results.

The beauty of natural appetite suppressants and fat burners is that they don't involve harsh chemicals or dangerous supplements. They come from everyday ingredients that you can easily incorporate into your meals and daily habits. Whether it's starting your day with a protein-packed breakfast, sipping on green tea, or adding a sprinkle of cayenne to your dinner, these small changes can make a big difference in your weight loss journey.

Herbs for Supporting Metabolic Function

When it comes to weight loss and overall health, your metabolism plays a starring role. It's the engine that keeps your body running, converting the food you eat into energy and determining how efficiently you burn calories. While genetics, age, and lifestyle all influence your metabolic rate, there are natural ways to give it a helpful boost. One of the gentlest and most effective ways to support your metabolism is through the use of herbs. These natural remedies have been used for centuries to enhance metabolic function, aid digestion, and promote overall wellness.

Ginger is one of the most well-known herbs for boosting metabolism. Its warming properties can slightly raise your body temperature, a process known as thermogenesis, which helps your body burn more calories. Beyond that, ginger is great for digestion, helping to soothe the stomach, reduce bloating, and promote better nutrient absorption. A cup of ginger tea in the morning or adding fresh ginger to your meals can be an easy way to take advantage of its metabolism-boosting benefits.

Green tea is packed with antioxidants, particularly catechins, which have been shown to help increase fat burning and improve metabolic health. The caffeine in green tea also works to stimulate the nervous system, encouraging your body to use stored fat for energy. Drinking a few cups of green tea each day can help boost your metabolism naturally, without the jittery side effects that come from stronger stimulants. It's a simple, soothing way to support your metabolic function and enhance fat oxidation.

Cinnamon is not just a warming spice; it's also a great herb for helping regulate blood sugar levels, which is key for maintaining a healthy metabolism. When your blood sugar is stable, your body is less likely to store fat, and you're less prone to energy crashes and cravings. Adding a sprinkle of cinnamon to your morning coffee, oatmeal, or smoothies can help keep your blood sugar balanced and your metabolism steady. It's a delicious, easy-to-incorporate herb that can help with weight management and metabolic health.

Turmeric is a golden herb known for its anti-inflammatory properties, and it can also play a role in supporting metabolic health. Inflammation in the body can slow down metabolism and make it harder to lose weight. By reducing inflammation, turmeric helps your body function more efficiently, including your metabolism. The active compound in turmeric, curcumin, has been shown to aid in fat metabolism and prevent fat accumulation. You can add turmeric to soups, stews, or even golden milk lattes for a comforting way to support your metabolism.

If you're looking for a fiery kick to your metabolism, cayenne pepper is the herb for you. Cayenne contains capsaicin, a compound that has been shown to increase thermogenesis and boost calorie burning.

By raising your body's temperature, capsaicin helps your body burn more energy even when at rest. Sprinkling cayenne pepper onto your meals or adding it to sauces and marinades can provide that extra metabolic push. Just be careful with the spice level—it's powerful!

Ginseng is an adaptogenic herb, which means it helps your body adapt to stress, and it's also known to enhance energy levels and support metabolism. Panax ginseng, in particular, has been studied for its ability to improve fat metabolism and assist with weight loss. Ginseng helps balance blood sugar levels and improves insulin sensitivity, which is crucial for maintaining a healthy metabolism. Whether in tea form, supplements, or added to meals, ginseng can be a gentle, effective herb for supporting metabolic function.

Often considered a weed, dandelion is actually a powerhouse herb for your metabolism and digestion. Dandelion root is known to stimulate bile production, which helps break down fats more efficiently. It's also a natural diuretic, which means it helps reduce water retention and bloating, making you feel lighter and more energized. Dandelion tea is a simple way to enjoy the benefits of this herb, and it can easily be added to your daily routine to support better digestion and metabolic health.

Ashwagandha is another adaptogenic herb that helps balance hormones and reduce stress, both of which are key factors in supporting a healthy metabolism. When you're stressed, your body produces cortisol, a hormone that can slow down your metabolism and lead to weight gain, especially around the belly. Ashwagandha helps regulate cortisol levels, promoting a more balanced metabolic function. This herb can be taken as a supplement or added to smoothies or teas for a calming, stress-reducing effect.

Fenugreek is a herb traditionally used in Ayurvedic medicine to help regulate blood sugar levels and improve digestion. Its seeds are particularly rich in soluble fiber, which helps control appetite and promote feelings of fullness. By helping stabilize blood sugar and curbing cravings, fenugreek supports metabolic health and makes it easier to manage weight. You can soak fenugreek seeds in water overnight and drink the infused water in the morning, or use ground fenugreek as a spice in cooking.

Rosemary is a fragrant herb that not only adds flavor to your dishes but also supports digestive health and metabolism. It has been used traditionally to aid in the breakdown of fats and to stimulate circulation, which can support metabolic function. Rosemary also has antioxidant properties that help protect the body from oxidative stress, which can slow down metabolism. Adding fresh rosemary to roasted vegetables, meats, or soups is a flavorful way to incorporate this herb into your diet.

Oregano is more than just a flavorful herb for your pasta sauce—it's also rich in antioxidants and compounds that support metabolic health. Oregano contains carvacrol, a compound that has been shown to help regulate fat metabolism and reduce the formation of fat cells. Using oregano as a seasoning in your cooking is an easy way to add this herb to your meals, helping your body burn fat more effectively.

Balancing Blood Sugar for Weight Control

When it comes to managing your weight, balancing your blood sugar is one of the most important steps you can take. Stable blood sugar levels help you maintain steady energy throughout the day, reduce cravings, and prevent those energy crashes that often lead to overeating. By keeping your blood sugar balanced, you can create a healthy foundation for weight control, making it easier to achieve your goals without feeling deprived or constantly battling hunger.

Blood sugar, or glucose, is your body's primary source of energy. When you eat, your body breaks down carbohydrates into glucose, which enters your bloodstream and fuels your cells. The hormone insulin helps regulate this process by allowing your cells to absorb glucose. However, if your blood sugar spikes too high or drops too low, it can lead to issues like cravings, fatigue, and even weight gain. Frequent blood sugar spikes signal your body to store excess glucose as fat, while dips in blood sugar can trigger cravings for sugary or high-calorie foods to quickly restore energy.

By keeping your blood sugar stable, you not only avoid these energy swings but also help your body burn fat more efficiently and curb the constant hunger that can make weight loss challenging.

One of the best ways to keep your blood sugar balanced is by choosing the right kinds of carbohydrates. Not all carbs are created equal! Simple carbs, like white bread, pastries, and sugary snacks, are quickly broken down by your body, causing rapid spikes in blood sugar followed by equally fast crashes. These quick shifts can leave you feeling tired and craving more food soon after eating.

On the other hand, complex carbohydrates, such as whole grains, vegetables, legumes, and fruits, are digested more slowly, providing a steady release of energy and keeping blood sugar levels more stable. These foods are also rich in fiber, which helps slow the absorption of glucose and promotes feelings of fullness, reducing the temptation to overeat. Incorporating fiber-rich, whole foods into your meals is a simple yet effective way to balance blood sugar and support weight loss.

While carbohydrates are important, pairing them with protein and healthy fats can make a big difference in balancing blood sugar. Protein helps slow down the digestion of carbs, preventing rapid spikes in blood sugar. It also helps you feel fuller for longer, making it easier to control portion sizes and avoid overeating. Including protein in every meal, such as eggs, lean meats, tofu, or beans, can stabilize your blood sugar and keep hunger at bay.

Healthy fats also play a crucial role in blood sugar control. Fats take longer to digest, which helps slow the absorption of glucose into your bloodstream. They also provide a steady source of energy and promote satiety, reducing the urge to snack between meals. Healthy fats like avocados, olive oil, nuts, and seeds can easily be incorporated into your diet to support balanced blood sugar and overall metabolic health.

When and how often you eat can significantly impact your blood sugar levels. Skipping meals or going too long without eating can cause your blood sugar to drop, leading to cravings and overeating later on. On the other hand, eating small, balanced meals or snacks throughout the day helps keep your blood sugar stable and your energy consistent.

Try not to go more than four to five hours between meals, and if you feel hungry in between, reach for a healthy snack that includes a mix of protein, fiber, and healthy fats. Something as simple as a handful of almonds, a piece of fruit with nut butter, or some veggies with hummus can help keep your blood sugar in check and prevent those mid-afternoon energy slumps.

Sugary drinks, like soda, sweetened coffee, and juice, can cause your blood sugar to spike quickly since they are absorbed almost immediately into your bloodstream. These quick spikes are often followed by sharp drops, which can lead to feelings of fatigue and increased cravings for sugary foods. Instead, opt for water, herbal teas, or drinks with no added sugar to keep your blood sugar more stable throughout the day.

If you enjoy flavored drinks, consider infusing your water with fresh fruits or herbs for a refreshing and healthy alternative. This way, you can stay hydrated without the risk of disrupting your blood sugar balance.

Stress and lack of sleep can also wreak havoc on your blood sugar levels. When you're stressed, your body releases cortisol, a hormone that can raise blood sugar levels and increase cravings for high-calorie, sugary foods. Chronic stress can make it harder to control your appetite and may lead to weight gain over time.

Similarly, poor sleep can affect how your body regulates blood sugar and insulin. When you're sleep-deprived, your body may become less efficient at processing glucose, leading to higher blood sugar levels and increased hunger. Prioritizing restful sleep and managing stress through relaxation techniques like deep breathing, meditation, or gentle exercise can help keep your blood sugar—and your weight—under control.

One natural way to help balance your blood sugar is by adding cinnamon to your diet. Studies have shown that cinnamon can improve insulin sensitivity, allowing your body to better regulate blood sugar levels. Sprinkling cinnamon on your morning oatmeal, yogurt, or smoothies is a simple and delicious way to support stable blood sugar throughout the day.

The Role of Detoxification in Weight Loss

Detoxification, or simply "detox," is a concept that has gained significant attention when it comes to weight loss. But what does detoxification really mean, and how can it support your weight loss goals? At its core, detoxification is the body's natural process of eliminating toxins, waste, and harmful substances. When you give your body the right support to detoxify effectively, it can enhance your overall health and even play a pivotal role in helping you shed unwanted pounds.

Every day, your body is exposed to toxins from the food you eat, the air you breathe, and even the products you use on your skin. These toxins can accumulate in your system, making it harder for your body to function optimally. When your body is overwhelmed with toxins, it may hold onto excess fat, as fat cells can act as storage sites for harmful substances. This can slow down your metabolism, making weight loss more difficult.

Supporting your body's natural detox processes helps it rid itself of these toxins more efficiently. By doing so, you create an environment that encourages fat loss, boosts metabolism, and promotes overall well-being. Think of detoxification as clearing out the clutter, allowing your body to focus on burning fat and maintaining a healthy weight.

Detoxification and weight loss go hand in hand for several reasons. First, when your body is bogged down by toxins, your liver, kidneys, and other organs responsible for detoxifying your system have to work overtime. This extra burden can lead to a sluggish metabolism, which makes burning fat more challenging. By supporting your body's natural detox systems, you allow these organs to function more effectively, which in turn can boost your metabolic rate and help you burn more calories.

Additionally, detoxing can help reduce bloating, water retention, and inflammation—all factors that can contribute to weight gain. By flushing out toxins and excess waste, your body can release stored water weight, making you feel lighter and more energized. Plus, when your body isn't working as hard to process toxins, you'll often experience improved digestion, which is another key element of weight loss.

Detoxing doesn't have to be extreme or involve harsh cleanses. In fact, gentle and natural methods are often the most sustainable and effective. Here are a few ways you can support your body's detoxification process while working toward your weight loss goals:

Hydration: Drinking plenty of water is one of the simplest and most effective ways to support detoxification. Water helps flush toxins from your system, supports kidney function, and aids digestion. Aim for at least 8 cups of water a day, and consider starting your morning with a glass of warm water and lemon to kickstart your liver's detox process.

Fiber-Rich Foods: Fiber is your friend when it comes to detoxing and weight loss. Foods high in fiber, such as fruits, vegetables, whole grains, and legumes, help move waste through your digestive system more efficiently. This not only supports detoxification but also keeps you feeling full, reducing overeating and aiding weight control.

Herbal Teas: Certain herbs, like dandelion, milk thistle, and burdock root, are known for their liver-supporting properties. These herbs can help cleanse your liver, the body's primary detoxification organ, and improve its ability to process toxins and fats. Drinking detoxifying herbal teas can be a gentle way to support your body's natural cleansing process.

Sweating It Out: Exercise is not only great for burning calories but also for detoxification. When you sweat, your body releases toxins through your skin, one of its largest detox organs. Regular physical activity, whether it's a brisk walk, yoga, or strength training, promotes circulation and helps your body flush out harmful substances.

Eating Clean: Supporting detoxification isn't just about removing toxins—it's also about reducing the intake of harmful substances in the first place. Eating a clean, whole-foods-based diet with plenty of fruits, vegetables, lean proteins, and healthy fats helps reduce your exposure to toxins while providing essential nutrients that support your body's detox processes. Avoiding processed foods, artificial additives, and excessive sugar can make a significant difference in how your body detoxifies.

Gut Health: Your gut plays a crucial role in detoxification. A healthy gut helps eliminate toxins through bowel movements, and having regular, healthy digestion is essential for weight loss. Probiotics from fermented foods like yogurt, sauerkraut, and kimchi, along with prebiotic-rich foods like garlic, onions, and bananas, can promote a healthy gut environment that supports detoxification and weight management.

The benefits of detoxification extend far beyond just weight loss. When your body is effectively detoxifying, you're likely to notice improvements in your energy levels, digestion, skin health, and even mental clarity. A well-functioning detox system supports better sleep, reduces inflammation, and enhances your body's ability to burn fat more efficiently.
By taking a balanced, natural approach to detoxing, you're not only setting yourself up for success in weight loss but also for a healthier, more vibrant lifestyle overall.

It's important to keep in mind that not all detox programs are created equal. Many fad detox diets promise rapid weight loss through extreme methods like juice fasting or taking expensive supplements. While these approaches may lead to quick weight loss, they are often unsustainable and can deprive your body of essential nutrients. Instead of relying on short-term fixes, focus on gentle, natural methods that support your body's detox process in the long term.

Remember, your body is already equipped with a powerful detox system—your liver, kidneys, skin, and digestive system are working constantly to eliminate toxins. The goal is to support these organs with healthy habits, not overburden them with drastic detox plans that may do more harm than good.

Managing Emotional Eating with Natural Remedies

Managing emotional eating can be a challenge, but it's something that can be addressed naturally and effectively. Emotional eating happens when we turn to food to cope with feelings like stress, sadness, boredom, or even happiness. This type of eating often leads to cravings for high-calorie, sugary, or salty foods, which can interfere with our health and weight loss goals. The key to managing emotional eating is to understand its triggers and find healthier ways to respond to our emotions.

When we eat due to emotions, it's not about satisfying physical hunger. Instead, it's a response to feelings that can be overwhelming. Stress from work, personal challenges, or even minor frustrations can trigger the urge to snack, especially on foods that offer temporary comfort but don't serve our long-term goals. Acknowledging these triggers is the first step in breaking the emotional eating cycle. Once we understand the emotional root of our cravings, we can begin to manage them in a healthier way.

One of the most effective ways to reduce emotional eating is by using natural remedies that help calm the mind and body. Certain herbs have long been known for their ability to ease stress and anxiety, which are common causes of emotional eating. Chamomile, for example, is a gentle herb that promotes relaxation. A warm cup of chamomile tea at the end of a stressful day can provide a sense of calm, helping to reduce the urge to reach for comfort food.

Another useful herb is ashwagandha, which helps the body manage stress by balancing cortisol levels. High cortisol, often referred to as the "stress hormone," can lead to cravings for unhealthy foods. By helping to regulate cortisol, ashwagandha makes it easier to stay in control of your eating habits. Lavender, whether used in tea or as an essential oil, is another calming herb that can help reduce emotional eating by soothing anxiety and promoting relaxation.

Lemon balm is another excellent herb for emotional well-being. It's known for its calming effects and can be particularly helpful in reducing feelings of stress or nervousness that often lead to overeating. Holy basil, also called tulsi, is a powerful adaptogen that helps the body cope with stress and balance mood, making it easier to avoid stress-induced eating.

Mindfulness is another key tool for managing emotional eating. Being mindful means paying close attention to your thoughts, feelings, and physical sensations. When it comes to eating, mindfulness helps you recognize the difference between true physical hunger and emotional hunger. Before reaching for food, take a moment to check in with yourself. Are you actually hungry, or are you eating because you're feeling anxious, bored, or stressed? By pausing and reflecting, you give yourself the opportunity to make a conscious choice rather than reacting automatically to emotions.

Mindful eating also encourages you to slow down and truly savor your food when you do eat. Paying attention to the flavors, textures, and smells of each bite helps you enjoy your meal more and feel satisfied with less. This can help prevent overeating and create a more positive relationship with food. In addition to herbs and mindfulness, finding healthier alternatives to traditional comfort foods can make a big difference. When cravings strike, try reaching for a small piece of dark chocolate instead of sugary treats. Dark chocolate can boost your mood without the sugar crash. Nuts and seeds are another great option because they provide healthy fats and protein, keeping you satisfied for longer.

Sometimes, simply sipping on a warm, soothing drink can be enough to calm your mind and reduce the urge to snack. Herbal teas like peppermint, chamomile, or cinnamon can help you relax and provide comfort without extra calories. If you crave something crunchy or sweet, try a homemade mix of dried fruit and nuts, which offers natural sweetness and satisfying texture without the added sugars or unhealthy fats of processed snacks.

Incorporating emotional wellness practices into your routine can also help manage emotional eating. Deep breathing exercises and meditation are effective ways to calm your mind and reduce stress. Just a few minutes of focusing on your breath can help you feel more centered and less likely to turn to food for comfort.

Physical activity is another powerful tool for managing emotions. Exercise releases endorphins, which improve mood and relieve stress. Whether it's a short walk, yoga, or a dance session, moving your body can help shift your focus away from food and towards healthier coping mechanisms.

Journaling is another great way to process emotions without reaching for food. Writing down your thoughts and feelings can help you gain clarity and understand the emotional triggers that lead to overeating. It's a therapeutic practice that allows you to release tension and address the underlying issues behind your emotional eating.

Engaging in creative activities, such as painting, drawing, or playing music, can also provide a healthy outlet for emotional energy. Creativity helps redirect your focus and provides fulfillment without turning to food. This can be especially helpful when you're feeling bored or restless, which are common triggers for emotional eating.

Having a strong support system is crucial for managing emotional eating. Talking to friends, family, or a counselor about your emotions can help you feel less isolated and overwhelmed. Sometimes, just having someone to listen can make a big difference in how you cope with stress. Joining a community or support group, whether online or in-person, can also provide accountability and encouragement as you work through emotional eating challenges.

Nutritional Strategies for Sustainable Weight Loss

Achieving sustainable weight loss is not about following a strict diet for a few weeks or months. It's about making long-term changes that you can stick with, ensuring that your body gets the nutrients it needs while supporting a healthy weight. The goal is to nourish your body, not deprive it, so that you can lose weight in a way that feels natural and maintainable. In this section, we'll explore some key nutritional strategies that can help you manage your weight effectively and in a way that lasts.

One of the most important aspects of sustainable weight loss is focusing on whole, unprocessed foods. These foods are packed with nutrients, which means your body can function optimally while you lose weight. Fresh fruits and vegetables, whole grains, lean proteins, and healthy fats should be the foundation of your meals. They not only provide essential vitamins and minerals but also help you feel fuller for longer, reducing the urge to snack on less healthy options.

A diet rich in fiber is essential for weight management. Foods high in fiber, such as vegetables, fruits, beans, and whole grains, help keep you feeling full by slowing digestion and stabilizing blood sugar levels.

Fiber also supports healthy digestion, which is key to your body efficiently processing nutrients and eliminating waste. By including more fiber-rich foods in your diet, you can naturally reduce calorie intake without feeling deprived.

Protein is another critical component for sustainable weight loss. It helps build and maintain muscle, which boosts your metabolism, meaning you burn more calories throughout the day. Protein also keeps you feeling full, reducing hunger and cravings. Including sources of lean protein like chicken, turkey, fish, eggs, beans, and plant-based options like lentils or tofu in each meal can make a big difference in your weight loss journey.

Healthy fats are often misunderstood, but they play a crucial role in a balanced diet and can aid in weight loss. Rather than cutting out fats completely, focus on incorporating sources of healthy fats like avocados, nuts, seeds, olive oil, and fatty fish. These fats are not only satisfying but also essential for nutrient absorption and hormone regulation, both of which support weight management.

Meal timing can also play a role in sustainable weight loss. Many people find success with strategies like eating smaller, more frequent meals or spacing out meals to avoid snacking too often. Another popular approach is intermittent fasting, which involves eating within a certain window each day, giving the body time to burn fat while not actively digesting food. However, it's important to find a routine that works for your body and lifestyle. The key is consistency.

Another useful tip for managing your weight is to keep an eye on portion sizes. Even when you're eating healthy foods, it's easy to overeat if you're not mindful of portions. Using smaller plates, paying attention to hunger cues, and stopping when you're satisfied, not stuffed, can help you stay on track without counting calories obsessively.

Hydration is often overlooked, but it's essential for both weight loss and overall health. Drinking plenty of water helps keep your metabolism running smoothly and can help you avoid mistaking thirst for hunger. Sometimes, we reach for snacks when our bodies are actually just dehydrated. Starting your day with a glass of water and staying hydrated throughout the day can support your weight loss efforts in a big way.

Sugar and refined carbs are two of the biggest obstacles to sustainable weight loss. These foods cause spikes and crashes in blood sugar, leading to increased hunger and cravings for more unhealthy foods. By reducing or eliminating added sugars and processed carbs like white bread, pastries, and sugary drinks, you can keep your blood sugar stable and reduce your overall calorie intake without feeling deprived.

Instead, focus on complex carbohydrates like whole grains, sweet potatoes, and legumes. These foods provide steady energy and keep you feeling satisfied for longer, making it easier to avoid overeating. The fiber in these foods also supports healthy digestion and helps prevent the blood sugar spikes that lead to cravings.

One of the most helpful strategies for sustainable weight loss is planning and preparing meals ahead of time. When you have healthy meals and snacks ready to go, you're less likely to reach for convenience foods that don't align with your goals. Meal prepping at the start of the week or setting aside time each day to prepare nourishing meals can help you stay consistent and avoid last-minute unhealthy choices. Mindful eating is another powerful tool for weight management. By paying attention to what you're eating and how your body feels, you can avoid overeating and enjoy your food more.

This means slowing down, savoring each bite, and tuning into your body's hunger and fullness signals. Mindful eating helps prevent emotional eating and encourages a healthier relationship with food.

It's also important to allow yourself flexibility and balance. Strict diets that cut out entire food groups or drastically reduce calorie intake are often unsustainable in the long term. Instead, focus on moderation and making healthy choices most of the time, while allowing yourself the occasional treat. This approach helps prevent feelings of deprivation, which can lead to overeating or bingeing later on.

A sustainable approach to weight loss also includes addressing emotional and mental well-being. Stress, lack of sleep, and emotional eating can all contribute to weight gain or make it harder to lose weight. Incorporating stress-management techniques, such as meditation, exercise, or relaxation practices, can support both your mental health and your weight loss goals. Getting enough sleep is also crucial, as sleep deprivation can lead to increased hunger and cravings for high-calorie foods.

Book 24: Skin Healing and Beauty from Within

The Importance of Nutrition for Skin Health

Maintaining healthy, radiant skin is often viewed as a matter of external care—cleansing, moisturizing, and using sunscreen. However, the foundation of great skin starts from within. Nutrition plays a fundamental role in skin health, influencing everything from texture and elasticity to overall appearance. Your skin is a dynamic organ that reflects the state of your internal environment, making it essential to provide it with the right nutrients to keep it vibrant and resilient.

To truly understand the importance of nutrition for skin health, it's helpful to view your skin as a living organ that requires a balanced supply of essential nutrients to function optimally. Just as a well-maintained garden thrives with proper nourishment, your skin flourishes when it receives the right vitamins, minerals, and antioxidants from your diet.

One of the cornerstones of skin health is vitamin A. This vitamin is crucial for the maintenance and repair of skin tissues. It supports the process of cell turnover, where old, dead skin cells are replaced by new, healthy ones. This process is vital for maintaining a smooth, even complexion and for preventing issues like acne and dryness. Foods rich in vitamin A, such as sweet potatoes, carrots, spinach, and kale, are particularly beneficial. They help to strengthen the skin's natural barrier, promoting a healthy, glowing appearance.

Similarly, vitamin C is a powerhouse nutrient with significant benefits for skin health. As a potent antioxidant, vitamin C helps to neutralize harmful free radicals that can damage skin cells and accelerate aging. It also plays a crucial role in collagen synthesis. Collagen is a structural protein that provides your skin with firmness and elasticity. Without adequate collagen, skin can become saggy and wrinkled. Citrus fruits like oranges and grapefruits, along with strawberries, bell peppers, and broccoli, are excellent sources of vitamin C. Including these in your diet can enhance your skin's resilience and maintain its youthful appearance.

Vitamin E, another vital nutrient, works synergistically with vitamin C to protect the skin from oxidative damage. It acts as a powerful antioxidant, helping to reduce inflammation and support the skin's natural healing processes. Vitamin E is found in nuts, seeds, avocados, and leafy greens. Regular consumption of these foods can improve your skin's ability to repair itself and reduce the appearance of fine lines and wrinkles.

Omega-3 fatty acids, found in fatty fish like salmon, as well as flaxseeds and walnuts, are essential for maintaining skin hydration. These healthy fats help to strengthen the skin's lipid barrier, which is crucial for retaining moisture and preventing dryness. Omega-3s also possess anti-inflammatory properties that can help soothe irritated skin and reduce the risk of inflammatory skin conditions such as acne and eczema.

Zinc is another critical mineral that supports skin health. It plays a role in cell growth, repair, and the regulation of oil production. Zinc deficiency can lead to various skin issues, including acne, delayed wound healing, and overall poor skin condition. Foods rich in zinc, such as pumpkin seeds, lentils, chickpeas, and whole grains, can help ensure that your skin remains healthy and resilient.

Hydration is a fundamental aspect of skin care that should not be overlooked. Drinking adequate amounts of water throughout the day is essential for maintaining skin moisture and flushing out toxins. Proper hydration supports the skin's natural elasticity and helps to prevent dryness and dullness.

A balanced diet that includes a variety of colorful fruits and vegetables, whole grains, lean proteins, and healthy fats is key to supporting skin health. Each food group offers unique nutrients that contribute to the overall well-being of your skin. For example, leafy greens provide vitamins and minerals essential for skin repair, while lean proteins supply the amino acids necessary for collagen production.

Herbal Remedies for Acne and Blemishes

Dealing with acne and blemishes can be frustrating, but nature offers a range of gentle and effective remedies to help soothe and clear your skin. Herbs have been used for centuries to treat skin issues, and many of these natural solutions can be surprisingly effective in addressing acne and blemishes.

Tea tree oil is a well-known remedy for acne due to its powerful antibacterial properties. It helps to kill the bacteria responsible for acne and reduces inflammation. To use tea tree oil, dilute a few drops with a carrier oil like coconut or jojoba oil and apply it directly to the affected areas. Be sure to do a patch test first to ensure your skin doesn't have an adverse reaction.

Aloe vera is celebrated for its soothing and healing properties. It helps to reduce redness and inflammation while promoting skin repair. You can apply fresh aloe vera gel directly from the plant to your skin or use a store-bought gel with minimal additives. Apply it as a moisturizer or spot treatment to help calm irritated skin and reduce blemishes.

Chamomile is not just for tea; it's also great for your skin. It has anti-inflammatory and antioxidant properties that can help soothe irritated skin and reduce redness. You can make a chamomile tea and use it as a facial toner by letting it cool and applying it with a cotton pad. For a more concentrated treatment, steep chamomile tea bags, let them cool, and place them on your blemishes for a calming effect.

Witch hazel is a natural astringent that can help tighten the skin and reduce the appearance of pores. It also has anti-inflammatory properties that can soothe irritation. Apply witch hazel to your skin using a cotton ball, focusing on areas prone to breakouts. It's a great addition to your skincare routine to help control oil and reduce blemishes.

Lavender oil is another excellent herb for acne-prone skin. It has antibacterial and anti-inflammatory properties that help reduce acne and promote healing. Dilute lavender oil with a carrier oil and apply it to the affected areas. Its calming scent also makes it a relaxing addition to your skincare regimen.

Neem is known for its powerful antibacterial and antifungal properties. It can help clear up acne and reduce inflammation. You can use neem oil or make a neem paste by grinding neem leaves and applying it to your skin. Leave it on for about 10-15 minutes before rinsing off. Neem is particularly useful for treating stubborn acne and promoting clearer skin.

Turmeric contains curcumin, which has anti-inflammatory and antioxidant properties. It can help reduce redness and swelling associated with acne. Create a turmeric paste by mixing turmeric powder with a little water or honey, and apply it to the affected areas. Leave it on for about 10 minutes before rinsing off. Be cautious, as turmeric can sometimes leave a temporary yellow stain on your skin.

Green tea is rich in antioxidants and has anti-inflammatory properties that can help with acne. You can use green tea both topically and internally. For topical use, brew a strong cup of green tea, let it cool, and apply it to your skin with a cotton ball. Drinking green tea regularly can also help reduce inflammation and support overall skin health.

Peppermint has cooling and soothing effects on the skin. Its menthol content can help reduce itching and inflammation. You can make a peppermint tea and use it as a facial rinse or apply diluted peppermint oil to affected areas. Peppermint helps to refresh your skin and provides a cooling sensation.

Rosewater is known for its gentle and soothing properties. It helps to balance the skin's pH and reduce redness. Use rosewater as a toner by applying it with a cotton pad after cleansing. It can also be used as a refreshing facial mist throughout the day to help maintain skin hydration.

Essential Oils for Skin Radiance

When it comes to achieving glowing, radiant skin, essential oils can be a game-changer. These concentrated plant extracts are packed with powerful nutrients that can transform your skin care routine. They not only offer a natural alternative to commercial products but also bring a touch of luxury and indulgence to your daily regimen.
Here's a guide to some of the best essential oils for enhancing skin radiance, each with its unique benefits:

Lavender oil is a versatile essential oil with a reputation for its soothing and calming effects. It helps to balance skin tone, reduce redness, and promote healing. Lavender's gentle nature makes it suitable for all skin types, including sensitive skin. You can add a few drops to your moisturizer or face oil, or use it in a calming facial steam to enhance your skin's natural glow.

Rose geranium oil is known for its ability to balance oil production and improve skin texture. It helps to even out skin tone, reduce the appearance of blemishes, and enhance overall radiance. Its sweet, floral scent adds a touch of luxury to your skincare routine. Dilute rose geranium oil with a carrier oil and apply it to your face or mix it into your daily moisturizer for a beautiful, radiant complexion.

Frankincense oil has been prized for centuries for its rejuvenating properties. It helps to reduce the appearance of fine lines and wrinkles, promote cell regeneration, and improve skin tone. Its warm, earthy aroma is also incredibly grounding and calming. You can blend frankincense oil with a carrier oil and gently massage it into your skin to enhance its elasticity and glow.

Sandalwood oil is known for its soothing and hydrating properties. It helps to calm inflammation, reduce dryness, and promote a healthy, radiant complexion. Its rich, woody scent also provides a sense of relaxation. Add a few drops of sandalwood oil to your nighttime skincare routine by mixing it with a carrier oil or your favorite moisturizer to help maintain soft, glowing skin.

Tea tree oil is renowned for its powerful antibacterial and antifungal properties, making it a great choice for managing blemishes and promoting clear skin. While it's best known for its acne-fighting benefits, tea tree oil also helps to balance the skin's oil production, leading to a more even complexion. Dilute tea tree oil with a carrier oil and apply it to problem areas or mix it into your daily skincare products for clearer, healthier skin.

Ylang-ylang oil is celebrated for its ability to balance oil production and improve skin elasticity. It has a sweet, exotic fragrance that makes it a delightful addition to your skincare routine. Ylang-ylang oil can help reduce the appearance of fine lines and promote a youthful glow. Mix a few drops with a carrier oil and gently massage it into your skin to enjoy its radiant effects.

Carrot seed oil is rich in antioxidants and essential vitamins that help rejuvenate and revitalize the skin. It promotes cell regeneration and helps to even out skin tone, making it a great choice for achieving a radiant complexion. The oil has a slightly earthy aroma and can be blended with a carrier oil and applied to your skin to boost its natural glow.

Neroli oil, derived from orange blossoms, is known for its brightening and rejuvenating properties. It helps to improve skin texture, reduce the appearance of dark spots, and enhance overall radiance. Neroli oil has a beautiful, floral scent that adds a touch of elegance to your skincare routine. Incorporate it into your routine by blending it with a carrier oil and applying it to your face for a radiant, youthful appearance.

Though technically a carrier oil, jojoba oil is often included in essential oil blends for its remarkable similarity to the skin's natural sebum. It helps to moisturize and balance the skin, enhancing its natural glow. Jojoba oil can be used on its own or as a base for other essential oils. It's perfect for creating a nourishing blend that leaves your skin feeling soft and radiant.

Patchouli oil is known for its grounding and calming effects. It helps to improve skin texture, reduce the appearance of scars, and promote a healthy, glowing complexion. Its rich, earthy aroma adds a sense of luxury to your skincare routine. Blend patchouli oil with a carrier oil and apply it to your skin to enjoy its radiant benefits.

Healing Eczema and Psoriasis Naturally

Dealing with eczema and psoriasis can be challenging, but nature offers a wealth of soothing remedies that can help manage and alleviate these conditions. Both eczema and psoriasis are chronic skin conditions that cause inflammation, redness, and irritation. While they require a comprehensive approach to manage, incorporating natural remedies can make a significant difference in soothing symptoms and supporting overall skin health.

Coconut oil is a fantastic natural moisturizer that can help soothe dry, itchy skin associated with eczema and psoriasis. Its rich, fatty acid content provides deep hydration and creates a protective barrier to lock in moisture. Coconut oil also has anti-inflammatory and antimicrobial properties that can help reduce irritation and prevent infections. Simply apply a thin layer of pure coconut oil to the affected areas several times a day to keep your skin hydrated and calm.

Aloe vera is well-known for its soothing and healing properties. It helps to reduce inflammation, alleviate itching, and promote skin repair. You can use fresh aloe vera gel directly from the plant or opt for a store-bought product with minimal additives. Apply aloe vera gel to the affected areas as needed to cool and calm the skin.

Oatmeal baths are a time-tested remedy for soothing irritated skin. Oats contain anti-inflammatory compounds that help to reduce itching and inflammation. To prepare an oatmeal bath, add a cup of colloidal oatmeal (finely ground oats) to lukewarm bathwater and soak for 15-20 minutes. Pat your skin dry with a soft towel and apply a moisturizer immediately afterward to lock in the benefits.

Apple cider vinegar has natural antibacterial and anti-inflammatory properties that can help soothe eczema and psoriasis flare-ups. It can be used as a diluted topical treatment or added to a bath. To use it topically, dilute apple cider vinegar with an equal amount of water and apply it to the affected areas using a cotton ball. For a bath, add a cup of apple cider vinegar to lukewarm water and soak for 15 minutes. Be cautious if you have open wounds or very sensitive skin, as vinegar can cause irritation.

Certain essential oils can offer soothing and anti-inflammatory benefits for eczema and psoriasis. Lavender oil is known for its calming effects and can help reduce itching and irritation. Chamomile oil has anti-inflammatory properties that can soothe inflamed skin. Always dilute essential oils with a carrier oil, such as coconut or jojoba oil, before applying them to your skin. Apply a small amount to the affected areas once or twice daily.

Honey is a natural humectant, meaning it attracts and retains moisture. It also has antimicrobial properties that can help prevent infection in damaged skin. Apply raw honey to the affected areas and leave it on for 15-20 minutes before rinsing off with lukewarm water. Honey can help keep the skin moisturized and support the healing process.

Calendula, also known as marigold, has been used for centuries to treat skin conditions due to its anti-inflammatory and healing properties. Calendula oil or creams can help reduce redness and promote healing. Apply calendula oil or an ointment containing calendula extract to the affected areas as needed.

Epsom salt is rich in magnesium, which can help reduce inflammation and ease discomfort. Adding Epsom salt to your bath can help soothe itchy, irritated skin. Dissolve 1-2 cups of Epsom salt in a warm bath and soak for 15-20 minutes. Rinse off with clean water and follow up with a moisturizer.

What you eat can also impact your skin health. Incorporating anti-inflammatory foods such as fatty fish (rich in omega-3 fatty acids), leafy greens, nuts, and seeds can support overall skin health. Avoiding triggers such as processed foods, excessive sugar, and dairy may also help reduce flare-ups.

Stress can exacerbate both eczema and psoriasis. Finding ways to manage stress, such as through mindfulness practices, yoga, or regular exercise, can help keep symptoms under control. A holistic approach that includes stress management, along with natural remedies, can make a big difference in your overall well-being.

Detoxifying the Skin Through Natural Methods

Our skin is not just a protective barrier; it's also a reflection of our overall health. To maintain a vibrant, healthy complexion, it's essential to support your skin's natural detoxification processes. Luckily, there are many natural methods you can use to help your skin clear out impurities and achieve a radiant glow. One of the simplest and most effective ways to detoxify your skin is by staying well-hydrated. Drinking plenty of water throughout the day helps flush out toxins from your body and keeps your skin hydrated. Aim for at least eight glasses of water daily. You can also enhance your hydration routine by adding slices of lemon or cucumber to your water, which not only makes it more refreshing but also provides additional detoxifying benefits.

Incorporating green tea into your daily routine is another excellent way to support your skin's detoxification. Green tea is rich in antioxidants, which help combat oxidative stress and inflammation.

Drinking a cup of green tea each day or using it as a facial toner can help clear out impurities and protect your skin from damage. To use green tea as a toner, simply brew a strong cup, let it cool, and then apply it to your face with a cotton pad.

Activated charcoal is another powerful natural detoxifier for the skin. It works by drawing out impurities and toxins from your pores, leaving your skin feeling clean and refreshed. You can use an activated charcoal mask once a week to help purify your skin. Apply the mask according to the product instructions, and make sure to follow up with a moisturizer to keep your skin from drying out.

Exfoliation is key to maintaining healthy, glowing skin. Regularly removing dead skin cells helps promote new cell growth and keeps your skin looking fresh. Natural exfoliants, such as oatmeal, sugar, or coffee grounds, can be mixed with ingredients like honey or yogurt to create a gentle scrub. Use the scrub once or twice a week to slough off dead skin and reveal a smoother, more radiant complexion.

Eating a diet rich in detoxifying foods can also support your skin's natural cleansing process. Leafy greens, beets, and citrus fruits are packed with vitamins and antioxidants that help cleanse the body and improve skin clarity. Including these foods in your meals can enhance your skin's ability to detoxify from within.

Clay masks, such as bentonite or French green clay, are excellent for deep cleansing the skin. These masks work by binding to toxins and drawing them out of your pores. Apply a clay mask once a week to help remove impurities and excess oil, and rinse it off once it's dry for a cleaner, clearer complexion.

Herbal steams provide a soothing way to open up your pores and release trapped toxins. To prepare a herbal steam, boil a pot of water and add a handful of dried herbs like chamomile, mint, or rosemary. Position your face over the steam with a towel draped over your head to trap the steam. Steam your face for about 5 to 10 minutes, then rinse with cool water and follow up with a toner and moisturizer.

Apple cider vinegar is a versatile natural remedy that can help balance your skin's pH and remove impurities. As a facial toner, dilute apple cider vinegar with equal parts water and apply it to your skin with a cotton pad. Alternatively, you can add a cup of apple cider vinegar to your bathwater for a detoxifying soak.

Adopting a healthy lifestyle can also greatly benefit your skin. Regular exercise boosts circulation and helps flush out toxins through sweating. A balanced diet full of fruits, vegetables, and whole grains supports overall skin health. Additionally, avoiding excessive alcohol, smoking, and high-sugar foods can contribute to a clearer complexion.

Lastly, don't underestimate the power of a good night's sleep. Your skin rejuvenates and repairs itself while you sleep, so aim for 7 to 9 hours of restful sleep each night. Establishing a calming bedtime routine, such as using a soothing lavender essential oil or reading a book, can help you unwind and support your skin's natural detoxification process.

Preventing Premature Aging with Natural Products

As we age, our skin undergoes changes that are often influenced by various factors like sun exposure, lifestyle, and environmental stressors. While aging is a natural process, there are several natural ways to help slow it down and keep your skin looking youthful and vibrant.

Embracing natural products in your skincare routine can be a gentle yet effective approach to preventing premature aging. Here's how you can do it.

Hydration is fundamental for maintaining youthful skin. One of the most beneficial ways to keep your skin hydrated is by using natural oils. Oils such as argan oil, jojoba oil, and rosehip oil are packed with essential fatty acids and vitamins that nourish and hydrate the skin. These oils help to maintain skin elasticity and reduce the appearance of fine lines. Applying a few drops of these oils to your face and neck daily can make a noticeable difference in your skin's texture and glow.

Antioxidants play a crucial role in protecting your skin from damage caused by free radicals. Free radicals are unstable molecules that can accelerate the aging process. Incorporating antioxidant-rich foods into your diet, such as berries, green tea, and nuts, can help combat oxidative stress. Additionally, skincare products containing antioxidants like vitamin C can brighten the skin and diminish dark spots, contributing to a more youthful appearance.

Aloe vera is another powerful natural ingredient that can help combat premature aging. Known for its soothing and healing properties, aloe vera helps to hydrate the skin and boost collagen production. Applying fresh aloe vera gel directly from the plant can promote skin renewal and improve texture. If you prefer, look for skincare products that feature aloe vera as a key ingredient for its rejuvenating effects.

Sun protection is crucial in preventing premature aging, as UV exposure is a major cause of wrinkles and age spots. Opt for natural sunscreens that contain ingredients like zinc oxide or titanium dioxide, which provide effective protection from harmful UV rays without the harsh chemicals found in some commercial sunscreens. Applying sunscreen daily, even on cloudy days, helps shield your skin from sun damage and maintains its youthful appearance.

Exfoliation is important for removing dead skin cells and encouraging the growth of new, healthy cells. Natural exfoliants, such as sugar, coffee grounds, or oatmeal, can be used to create a gentle scrub for your face. Mixing these exfoliants with honey or yogurt not only exfoliates but also provides added hydration. Regular exfoliation, about once or twice a week, helps keep your skin smooth and radiant. Green tea is not just beneficial when consumed; it also offers great benefits for your skin when used topically. Green tea's antioxidant and anti-inflammatory properties can help soothe the skin and reduce signs of aging. To make a green tea facial toner, brew a strong cup of green tea, let it cool, and apply it to your face with a cotton pad. This simple remedy refreshes your skin and helps reduce the appearance of fine lines.

Honey, known for its natural humectant properties, attracts and retains moisture, making it an excellent ingredient for hydration. Additionally, honey has antimicrobial properties that support skin health. Applying raw honey as a mask and leaving it on for 15-20 minutes before rinsing off can help keep your skin hydrated and assist in its natural healing process.

Vitamin E is a potent antioxidant that supports skin repair and protection. It can help reduce the appearance of scars and fine lines. You can apply vitamin E oil directly to your skin or choose skincare products enriched with this nutrient. Regular use of vitamin E helps improve skin texture and maintain a youthful look.

Incorporating a diet rich in fresh fruits and vegetables is another way to support skin health. These foods provide essential vitamins and antioxidants that help combat signs of aging.

Vitamins A, C, and E are particularly beneficial for preventing premature aging. Adding carrots, spinach, and citrus fruits to your meals can enhance your skin's natural glow and resilience.

Lastly, getting adequate rest is essential for maintaining youthful skin. While you sleep, your body repairs and regenerates, including your skin. Aiming for 7-9 hours of quality sleep each night allows your skin to recover and renew itself. Establishing a calming bedtime routine can improve sleep quality and contribute to a more youthful complexion.

DIY Natural Beauty Recipes for Radiant Skin

Creating your own natural beauty recipes at home can be both delightful and effective, offering you a way to nurture your skin with ingredients that are kind to your complexion. By embracing DIY beauty treatments, you can harness the power of nature to achieve glowing, radiant skin. Here's how you can use everyday ingredients to craft your own skin-loving treatments.

One of the simplest and most nourishing treatments you can make is an avocado face mask. Avocado is renowned for its rich content of healthy fats, vitamins E and C, and antioxidants. These nutrients work together to deeply moisturize and rejuvenate the skin. To prepare the mask, mash half an avocado until smooth, and mix it with a tablespoon of honey. Apply this creamy blend to your face, leave it on for 15-20 minutes, and then rinse off with warm water. This treatment will leave your skin feeling incredibly soft and revitalized.

Another excellent option for achieving radiant skin is a revitalizing green tea facial toner. Green tea is packed with antioxidants and has anti-inflammatory properties that can soothe the skin and protect it from damage. Brew a strong cup of green tea and allow it to cool completely. Once cooled, transfer the tea into a clean spray bottle. After cleansing your face, spritz the green tea toner onto your skin. Let it dry naturally, and then follow up with your favorite moisturizer. This toner refreshes and revitalizes the skin while offering antioxidant protection.

For those looking to hydrate and calm their skin, a cucumber and yogurt mask is a great choice. Cucumber is known for its soothing and hydrating properties, while yogurt provides gentle exfoliation and nourishment. To make the mask, blend half a cucumber with two tablespoons of plain yogurt until you have a smooth mixture. Apply this mask to your face and let it sit for 15-20 minutes before rinsing with cool water. Your skin will feel refreshed and deeply hydrated, with a noticeable glow.

If you're aiming to brighten your complexion, consider making a lemon and honey scrub. Lemon is known for its brightening effects, and when combined with honey, it creates an exfoliating scrub that helps even out skin tone. Mix one tablespoon of lemon juice with two tablespoons of honey and a tablespoon of sugar. Gently massage this mixture onto your face in circular motions, taking care to avoid the eye area. Rinse with lukewarm water to reveal a brighter, more radiant complexion.

For a refreshing and calming toner, you can create a rosewater and aloe vera blend. Rosewater is famous for its soothing and balancing effects, while aloe vera provides hydration and healing. Simply mix equal parts of rosewater and aloe vera gel. Apply this mixture to your face using a cotton pad or spray bottle after cleansing. This toner helps balance the skin's pH, reduce redness, and provide a calming effect.

Another effective DIY beauty treatment is an exfoliating coffee and coconut oil scrub. Coffee grounds offer natural exfoliation, while coconut oil provides deep moisturization. Combine two tablespoons of coffee grounds with one tablespoon of melted coconut oil.

Gently massage this scrub onto your face and body in circular motions, then rinse with warm water. This scrub helps remove dead skin cells and invigorates the skin, leaving it smooth and glowing.

For a soothing treatment, consider an oatmeal and honey mask. Oatmeal is gentle and calming, making it perfect for sensitive or irritated skin. Mix two tablespoons of finely ground oatmeal with one tablespoon of honey and a splash of warm water to create a paste. Apply this mask to your face and leave it on for about 15 minutes. Rinse with lukewarm water to soothe and hydrate your skin, reducing redness and irritation.

If you're looking to clarify your complexion, a diluted apple cider vinegar toner might be just what you need. Apple cider vinegar helps balance the skin's pH and acts as a natural astringent. To make this toner, dilute one part apple cider vinegar with two parts water. Apply this mixture to your face with a cotton pad after cleansing. It can help minimize pores and promote a clearer complexion. Be sure to follow with a moisturizer to keep your skin hydrated.

A honey and turmeric mask is another excellent option for brightening and healing the skin. Turmeric is known for its anti-inflammatory and antioxidant properties, while honey helps to moisturize. Mix one tablespoon of honey with a pinch of turmeric powder to create a paste. Apply this mask to your face and leave it on for 10-15 minutes. Rinse with warm water to brighten your skin and reduce inflammation.

Finally, a mint and yogurt face pack can be wonderfully refreshing. Mint has a cooling effect that rejuvenates tired skin, and yogurt provides gentle exfoliation. Blend a handful of fresh mint leaves with two tablespoons of plain yogurt. Apply this mixture to your face and leave it on for about 10-15 minutes before rinsing off. This face pack helps to revitalize your skin and give it a fresh, healthy glow.

Book 25: Natural Remedies for Allergies and Asthma

Understanding the Root Causes of Allergies

Allergies can feel like a mystery, often leaving us puzzled about why our bodies react so strongly to certain substances. Understanding the root causes of allergies can shed light on this complex issue and help you manage your symptoms more effectively. Let's explore what might be behind those allergy triggers and how they impact your body.

At its core, an allergy is an overreaction of the immune system to substances that are typically harmless. These substances, known as allergens, can include a wide range of things like pollen, pet dander, certain foods, or even dust mites. Your immune system's job is to protect you from harmful invaders, but sometimes it mistakenly identifies these harmless substances as threats.

When you come into contact with an allergen, your immune system responds by producing a type of antibody called immunoglobulin E (IgE). This antibody attaches to certain cells called mast cells and basophils, which are found in various tissues throughout your body. When the allergen reappears, these cells release chemicals like histamine into the bloodstream. Histamine is what causes many of the symptoms we associate with allergies, such as itching, swelling, and mucus production.

There are several factors that contribute to why some people develop allergies. Genetics play a significant role—if you have a family history of allergies, you may be more likely to develop them yourself. This genetic predisposition affects how your immune system reacts to allergens.

Environmental factors also play a crucial role in the development of allergies. Exposure to certain allergens during critical periods of development, such as childhood, can influence whether or not you develop an allergy. For instance, growing up in a highly sanitized environment may contribute to an increased risk of allergies because your immune system may not have been exposed to a variety of substances, leading it to overreact to harmless ones.

Moreover, lifestyle choices and environmental conditions can exacerbate allergic reactions. For example, exposure to pollution, cigarette smoke, and other irritants can increase the likelihood of developing allergies or worsen existing ones. Maintaining a clean living environment and avoiding irritants can help manage allergy symptoms more effectively.

Another aspect to consider is the role of the gut microbiome in immune function. Emerging research suggests that the balance of bacteria in your gut can influence your body's immune responses. A healthy, diverse gut microbiome may help regulate immune responses and reduce the likelihood of developing allergies. Consuming a diet rich in fiber and probiotics can support gut health and potentially play a role in allergy prevention.

It's also worth noting that allergies can develop at any stage of life, even if you have previously been unaffected. Sometimes, changes in the environment, diet, or lifestyle can trigger new allergies or cause existing ones to become more pronounced.

By understanding the root causes of allergies, you can take proactive steps to manage your symptoms and improve your quality of life. Identifying and avoiding specific allergens, maintaining a healthy lifestyle, and supporting your immune system with a balanced diet are all ways to help manage and reduce allergy symptoms.

Herbal Remedies for Respiratory Health

Taking care of your respiratory health is essential for overall well-being, especially if you're dealing with conditions like asthma or allergies. Herbal remedies can be a natural and effective way to support your respiratory system and ease breathing difficulties. Let's explore some wonderful herbs that can help you breathe easier and stay healthy.

One of the most popular herbs for respiratory health is peppermint. Peppermint contains menthol, a natural compound that acts as a decongestant, helping to clear mucus from the airways. It also has soothing properties that can ease coughing and open up the nasal passages. You can enjoy peppermint as a tea or use peppermint essential oil in a diffuser to help relieve congestion and promote easier breathing.

Eucalyptus is another fantastic herb for respiratory health. It's well-known for its ability to help clear the airways and reduce inflammation. Eucalyptus oil can be used in steam inhalation by adding a few drops to a bowl of hot water and breathing in the steam. This can help loosen mucus and ease congestion. You can also find eucalyptus in some chest rubs and inhalers for an added respiratory boost.

Thyme is not only a flavorful herb but also a powerful ally for respiratory health. It has antimicrobial properties that can help fight off infections and soothe the throat. Thyme tea can be a comforting way to ease coughing and promote respiratory wellness. To make thyme tea, steep a few sprigs of fresh thyme or a teaspoon of dried thyme in hot water for about 10 minutes. Drink this tea to help soothe your respiratory system and enjoy its beneficial effects.

For those dealing with chronic respiratory issues, licorice root may offer some relief. Licorice root has anti-inflammatory and soothing properties that can help reduce inflammation in the airways and ease coughing. You can enjoy licorice root as a tea or take it in supplement form. However, it's best to consult with a healthcare provider before using licorice root, especially if you have high blood pressure or other health conditions.

Ginger is another herb that supports respiratory health. It has anti-inflammatory and antioxidant properties that can help reduce inflammation in the airways and strengthen the immune system. Fresh ginger tea is a great way to enjoy its benefits. Simply slice a few pieces of fresh ginger and steep them in hot water for 10 minutes. This tea can help soothe your throat and support overall respiratory health.

Mullein is a lesser-known but effective herb for respiratory support. It has been used traditionally to treat coughs, bronchitis, and asthma. Mullein helps to soothe and clear the respiratory tract. You can find mullein in tea form or as an extract. Drinking mullein tea or using a mullein tincture can help alleviate respiratory discomfort and support lung health.

Elderberry is another herb that's gaining popularity for its immune-boosting and anti-inflammatory properties. Elderberry helps to support the immune system and may reduce the severity and duration of respiratory infections. Elderberry syrup or tea can be a tasty and effective way to incorporate this herb into your routine.

Lastly, slippery elm is known for its soothing properties, which can help relieve irritation in the throat and respiratory tract. Slippery elm contains mucilage, a gel-like substance that coats and soothes the mucous membranes. You can use slippery elm powder to make a soothing tea or lozenge, which can help calm coughing and throat irritation.

Managing Seasonal Allergies Naturally

Seasonal allergies can be a real challenge, especially when pollen counts are high and your nose starts to feel like a running faucet. But don't worry—there are plenty of natural remedies and lifestyle changes you can make to help manage those pesky symptoms and keep your seasonal allergies in check.

One of the simplest and most effective ways to manage seasonal allergies naturally is by incorporating local honey into your diet. The idea is that local honey contains trace amounts of local pollen, which might help your body build a tolerance to these allergens over time. Try adding a spoonful of local honey to your tea or yogurt daily. Just remember, it's best to start this remedy before allergy season begins for the most benefit.

Keeping your home environment allergen-free is also crucial. Consider using an air purifier with a HEPA filter to help trap pollen and other allergens in the air. Regularly cleaning your home, including vacuuming carpets and washing bedding in hot water, can also help reduce the presence of allergens. Make sure to also wash your hands and change your clothes after spending time outdoors to avoid bringing pollen inside.

Nasal irrigation is another great natural method for managing seasonal allergies. Using a saline solution or a neti pot to rinse your nasal passages can help flush out pollen and other irritants. This simple practice can reduce congestion and help you breathe easier. Just be sure to use sterile water and clean your neti pot thoroughly to avoid any risk of infection.

Incorporating anti-inflammatory foods into your diet can also provide relief from allergy symptoms. Foods rich in omega-3 fatty acids, like flaxseeds, chia seeds, and walnuts, have anti-inflammatory properties that can help reduce the inflammation caused by allergies. Additionally, incorporating fruits and vegetables high in antioxidants, such as berries, spinach, and kale, can support your immune system and help combat allergy symptoms.

Herbal teas can be both soothing and beneficial for seasonal allergy relief. Teas made from nettles or butterbur are known for their natural antihistamine properties. Drinking a cup of nettle tea or butterbur tea each day may help reduce allergy symptoms. Just be sure to consult with a healthcare professional before trying new herbs, especially if you are on other medications.

Essential oils can also play a role in managing seasonal allergies. Eucalyptus oil and peppermint oil are both known for their ability to help clear nasal congestion and soothe respiratory discomfort. You can use these oils in a diffuser or add a few drops to a bowl of hot water and inhale the steam. Essential oils can provide a natural way to alleviate symptoms and help you breathe easier.

Lastly, consider adding probiotics to your daily routine. A healthy gut microbiome can have a positive impact on your immune system and reduce allergic reactions. Probiotic-rich foods like yogurt, kefir, and fermented vegetables can support your digestive health and potentially help in managing seasonal allergies.

Preventing Asthma Attacks with Natural Approaches

Living with asthma can be challenging, but there are many natural approaches you can use to help prevent asthma attacks and manage your symptoms effectively. By incorporating some lifestyle changes and natural remedies into your routine, you can support your respiratory health and reduce the frequency and severity of asthma attacks.

One of the key strategies for preventing asthma attacks is to identify and avoid triggers. Common asthma triggers include allergens like pollen, dust mites, and pet dander, as well as irritants such as smoke, strong odors, and pollution. Keeping track of your symptoms and noting when they worsen can help you pinpoint what might be causing your attacks. Once you identify your triggers, you can take steps to minimize your exposure to them. For example, using an air purifier with a HEPA filter in your home can help reduce airborne allergens and irritants.

Incorporating anti-inflammatory foods into your diet can also support your respiratory health and help prevent asthma attacks. Foods rich in omega-3 fatty acids, such as flaxseeds, chia seeds, and walnuts, have anti-inflammatory properties that can help reduce airway inflammation. Fruits and vegetables high in antioxidants, like berries, oranges, and leafy greens, can also support lung health and boost your immune system.

Another helpful approach is to use herbal remedies that have been shown to support respiratory health. For instance, ginger and turmeric are both known for their anti-inflammatory properties. Adding fresh ginger to your meals or drinking turmeric tea can help reduce inflammation in the airways. Similarly, licorice root is traditionally used to soothe the respiratory tract and support lung health. You can enjoy licorice root tea, but make sure to consult with a healthcare provider before starting any new herbal treatments, especially if you are on other medications.

Breathing exercises can also play a significant role in managing asthma. Techniques such as diaphragmatic breathing and pursed-lip breathing can help improve lung function and increase oxygen intake. Regular practice of these exercises can strengthen your respiratory muscles and help you control your breathing during an asthma attack. Consider incorporating these exercises into your daily routine to enhance your lung capacity and overall respiratory health.

Maintaining a healthy weight is important for asthma management as well. Excess weight can put additional strain on your lungs and make asthma symptoms worse. A balanced diet and regular physical activity can help you achieve and maintain a healthy weight, which can, in turn, reduce asthma symptoms. However, be sure to choose activities that are suitable for your condition and avoid exercising in extreme temperatures or environments that could trigger your asthma.

Stress management is another key factor in preventing asthma attacks. Stress and anxiety can trigger asthma symptoms or make them worse. Incorporating relaxation techniques such as yoga, meditation, or deep-breathing exercises into your routine can help manage stress and promote overall well-being. Finding activities that help you relax and unwind can have a positive impact on your respiratory health.

Foods and Supplements for Allergy Relief

Dealing with allergies can sometimes feel like a never-ending battle, but there are some natural ways to ease your symptoms and find relief. A balanced diet and certain supplements can play a significant role in managing allergies and keeping those pesky symptoms at bay. Let's dive into some foods and supplements that can help support your body and reduce allergy-related discomfort.

When it comes to foods that can help with allergy relief, focusing on those with anti-inflammatory properties is key. Omega-3 fatty acids are known for their ability to reduce inflammation, which can be beneficial for managing allergy symptoms. You can find omega-3s in foods like flaxseeds, chia seeds, walnuts, and fatty fish such as salmon and sardines. Including these foods in your diet can help support your immune system and potentially lessen the severity of your allergic reactions.

Quercetin, a natural compound found in many fruits and vegetables, is another powerful ally against allergies. It acts as a natural antihistamine, helping to reduce the release of histamine in your body, which is responsible for many allergy symptoms. You can boost your quercetin intake by enjoying foods like apples, onions, berries, and leafy greens. Adding these to your meals can provide a tasty way to support your allergy relief efforts.

Vitamin C is also a great nutrient for allergy relief. It has antioxidant properties that help stabilize mast cells, which release histamine during allergic reactions. Foods rich in vitamin C, such as oranges, strawberries, bell peppers, and broccoli, can be a delicious and effective way to support your immune system and reduce allergy symptoms.

Incorporating probiotics into your diet can also be beneficial. Probiotics help maintain a healthy balance of bacteria in your gut, which plays a role in regulating your immune system. A healthy gut microbiome can help your body manage allergies more effectively. You can find probiotics in foods like yogurt, kefir, sauerkraut, and other fermented foods. If you're considering a probiotic supplement, look for one with a variety of strains for the best results.

Nettle is an herb that has been traditionally used to help manage allergy symptoms. It contains natural antihistamines that can help reduce sneezing and itching. You can find nettle in the form of tea or capsules. Drinking nettle tea or taking a nettle supplement may provide some relief from seasonal allergies.

Butterbur is another herbal supplement known for its potential to help with allergy relief. It has been shown to reduce symptoms of hay fever and other allergy-related conditions. Butterbur supplements should be taken with caution, as they can have side effects and may interact with other medications. Always consult with a healthcare provider before starting any new supplement.

Spirulina, a type of blue-green algae, is another supplement that may offer allergy relief. It has anti-inflammatory and immune-boosting properties that can help manage allergy symptoms. Spirulina is available in powder or tablet form and can be a great addition to smoothies or your daily supplement routine.

Zinc is an essential mineral that supports your immune system and may help reduce allergy symptoms. Foods rich in zinc, such as pumpkin seeds, nuts, and whole grains, can help ensure you're getting enough of this important nutrient. Zinc supplements can also be considered, but it's best to talk to a healthcare provider to determine the right dosage for you.

Detoxifying the Body to Reduce Allergic Reactions

When it comes to managing allergies, detoxifying your body can be a helpful strategy to reduce allergic reactions and support overall health. By focusing on natural ways to cleanse and support your body's detoxification processes, you can help minimize the impact of allergens and promote a healthier immune system. Let's explore some gentle and effective ways to detoxify your body and enhance your allergy management.

Hydration is one of the simplest and most effective ways to support your body's natural detoxification processes. Drinking plenty of water throughout the day helps flush out toxins and keeps your organs functioning optimally. Aim to drink at least eight glasses of water daily, and consider adding a splash of lemon juice for an extra boost. Lemon water can help stimulate digestion and promote the detoxification of the liver.

Incorporating fiber-rich foods into your diet is another great way to support your body's detoxification efforts. Fiber helps to keep your digestive system moving and aids in the elimination of waste products. Foods like fruits, vegetables, whole grains, and legumes are excellent sources of fiber. Try to include a variety of these foods in your daily meals to support healthy digestion and help your body remove toxins more effectively.

Green tea is a fantastic beverage to include in your detox regimen. Rich in antioxidants, particularly catechins, green tea helps to combat oxidative stress and support the liver's detoxification processes. Drinking a cup or two of green tea each day can provide a gentle boost to your body's natural cleansing mechanisms and help reduce inflammation.

Cruciferous vegetables, such as broccoli, cauliflower, Brussels sprouts, and kale, are excellent choices for supporting detoxification. These vegetables contain compounds that help the liver process and eliminate toxins. They also have anti-inflammatory properties that can benefit your overall health and help manage allergic reactions. Try to include these veggies in your meals a few times a week for optimal benefits.

Herbal teas can also play a role in detoxification. Herbs like dandelion root, milk thistle, and burdock root are known for their liver-supportive properties. Drinking herbal teas made from these herbs can help support your liver's function and promote overall detoxification. Dandelion root tea, in particular, is great for stimulating liver function and aiding digestion.

Sweating is another natural way your body detoxifies itself. Regular exercise can help you sweat out toxins and improve circulation. Activities like jogging, cycling, or even a brisk walk can promote sweating and support your body's natural detoxification processes. If you enjoy a sauna, spending some time there can also help you sweat and eliminate toxins through your skin.

Avoiding processed foods and refined sugars is crucial for supporting your body's detoxification efforts. These foods can contribute to inflammation and put additional strain on your liver. Instead, focus on whole, unprocessed foods that nourish your body and support healthy liver function. Fresh fruits, vegetables, lean proteins, and whole grains are all excellent choices.

Detoxifying the Body to Reduce Allergic Reactions

When it comes to managing allergies, detoxifying your body can be a helpful strategy to reduce allergic reactions and support overall health. By focusing on natural ways to cleanse and support your body's detoxification processes, you can help minimize the impact of allergens and promote a healthier immune system. Let's explore some gentle and effective ways to detoxify your body and enhance your allergy management.

Hydration is one of the simplest and most effective ways to support your body's natural detoxification processes. Drinking plenty of water throughout the day helps flush out toxins and keeps your organs functioning optimally. Aim to drink at least eight glasses of water daily, and consider adding a splash of lemon juice for an extra boost. Lemon water can help stimulate digestion and promote the detoxification of the liver.

Incorporating fiber-rich foods into your diet is another great way to support your body's detoxification efforts. Fiber helps to keep your digestive system moving and aids in the elimination of waste products. Foods like fruits, vegetables, whole grains, and legumes are excellent sources of fiber. Try to include a variety of these foods in your daily meals to support healthy digestion and help your body remove toxins more effectively.

Green tea is a fantastic beverage to include in your detox regimen. Rich in antioxidants, particularly catechins, green tea helps to combat oxidative stress and support the liver's detoxification processes. Drinking a cup or two of green tea each day can provide a gentle boost to your body's natural cleansing mechanisms and help reduce inflammation.

Cruciferous vegetables, such as broccoli, cauliflower, Brussels sprouts, and kale, are excellent choices for supporting detoxification. These vegetables contain compounds that help the liver process and eliminate toxins. They also have anti-inflammatory properties that can benefit your overall health and help manage allergic reactions. Try to include these veggies in your meals a few times a week for optimal benefits.

Herbal teas can also play a role in detoxification. Herbs like dandelion root, milk thistle, and burdock root are known for their liver-supportive properties. Drinking herbal teas made from these herbs can help support your liver's function and promote overall detoxification. Dandelion root tea, in particular, is great for stimulating liver function and aiding digestion.

Sweating is another natural way your body detoxifies itself. Regular exercise can help you sweat out toxins and improve circulation. Activities like jogging, cycling, or even a brisk walk can promote sweating and support your body's natural detoxification processes. If you enjoy a sauna, spending some time there can also help you sweat and eliminate toxins through your skin.

Avoiding processed foods and refined sugars is crucial for supporting your body's detoxification efforts. These foods can contribute to inflammation and put additional strain on your liver. Instead, focus on whole, unprocessed foods that nourish your body and support healthy liver function. Fresh fruits, vegetables, lean proteins, and whole grains are all excellent choices.

Reducing exposure to environmental toxins is also important for overall detoxification. Try to minimize your use of household chemicals, opt for natural cleaning products, and avoid smoking or excessive alcohol consumption. Creating a cleaner environment can reduce the burden on your body's detoxification systems and help manage allergic reactions more effectively.

Book 26: Digestive Health and Natural Solutions for IBS

Identifying the Causes of Irritable Bowel Syndrome (IBS)

Irritable Bowel Syndrome, or IBS, is a common digestive disorder that can cause a range of symptoms, from abdominal pain and bloating to diarrhea and constipation. While the exact cause of IBS isn't fully understood, there are several factors that can contribute to its development. Let's explore these potential causes and how they might play a role in IBS.

One of the most significant factors in IBS is diet. Certain foods can trigger IBS symptoms in some people. Common culprits include high-fat foods, dairy products, and foods rich in certain types of carbohydrates, known as FODMAPs (Fermentable Oligo-, Di-, Mono-saccharides, and Polyols). These carbohydrates can be hard for some people to digest, leading to symptoms like gas, bloating, and diarrhea. Keeping a food diary can help you identify which foods might be triggering your symptoms, allowing you to make adjustments to your diet.

Another important factor to consider is stress. Stress and anxiety can have a profound impact on your digestive system. They can affect gut motility, increase sensitivity to pain, and alter the balance of gut bacteria, all of which can contribute to IBS symptoms. Finding effective ways to manage stress, such as through mindfulness, relaxation techniques, or counseling, can be beneficial in alleviating IBS symptoms.

Hormonal changes also play a role in IBS, particularly in women. Many women notice that their IBS symptoms can fluctuate with their menstrual cycle. Hormones like estrogen and progesterone can influence gut function, which may explain why IBS symptoms can sometimes worsen during certain times of the month. Tracking your symptoms in relation to your menstrual cycle might help you identify patterns and manage your symptoms more effectively.

Gut microbiota is another area of interest when it comes to IBS. The gut is home to a complex community of microorganisms, including bacteria, viruses, and fungi. An imbalance in these microorganisms, known as dysbiosis, can affect digestion and contribute to IBS symptoms. Research into probiotics and prebiotics, which support healthy gut bacteria, is ongoing and shows promise in helping manage IBS.

Food intolerances are also a common factor in IBS. Unlike food allergies, which involve an immune response, food intolerances are typically related to difficulties in digesting certain foods. Lactose intolerance (difficulty digesting dairy products) and gluten sensitivity are two examples. If you suspect a food intolerance, working with a healthcare provider to get a proper diagnosis can help you manage your symptoms effectively.

Physical inactivity can also impact digestive health. Regular exercise helps maintain healthy digestion and can reduce symptoms of IBS. Incorporating physical activity into your routine, such as walking, swimming, or yoga, can promote better gut motility and overall well-being.

Lastly, genetics might play a role in IBS. While more research is needed, some studies suggest that IBS can run in families, indicating that genetic factors might contribute to its development. If IBS is common in your family, it might be helpful to discuss your symptoms with a healthcare provider, who can offer guidance on management strategies tailored to your needs.

Herbal Remedies for IBS Relief

Managing Irritable Bowel Syndrome (IBS) can be challenging, but incorporating herbal remedies into your routine might provide some much-needed relief. Nature offers a variety of herbs known for their soothing properties that can help ease IBS symptoms like bloating, abdominal pain, and irregular bowel movements. Let's explore some herbal options that might help you feel better.

Peppermint is one of the most well-known herbs for IBS relief. Its active compound, menthol, has natural antispasmodic properties, which means it can help relax the muscles of the digestive tract and alleviate cramping and pain. Peppermint tea is a simple way to incorporate this herb into your diet. If you prefer, enteric-coated peppermint oil capsules are also available, which can help reduce symptoms of IBS, particularly those related to bloating and gas.

Ginger is another powerful herb with a long history of use for digestive issues. It has anti-inflammatory and soothing properties that can help reduce nausea, bloating, and gas. Fresh ginger tea or ginger capsules can be a great addition to your daily routine. You can also add fresh ginger to your meals for a flavorful and beneficial boost.

Fennel seeds have been traditionally used to aid digestion and reduce bloating and gas. Fennel acts as a natural carminative, which helps relieve gas and promote smoother digestion. You can chew on a teaspoon of fennel seeds after meals or brew fennel tea for a gentle, soothing effect on your digestive system.

Chamomile is well-known for its calming effects and can also be helpful for IBS. It has anti-inflammatory and antispasmodic properties that can help soothe an upset stomach and reduce cramping. Drinking chamomile tea before bed or throughout the day can promote relaxation and help with digestion.

Slippery elm is an herb that has been used traditionally to soothe the digestive tract. It contains mucilage, a gel-like substance that coats and protects the lining of the intestines. This can help reduce irritation and inflammation, making it beneficial for managing IBS symptoms. Slippery elm is often available in powder form, which you can mix with water to make a soothing tea or drink.

Licorice root has been used for centuries to support digestive health. It contains compounds that can help soothe the digestive tract and reduce inflammation. However, it's important to use it in moderation, as excessive consumption can lead to side effects. Licorice root tea or capsules can be a gentle way to incorporate this herb into your regimen.

Turmeric is known for its anti-inflammatory properties and can be helpful for calming an irritated digestive system. Curcumin, the active compound in turmeric, may help reduce symptoms of IBS by decreasing inflammation and promoting overall gut health. You can add turmeric to your meals or take it as a supplement.

Caraway seeds are another herb that can aid digestion. They have been traditionally used to relieve symptoms like bloating and gas. Caraway seed tea or simply chewing on a small amount of caraway seeds can offer relief and improve digestive comfort.

When trying herbal remedies for IBS, it's essential to start with small amounts and monitor your body's response. Each person's digestive system is unique, so what works well for one individual might not be as effective for another. It's also a good idea to consult with a healthcare provider before starting any new herbal regimen, especially if you have other health conditions or are taking medications.

The Role of Probiotics in Digestive Health

When it comes to maintaining a healthy digestive system, probiotics often come into the spotlight. These beneficial bacteria are more than just a trendy topic; they play a crucial role in supporting your digestive health and overall well-being. Let's dive into what probiotics are, how they work, and how they can benefit you.

Probiotics are live microorganisms, primarily bacteria and yeast, that provide health benefits when consumed in adequate amounts. They're often referred to as "good" or "friendly" bacteria because they help maintain a balanced gut microbiome. Your gut is home to a complex community of microorganisms, and keeping this balance is essential for good digestive health.

One of the main roles of probiotics is to help maintain a healthy balance of gut flora. A balanced gut microbiome is crucial because it supports proper digestion, helps manage inflammation, and strengthens your immune system. When the balance is disrupted, which can happen due to stress, a poor diet, or illness, probiotics can help restore order and support your digestive health.

Probiotics can aid digestion in several ways. They help break down food, produce certain vitamins, and enhance nutrient absorption. For individuals with IBS, probiotics can be especially beneficial. Research has shown that certain strains of probiotics can help alleviate symptoms like bloating, gas, and diarrhea by promoting a healthier gut environment and reducing inflammation.

Different strains of probiotics offer various benefits, so choosing the right one is important. Common probiotic strains include Lactobacillus and Bifidobacterium, each with unique properties. For example, Lactobacillus acidophilus is known for supporting digestive health and preventing diarrhea, while Bifidobacterium bifidum helps maintain a healthy balance of gut bacteria.

You can find probiotics in a variety of foods and supplements. Yogurt is a popular source, especially those labeled with "live and active cultures." Kefir, a fermented dairy product, and fermented vegetables like sauerkraut and kimchi are also excellent sources of probiotics. For those who prefer supplements, probiotic capsules or powders are widely available and can be a convenient way to ensure you're getting a sufficient amount of beneficial bacteria.

Incorporating probiotics into your diet can be a simple yet effective way to support your digestive health. However, it's essential to remember that probiotics are not a one-size-fits-all solution. Different people may respond differently to various strains, so it might take some experimentation to find the one that works best for you. Additionally, if you have underlying health conditions or are on medication, it's a good idea to consult with a healthcare provider before starting any new probiotic regimen.

Maintaining a healthy digestive system involves more than just taking probiotics. It's important to complement probiotic use with a balanced diet rich in fiber, adequate hydration, and a healthy lifestyle. Probiotics can be a valuable part of your digestive health strategy, helping to keep your gut flora balanced and supporting overall well-being.

Nutritional Strategies for Soothing the Digestive System

Taking care of your digestive system can make a world of difference in how you feel day to day, especially if you're dealing with issues like IBS. The foods you eat and how you eat them play a crucial role in soothing your digestive system and maintaining overall gut health. Let's explore some friendly and effective nutritional strategies to help keep your digestive system calm and comfortable.

First, it's helpful to focus on a high-fiber diet. Fiber helps keep things moving through your digestive tract and can be particularly beneficial for managing IBS symptoms. Incorporate plenty of soluble fiber, which can help absorb excess fluid and form a gel-like substance that can soothe the gut. Foods rich in soluble fiber include oats, apples, carrots, and beans. Insoluble fiber, found in whole grains, nuts, and vegetables, is also important but should be balanced with soluble fiber to avoid aggravating symptoms.

Stay hydrated! Drinking plenty of water is essential for maintaining digestive health. Water helps dissolve nutrients and soluble fiber, allowing them to pass through your digestive system more easily. Aim for at least eight glasses of water a day, and consider herbal teas like ginger or peppermint, which can also provide soothing benefits for your digestive tract.

Eat smaller, more frequent meals instead of larger, heavier meals. This can help prevent overeating and reduce the pressure on your digestive system. Smaller meals are easier to digest and can help manage symptoms like bloating and discomfort. Focus on including a variety of nutrient-rich foods in each meal, such as lean proteins, healthy fats, and complex carbohydrates.

Include probiotics and prebiotics in your diet. Probiotics are beneficial bacteria that support a healthy gut microbiome, while prebiotics are foods that feed these good bacteria. Foods rich in probiotics include yogurt, kefir, and fermented vegetables, while prebiotics can be found in foods like bananas, onions, garlic, and asparagus. Together, they help maintain a balanced gut environment and improve digestion.

Limit trigger foods that can exacerbate digestive issues. Common triggers for IBS include high-fat foods, dairy products, and foods high in FODMAPs (certain fermentable carbohydrates). Pay attention to how your body responds to different foods and consider keeping a food diary to identify and manage any personal triggers. This can help you make informed choices and avoid discomfort.

Incorporate soothing herbs and spices into your meals. Herbs like ginger, peppermint, and fennel have natural anti-inflammatory and antispasmodic properties that can help calm your digestive system. Try adding fresh ginger to your smoothies, drinking peppermint tea, or using fennel seeds in your cooking for a gentle digestive boost.

Practice mindful eating. Eating slowly and chewing your food thoroughly can aid digestion and help prevent overeating. Mindful eating encourages you to pay attention to your hunger cues and savor each bite, which can improve digestion and reduce stress on your digestive system.

Avoid excessive caffeine and alcohol, as these can irritate the digestive tract and exacerbate symptoms. If you find that caffeine or alcohol affects your digestion, consider reducing your intake or opting for non-caffeinated and non-alcoholic alternatives.

Balance your diet with a variety of nutrient-dense foods. Include a wide range of fruits, vegetables, whole grains, lean proteins, and healthy fats to ensure you're getting all the essential nutrients your body needs. A balanced diet supports overall health and helps keep your digestive system functioning smoothly.

Managing Stress to Improve IBS Symptoms

When it comes to managing Irritable Bowel Syndrome (IBS), stress can play a significant role in exacerbating symptoms. The gut-brain connection is a powerful one, meaning that emotional and psychological stress can directly impact your digestive health. Learning how to manage stress effectively can be a game-changer for those dealing with IBS. Let's explore some friendly and practical strategies for managing stress to improve your IBS symptoms.

Recognize the Connection: Understanding that stress can trigger or worsen IBS symptoms is an essential first step. Stress can lead to increased gut sensitivity, changes in bowel movements, and a heightened perception of pain. By acknowledging this connection, you can take proactive steps to manage stress and, in turn, support your digestive health.

Practice Mindfulness and Meditation: Mindfulness and meditation are excellent tools for reducing stress and promoting relaxation. These practices help you focus on the present moment and calm your mind, which can have a positive effect on your digestive system. Even just a few minutes of mindfulness each day can help reduce stress levels and improve your overall sense of well-being.

Incorporate Deep Breathing Exercises: Deep breathing exercises are a simple yet effective way to manage stress. When you take slow, deep breaths, you activate the body's relaxation response, which can help soothe your nervous system and reduce stress. Try incorporating deep breathing exercises into your daily routine or whenever you feel stressed. A quick breathing exercise might involve inhaling deeply through your nose, holding the breath for a few seconds, and then exhaling slowly through your mouth.

Engage in Regular Physical Activity: Exercise is a fantastic way to reduce stress and improve overall health. Physical activity stimulates the release of endorphins, which are natural mood enhancers. Regular exercise can also help regulate your digestive system and reduce symptoms of IBS. Aim for at least 30 minutes of moderate exercise most days of the week. Activities like walking, swimming, or yoga can be particularly beneficial for managing stress and supporting digestive health.

Establish a Relaxing Routine: Creating a calming routine can help manage stress and improve your digestive health. Consider incorporating relaxing activities into your daily schedule, such as reading, taking a warm bath, or listening to soothing music. Establishing a consistent routine, especially before bed, can also improve your sleep quality, which is crucial for managing stress and supporting overall health.

Connect with Supportive People: Having a strong support network can make a big difference when managing stress. Talking to friends, family members, or support groups can provide emotional support and practical advice for dealing with IBS. Sharing your experiences and feelings with others who understand can help reduce stress and improve your overall well-being.

Set Realistic Goals and Prioritize Self-Care: It's important to set realistic goals and prioritize self-care to manage stress effectively. Avoid overloading yourself with responsibilities and make time for activities that you enjoy and that help you relax. Taking care of yourself and setting boundaries can help reduce stress and improve your overall quality of life.

Practice Stress-Relief Techniques: In addition to mindfulness and exercise, there are other stress-relief techniques you might find helpful. Techniques such as progressive muscle relaxation, guided imagery, and aromatherapy can help promote relaxation and reduce stress. Experiment with different methods to find what works best for you.

Seek Professional Help if Needed: If you find that stress is significantly impacting your IBS symptoms or overall well-being, consider seeking professional help. A therapist or counselor can provide support and strategies for managing stress and addressing any underlying issues. Cognitive-behavioral therapy (CBT) and other therapeutic approaches can be particularly effective in helping individuals manage stress and improve their quality of life.

Daily Practices for Long-Term Digestive Wellness

Maintaining a healthy digestive system is essential for overall well-being, and incorporating simple daily practices can make a big difference in promoting long-term digestive wellness. By adopting these habits into your routine, you can support your digestive health and feel your best every day. Let's explore some friendly and effective daily practices that can help keep your digestive system in top shape.

Start Your Day with Hydration: Begin your morning by drinking a glass of water. Hydration is key to supporting healthy digestion, as water helps break down food and move it through your digestive tract. Adding a splash of lemon to your water can also offer a gentle detoxifying boost and stimulate your digestive system.

Eat a Balanced Breakfast: A nutritious breakfast sets the tone for the rest of your day. Opt for a meal that includes fiber-rich foods like whole grains, fruits, and vegetables, along with a source of protein. This combination helps keep you full, supports healthy digestion, and provides sustained energy throughout the day.

Incorporate Fiber-Rich Foods: Aim to include a variety of fiber-rich foods in your daily diet. Fiber aids in digestion by promoting regular bowel movements and preventing constipation. Foods like leafy greens, berries, beans, and whole grains are excellent sources of fiber. Gradually increase your fiber intake to avoid any digestive discomfort.

Chew Your Food Thoroughly: Taking the time to chew your food well can greatly benefit your digestive system. Chewing breaks down food into smaller particles, making it easier for your stomach to digest and absorb nutrients. Practice mindful eating by focusing on each bite and chewing slowly to aid digestion.

Practice Portion Control: Eating large meals can put extra strain on your digestive system. Instead, opt for smaller, more frequent meals throughout the day. This approach can help prevent overeating and reduce digestive discomfort. Pay attention to your hunger cues and try to eat until you're satisfied, not stuffed.

Include Probiotics and Prebiotics: Probiotics and prebiotics play a vital role in maintaining a healthy gut microbiome. Probiotics are beneficial bacteria found in fermented foods like yogurt, kefir, and sauerkraut. Prebiotics, found in foods like bananas, garlic, and onions, help feed these good bacteria. Incorporating both into your daily diet can support digestive health and improve overall gut function.

Stay Active: Regular physical activity is important for digestive wellness. Exercise helps stimulate digestion and promotes regular bowel movements. Aim for at least 30 minutes of moderate exercise most days of the week. Activities like walking, cycling, or yoga can be particularly beneficial for supporting digestive health.

Manage Stress: Chronic stress can negatively impact your digestive system, so finding ways to manage stress is essential. Incorporate relaxation techniques into your daily routine, such as deep breathing exercises, meditation, or yoga. Prioritizing self-care and setting aside time for activities that you enjoy can also help reduce stress levels.

Listen to Your Body: Pay attention to how your body responds to different foods and eating habits. Keeping a food diary can help you identify any triggers or patterns that affect your digestive health. By understanding your body's needs and preferences, you can make informed choices that support long-term digestive wellness.

Get Adequate Sleep: Quality sleep is crucial for overall health, including digestive health. Aim for 7-9 hours of restful sleep each night. Establishing a consistent sleep routine and creating a relaxing bedtime environment can help improve sleep quality and support your body's natural healing processes.

Practice Mindful Eating: Mindful eating involves paying attention to your food and the eating experience. This practice can help you enjoy your meals more fully, prevent overeating, and improve digestion. Focus on savoring each bite, eating slowly, and being aware of your body's hunger and fullness cues.

Stay Consistent: Consistency is key when it comes to maintaining digestive wellness. By incorporating these daily practices into your routine and making them a regular part of your life, you'll support your digestive system and promote long-term health.

Book 27: Strengthening the Immune System with Natural Approaches

Understanding the Immune System's Role in Health

Imagine your body as a bustling city, and the immune system as the vigilant security force working 24/7 to protect it. This sophisticated network of cells, tissues, and organs is always on alert, ready to defend against threats like bacteria, viruses, and toxins. Understanding how the immune system works can help you appreciate its vital role in maintaining your health and well-being.

At its core, the immune system is your body's primary defense mechanism. It consists of various components, each with a specific function. White blood cells, for example, are the foot soldiers of this system. They patrol your body, identify potential threats, and neutralize them. Among these white blood cells, you have different types, such as macrophages that engulf and destroy pathogens and lymphocytes that target specific invaders.

When a harmful substance enters your body, the immune system springs into action. White blood cells detect the intruder and respond accordingly. Antibodies, which are special proteins produced by B-cells, come into play by specifically targeting and neutralizing the invading pathogen. This process ensures that the harmful substance is eliminated before it can cause significant damage. What's remarkable is that the immune system has a memory function. It remembers past invaders and can respond more quickly and effectively if they reappear.

The immune system also relies on various organs and tissues to perform its duties. The spleen, for example, helps filter the blood, removing old or damaged cells while storing white blood cells. The lymphatic system, a network of vessels and nodes, transports immune cells throughout the body and helps filter out harmful substances. Together, these components create a comprehensive defense network designed to keep you healthy.

Maintaining a healthy immune system is crucial for overall well-being. When it functions optimally, it helps prevent infections, reduces the risk of chronic diseases, and supports your body's ability to recover from illness. Conversely, a compromised immune system can make you more susceptible to diseases and infections. Therefore, supporting your immune system naturally can have a significant impact on your health.

You can support your immune system in several natural ways. For starters, a balanced diet plays a key role. Including a variety of fruits, vegetables, whole grains, and lean proteins in your meals provides essential vitamins and minerals that boost immune function. Staying hydrated by drinking plenty of water helps maintain the body's systems and supports the immune response. Regular exercise is also beneficial, as it improves circulation and reduces inflammation, which in turn supports overall immune health.

Prioritizing quality sleep is another important factor. Aim for 7-9 hours of restful sleep each night to allow your body to repair and rejuvenate. Managing stress is equally important, as chronic stress can weaken the immune system. Engaging in relaxation techniques such as mindfulness, deep breathing exercises, or pursuing enjoyable hobbies can help manage stress levels.

Good hygiene practices, such as regular handwashing and avoiding close contact with sick individuals, can also contribute to a stronger immune system. By incorporating these practices into your daily routine, you can enhance your body's natural defenses and promote overall health.

Herbal Immune Boosters

When it comes to fortifying your immune system, nature has gifted us with a variety of herbs that can play a crucial role in keeping your defenses strong. Herbal immune boosters have been used for centuries in traditional medicine and are celebrated for their ability to enhance immune function and support overall health. Let's take a friendly journey through some of these natural wonders and discover how they can benefit your immune system.

Echinacea is one of the most well-known herbs for boosting the immune system. Often used at the first sign of a cold or infection, Echinacea is believed to help stimulate the production of white blood cells, which are essential for fighting off invaders. It also has anti-inflammatory and antioxidant properties that contribute to overall immune health. You can find Echinacea in various forms, including teas, capsules, and tinctures.

Elderberry is another powerful herbal ally. Known for its rich antioxidant content, elderberry is thought to enhance immune response and reduce the severity and duration of cold and flu symptoms. Elderberry syrup is a popular choice and can be taken as a preventative measure or at the onset of symptoms. It's not just about the berries, though—elderflower, the blossom of the elderberry plant, also has immune-boosting properties.

Astragalus is a staple in traditional Chinese medicine and is revered for its ability to strengthen the immune system and improve overall vitality. This herb is known for its adaptogenic properties, meaning it helps the body adapt to stress and boosts the immune response. Astragalus root can be enjoyed in teas, capsules, or as a tincture.

Ginger, often found in our kitchens, is not just a flavorful spice but also a powerful immune booster. It has anti-inflammatory and antioxidant effects that can help enhance immune function and fight off infections. Ginger tea is a soothing way to incorporate this herb into your daily routine, especially during the colder months or when you're feeling under the weather.

Turmeric is another kitchen staple with impressive immune-boosting properties. Curcumin, the active compound in turmeric, has potent anti-inflammatory and antioxidant effects that support the immune system and help protect against diseases. You can enjoy turmeric in your cooking, or opt for turmeric supplements or golden milk for a healthful boost.

Garlic has been celebrated for its medicinal properties for centuries. It contains allicin, a compound known for its antibacterial, antiviral, and antifungal properties. Incorporating garlic into your diet can help strengthen your immune system and combat infections. For those who prefer not to eat raw garlic, garlic supplements are a convenient alternative.

Reishi mushroom is a staple in traditional Eastern medicine and is known for its immune-enhancing properties. It's often referred to as the "mushroom of immortality" due to its ability to support immune health and overall well-being. Reishi mushrooms can be consumed in various forms, including teas, capsules, and powders.

Licorice root is valued for its immune-boosting and anti-inflammatory properties. It's often used in traditional herbal medicine to help fight off infections and support respiratory health. Licorice root can be taken as a tea, tincture, or supplement, but it's best used in moderation, especially for those with high blood pressure.

Nutritional Support for Immune Strength

When it comes to supporting your immune system, what you eat plays a crucial role. The right nutrients can help your body fend off illnesses, stay energized, and maintain overall health. Think of your diet as the foundation upon which your immune system builds its defenses. By incorporating a variety of nutrient-rich foods into your meals, you can give your body the best possible support. Let's explore how you can use nutrition to boost your immune strength in a way that's both enjoyable and beneficial.

Vitamins and Minerals: The Immune System's Best Friends
First up are the vitamins and minerals that are essential for a healthy immune system. Vitamin C is one of the most celebrated nutrients for immune support. Found in citrus fruits like oranges and grapefruits, as well as in vegetables such as bell peppers and broccoli, Vitamin C helps stimulate the production of white blood cells, which are vital for fighting infections.

Vitamin D is another important player. Often referred to as the "sunshine vitamin," it helps regulate immune function and supports the body's ability to ward off pathogens. You can get Vitamin D from sunlight exposure, but it's also found in foods like fatty fish (salmon, mackerel), fortified dairy products, and egg yolks. In some cases, a supplement might be necessary, especially during the winter months or for those who have limited sun exposure.

Zinc is a mineral that supports immune function by helping your body produce and activate T-cells, which are critical for immune defense. You can find zinc in foods like nuts, seeds, whole grains, and legumes. Adding a handful of pumpkin seeds or a serving of chickpeas to your meals can give your immune system a boost.

Antioxidants: Fighting Free Radicals
Antioxidants are compounds that help protect your cells from damage caused by free radicals. These unstable molecules can contribute to inflammation and chronic disease if not neutralized. Fruits and vegetables are excellent sources of antioxidants. Berries, such as blueberries, strawberries, and raspberries, are particularly rich in antioxidants and can be a tasty addition to your diet. Spinach, kale, and sweet potatoes are also packed with antioxidant-rich vitamins and minerals that support immune health.

Healthy Fats: The Good Guys
Not all fats are created equal. Healthy fats, such as those found in avocados, nuts, seeds, and olive oil, play a significant role in maintaining immune function. Omega-3 fatty acids, in particular, are known for their anti-inflammatory properties and can be found in fatty fish like salmon, walnuts, and flaxseeds. These healthy fats help regulate immune responses and support overall cellular health.

Probiotics: The Good Bacteria
Probiotics are beneficial bacteria that support a healthy gut, which in turn plays a crucial role in immune health. A balanced gut microbiome helps regulate immune responses and protects against harmful pathogens. You can support your gut health by including probiotic-rich foods in your diet, such as yogurt, kefir, sauerkraut, and kombucha. These foods help maintain a healthy balance of gut bacteria and support your immune system.

Hydration: The Unsung Hero
Staying hydrated is often overlooked but is essential for maintaining overall health, including immune function. Water helps flush out toxins, supports nutrient absorption, and keeps your body's systems running smoothly. Aim to drink plenty of water throughout the day and include hydrating foods like cucumbers, watermelon, and oranges in your diet.

Balanced Meals: Building Immune Strength
Creating balanced meals that include a variety of nutrients can help support your immune system. Focus on incorporating a colorful array of fruits and vegetables, lean proteins, whole grains, and healthy fats into your daily diet. Eating a diverse range of foods ensures that you're getting a broad spectrum of vitamins, minerals, and antioxidants that are essential for optimal immune function.

The Role of Probiotics in Immune Function

When it comes to maintaining a robust immune system, probiotics are unsung heroes that deserve a closer look. These beneficial bacteria, often found in fermented foods and supplements, play a crucial role in supporting and enhancing your immune function. While they may seem like small players in the grand scheme of health, their impact on your well-being is profound and multifaceted.

Probiotics are live microorganisms, primarily bacteria and yeast, that offer numerous health benefits when consumed in adequate amounts. Their primary role is to maintain a healthy balance of gut bacteria, which is essential for optimal immune function. The gut is home to a vast community of microorganisms, collectively known as the gut microbiome. This delicate balance between beneficial and harmful bacteria is crucial for overall health, including the effectiveness of your immune system.

One of the key ways probiotics support immune function is by promoting a balanced gut microbiome. A healthy gut microbiome is essential for a well-functioning immune system. When the balance is disrupted, it can lead to inflammation and an increased susceptibility to infections. Probiotics help maintain this balance by encouraging the growth of beneficial bacteria and suppressing harmful ones. This helps ensure that your immune system is not overwhelmed and can effectively respond to threats. Probiotics also enhance your body's immune response by interacting with immune cells in the gut. They stimulate the production of antibodies and activate immune cells such as T-cells and macrophages. This heightened immune response helps your body recognize and combat pathogens more efficiently. By boosting the activity of these immune cells, probiotics contribute to a more robust defense against infections.

Reducing inflammation is another critical function of probiotics. Chronic inflammation is linked to various health issues, including weakened immune function. Probiotics help modulate the immune response and decrease inflammation by producing substances that inhibit harmful bacteria and promote anti-inflammatory processes. This reduction in inflammation supports overall immune health and helps maintain a balanced immune system.

The gut barrier plays a vital role in preventing harmful substances from entering your bloodstream. Probiotics support the integrity of this barrier by promoting the production of mucin, a protective mucus layer, and maintaining the health of the intestinal lining. A strong gut barrier helps prevent leaks of potentially harmful substances that could trigger immune responses and contribute to inflammation.

Probiotics also play a role in preventing infections. They do this by competing with harmful bacteria for resources and attachment sites in the gut. Additionally, probiotics produce substances like acids and antimicrobial peptides that inhibit the growth of pathogenic microbes. This protective effect helps reduce the risk of infections and supports a healthy immune system.

Incorporating probiotics into your diet is both simple and enjoyable. Many probiotic-rich foods are readily available and can easily be added to your daily routine. Yogurt, kefir, sauerkraut, kimchi, miso, and kombucha are excellent sources of probiotics. These foods not only offer the benefits of probiotics but also provide a variety of flavors and textures to enhance your meals.

Managing Autoimmune Disorders Naturally

Autoimmune disorders can be challenging to navigate, as they involve the immune system mistakenly attacking the body's own tissues. While conventional treatments often focus on managing symptoms and suppressing the immune system, incorporating natural approaches can complement these treatments and help support overall well-being. Let's explore some natural strategies that can be helpful in managing autoimmune disorders and enhancing your quality of life.

Autoimmune disorders occur when the immune system, which is designed to protect the body from invaders like viruses and bacteria, begins to target its own cells. This can lead to inflammation, pain, and damage in various parts of the body. Common autoimmune conditions include rheumatoid arthritis, lupus, multiple sclerosis, and Hashimoto's thyroiditis. Managing these conditions involves a combination of medical treatment and lifestyle adjustments.

One of the most impactful ways to manage autoimmune disorders naturally is through diet. Adopting an anti-inflammatory diet can help reduce inflammation and support overall health. Focus on incorporating whole, nutrient-dense foods into your meals. Fruits, vegetables, lean proteins, and healthy fats can all contribute to reducing inflammation and supporting the immune system.

Certain foods have been shown to have anti-inflammatory properties. For example, omega-3 fatty acids, found in fatty fish like salmon, flaxseeds, and walnuts, can help reduce inflammation. Turmeric, with its active compound curcumin, is another powerful anti-inflammatory spice that can be included in your diet. Ginger, garlic, and green tea also offer anti-inflammatory benefits.

Conversely, it's important to identify and avoid foods that may trigger inflammation or worsen symptoms. Common culprits include refined sugars, processed foods, and excessive consumption of red meat. Some individuals with autoimmune disorders find relief by following an elimination diet to pinpoint specific food sensitivities or intolerances.

Chronic stress can exacerbate autoimmune symptoms and contribute to flare-ups. Managing stress through relaxation techniques can be beneficial for those with autoimmune disorders. Practices such as mindfulness meditation, deep breathing exercises, yoga, and tai chi can help reduce stress and promote overall well-being. Finding time for activities that bring you joy and relaxation is also crucial for managing stress levels.

Several herbs have been studied for their potential benefits in managing autoimmune disorders. For instance, adaptogenic herbs like ashwagandha and rhodiola may help support the body's stress response and enhance resilience. Licorice root is another herb that has been traditionally used to support adrenal health and reduce inflammation.

Always consult with a healthcare provider before starting any new herbal supplements, especially if you're already on medication or have specific health concerns. They can help ensure that the herbs are safe and appropriate for your individual situation.

Regular physical activity is an essential part of managing autoimmune disorders. Exercise can help improve joint function, reduce fatigue, and enhance overall mood. Low-impact activities such as swimming, walking, and gentle stretching can be particularly beneficial. It's important to listen to your body and choose exercises that you enjoy and can sustain.

Adequate sleep is crucial for immune function and overall health. Establishing a regular sleep routine and creating a restful sleep environment can improve sleep quality. Aim for 7-9 hours of quality sleep each night and incorporate relaxing pre-sleep rituals, such as reading or taking a warm bath.

A healthy gut plays a significant role in overall immune function. Since autoimmune disorders are often linked to gut health, focusing on maintaining a balanced gut microbiome can be helpful. Probiotics, found in fermented foods like yogurt, kefir, and sauerkraut, can support gut health. Additionally, a diet high in fiber from fruits, vegetables, and whole grains can nourish beneficial gut bacteria.

Managing an autoimmune disorder can be challenging, both physically and emotionally. Building a support network of friends, family, and healthcare professionals can provide valuable emotional support and practical advice. Consider joining support groups or seeking counseling if needed to help navigate the emotional aspects of living with an autoimmune condition.

Daily Habits to Maintain a Strong Immune System

Keeping your immune system in top shape is essential for staying healthy and feeling your best. While it might seem like a big task, incorporating a few simple daily habits into your routine can make a significant difference in supporting your immune health. Here are some friendly and effective habits to consider for maintaining a strong immune system every day:

Fueling your body with the right nutrients is key to a strong immune system. Aim for a balanced diet rich in fruits, vegetables, whole grains, lean proteins, and healthy fats. Foods high in vitamins and minerals, such as vitamin C-rich citrus fruits, vitamin A-packed sweet potatoes, and zinc-rich nuts and seeds, can provide your immune system with the support it needs to function effectively. Don't forget to include probiotics from sources like yogurt or fermented vegetables to help maintain a healthy gut microbiome.

Water is vital for overall health, including immune function. Staying hydrated helps your body flush out toxins and keeps your mucous membranes, such as those in your respiratory tract, moist and effective at trapping germs. Aim to drink plenty of water throughout the day, and consider adding herbal teas like ginger or chamomile for additional immune-supporting benefits.

Physical activity is not just good for your heart and muscles—it's also great for your immune system. Regular exercise helps boost your immune response by promoting healthy circulation and reducing inflammation. Activities like walking, jogging, cycling, or even dancing can enhance your overall health and keep your immune system functioning optimally. Just remember to listen to your body and choose activities you enjoy.

Quality sleep is crucial for a well-functioning immune system. During sleep, your body repairs itself and produces important immune cells and proteins. Aim for 7-9 hours of restful sleep each night. Establish a calming bedtime routine, keep a consistent sleep schedule, and create a comfortable sleep environment to improve your sleep quality.

Chronic stress can take a toll on your immune system, making you more susceptible to illness. Incorporate stress-reducing activities into your daily routine, such as mindfulness meditation, deep breathing exercises, or yoga. Even simple practices like taking a walk in nature or enjoying a hobby can help lower stress levels and support your immune health.

Good hygiene habits are essential for preventing the spread of germs and infections. Wash your hands regularly with soap and water, especially before eating or after being in public places. Keeping your living spaces clean and avoiding touching your face can also help reduce your risk of illness.

Maintaining social connections can have a positive impact on your overall well-being, including your immune health. Engaging with friends and family, participating in community activities, or joining social groups can help boost your mood and provide emotional support, which in turn can benefit your immune system.

Smoking and excessive alcohol consumption can weaken your immune system and increase your risk of infections. If you smoke, seek support to quit, and try to limit alcohol intake to moderate levels. By avoiding these habits, you'll be giving your immune system a better chance to stay strong and resilient.

Getting outside and enjoying nature can be beneficial for your immune health. Fresh air and sunlight help your body produce vitamin D, which is important for immune function. Aim to spend time outdoors each day, whether it's gardening, taking a walk, or simply relaxing in your backyard.

Your mental and emotional health is closely linked to your immune system. Practicing mindfulness, gratitude, and positive thinking can help reduce stress and improve your overall outlook on life. Incorporate practices that promote a positive mindset, such as journaling, affirmations, or spending time with loved ones.

Preventing Infections with Natural Remedies

When it comes to keeping infections at bay, natural remedies offer a gentle yet effective approach to bolster your body's defenses. While conventional medicine is crucial for treating infections, incorporating natural remedies into your daily routine can provide added support and help prevent illness. Let's explore some friendly and practical natural remedies that can help you stay healthy and prevent infections.

Garlic is often hailed as a superfood for its immune-boosting properties. It contains allicin, a compound with antibacterial and antiviral effects. Including garlic in your diet can help strengthen your immune system and reduce the risk of infections.

You can add fresh garlic to your meals, make garlic-infused oil, or take garlic supplements if you prefer. Just remember that a little goes a long way, so start with small amounts to see what works best for you.

Ginger is another powerful natural remedy with antimicrobial and anti-inflammatory properties. It can help support your immune system and reduce the severity of infections. Adding fresh ginger to your tea, smoothies, or stir-fries is an easy way to incorporate it into your diet. You can also make a soothing ginger tea by simmering fresh ginger slices in hot water.

Echinacea is well-known for its ability to enhance immune function and help ward off infections. This herb can be taken as a tea, tincture, or supplement. Research suggests that echinacea can help reduce the duration and severity of colds and other respiratory infections. It's a great option to keep on hand, especially during cold and flu season.

Honey, particularly raw honey, has natural antimicrobial properties that can help prevent infections. It's often used as a soothing remedy for sore throats and coughs. You can add honey to your tea, spread it on toast, or simply take a spoonful to reap its benefits. Be sure to choose high-quality, raw honey for the most effective results.

Vitamin C is essential for a healthy immune system and can help prevent infections by supporting the production of white blood cells. Citrus fruits like oranges, grapefruits, and lemons are excellent sources of vitamin C. Additionally, vegetables like bell peppers and broccoli are rich in this vital nutrient. Including a variety of vitamin C-rich foods in your diet can help keep your immune system strong.

Staying hydrated is crucial for maintaining overall health and preventing infections. Herbal teas, such as those made from chamomile, peppermint, or elderberry, not only keep you hydrated but also offer additional immune-supporting benefits. These teas can help soothe the throat, ease congestion, and provide antioxidants that support your body's defenses.

Maintaining good oral hygiene is an important part of preventing infections. The mouth is a gateway for bacteria and viruses, so brushing your teeth twice a day, flossing regularly, and using an antibacterial mouthwash can help reduce the risk of oral infections. Additionally, staying hydrated and eating a balanced diet supports oral health and overall immune function.

Essential oils, such as tea tree oil, eucalyptus oil, and oregano oil, have natural antibacterial and antiviral properties that can help prevent infections. You can use essential oils in a diffuser, add them to a carrier oil for topical application, or incorporate them into homemade cleaning solutions. Just be sure to use essential oils safely and follow the recommended dilution guidelines.

A healthy lifestyle plays a significant role in preventing infections. Eating a balanced diet, exercising regularly, getting adequate sleep, and managing stress all contribute to a strong immune system. By focusing on these foundational aspects of health, you create a solid defense against infections and support your body's natural ability to stay well.

Regular hand washing and cleanliness are fundamental in preventing infections. Wash your hands with soap and water, especially before eating or after being in public spaces. Keep your living environment clean by disinfecting commonly-touched surfaces and avoiding close contact with sick individuals. These simple hygiene practices can significantly reduce your risk of infection.

Book 28: Detoxing the Body for Optimal Health

The Importance of Regular Detoxification

In our fast-paced world, our bodies are constantly exposed to various toxins—whether from processed foods, environmental pollutants, or stress. Regular detoxification plays a crucial role in helping our bodies maintain balance and stay healthy. It's not just about trendy cleanses or fad diets; it's about giving your body the support it needs to keep its natural detoxification systems running smoothly. Let's dive into why regular detoxification is so important and how it can benefit your overall health.

Our bodies have incredible built-in detoxification systems, primarily the liver, kidneys, and digestive tract. These organs work tirelessly to filter out harmful substances and eliminate waste. However, when we're bombarded with excessive toxins, these organs can become overwhelmed, leading to a buildup of toxins in the body. Regular detoxification helps to ease the burden on these organs and keeps them functioning at their best.

The liver is the body's primary detoxifier, processing and breaking down toxins so they can be safely eliminated. When the liver is overloaded, it can struggle to keep up with its detoxification duties. Regular detox practices, such as consuming liver-supporting foods like leafy greens, garlic, and beets, can help keep your liver in tip-top shape. By supporting liver health, you help your body efficiently process and remove toxins.

Your kidneys play a vital role in filtering blood and removing waste through urine. They also help regulate fluid balance and electrolyte levels. By staying hydrated and consuming kidney-friendly foods like cranberries, apples, and cucumbers, you can support your kidneys in their detoxification role. Regular detoxification helps ensure your kidneys can perform their crucial functions effectively.

A healthy digestive system is essential for effective detoxification. The digestive tract is responsible for breaking down food, absorbing nutrients, and eliminating waste. Regular detox practices can support digestive health by promoting regular bowel movements, reducing bloating, and improving nutrient absorption. Foods high in fiber, such as fruits, vegetables, and whole grains, are excellent for keeping your digestive system running smoothly.

A well-functioning detoxification system supports a strong immune system. When your body is less burdened by toxins, your immune system can focus on defending against pathogens and maintaining overall health. Incorporating detoxifying foods, such as antioxidant-rich berries and green tea, can help support your immune function and improve your body's ability to fight off illness.

Feeling sluggish and tired? Toxins can contribute to fatigue and low energy levels. Regular detoxification helps remove these toxins, allowing your body to use its energy more efficiently. By eating a balanced diet, staying hydrated, and incorporating gentle detox practices like herbal teas and light exercise, you can boost your energy levels and feel more vibrant throughout the day.

Toxins can also impact mental clarity and cognitive function. Regular detoxification supports brain health by reducing the overall toxic load on your body. Foods rich in omega-3 fatty acids, such as flaxseeds and walnuts, along with hydration and adequate sleep, can help improve mental clarity and focus.

Your skin is your body's largest organ and plays a significant role in detoxification through sweating. A regular detox can help clear up your skin by removing toxins that may contribute to issues like acne or dullness. Eating skin-friendly foods like avocados, nuts, and green leafy vegetables can support healthy, glowing skin.

Detoxification isn't just about short-term benefits; it's a key component of long-term health and wellness. Regular detox practices can help prevent the buildup of toxins, support healthy organ function, and reduce the risk of chronic diseases. By making detoxification a regular part of your routine, you're investing in your long-term health and well-being.

Liver and Kidney Cleansing Protocols

Your liver and kidneys are your body's natural detoxifiers, working tirelessly to filter out toxins and keep you healthy. Given the demands placed on them by our modern lifestyles, regular support for these organs can make a big difference in how effectively they perform their essential functions. Let's explore some practical and effective ways to enhance liver and kidney health through cleansing protocols.

Starting with your liver, it's crucial to support this hardworking organ to maintain its efficiency. One simple yet effective practice is to begin your day with a glass of warm lemon water. Lemon juice, packed with vitamin C, helps stimulate the production of detoxifying enzymes in the liver and encourages bile flow, which is essential for digestion and the elimination of toxins. Squeezing half a lemon into a glass of warm water and drinking it first thing in the morning sets a positive tone for your liver's daily detox activities.

Incorporating liver-supportive foods into your diet can also be highly beneficial. Foods such as beets, carrots, and leafy greens play a significant role in liver health. Beets are known for their high betaine content, which helps the liver process fats more efficiently. Carrots, rich in beta-carotene, contribute to liver health by supporting its natural detoxification processes. Leafy greens like spinach and kale aid in detoxification and enhance bile production, further supporting liver function.

Herbal teas can provide additional support for liver health. Herbs such as milk thistle, dandelion root, and turmeric are known for their beneficial effects on the liver. Milk thistle contains silymarin, an antioxidant that helps protect liver cells from damage. Dandelion root is helpful for improving liver function and stimulating bile production, while turmeric offers anti-inflammatory benefits that support overall liver health. Enjoying these herbs as teas can be a soothing and effective way to bolster your liver's detoxification efforts.

Limiting exposure to toxins is another important aspect of supporting liver health. This means moderating alcohol consumption, reducing intake of processed foods, and minimizing exposure to environmental pollutants. Opting for a diet rich in organic fruits and vegetables, lean proteins, and healthy fats can help reduce the toxic load on your liver and support its natural detoxification processes.

Turning to kidney health, proper hydration is one of the simplest yet most effective ways to support these vital organs. Drinking plenty of water helps flush out toxins and prevents the formation of kidney stones. Aim for at least eight glasses of water a day, and consider adding a splash of lemon or lime for extra benefits. Keeping hydrated ensures that your kidneys can efficiently filter waste and maintain fluid balance in your body.

Including kidney-friendly foods in your diet can also be advantageous. Cranberries, apples, and cucumbers are all beneficial for kidney health. Cranberries are known for their role in preventing urinary tract infections, while apples offer anti-inflammatory properties that can benefit kidney function. Cucumbers, being highly hydrating, help flush out toxins and support overall kidney health. Integrating these foods into your meals can support your kidneys' natural detoxification efforts.

Herbal support for the kidneys can be very effective as well. Herbs such as nettle leaf, horsetail, and parsley have natural diuretic properties, which can help increase urine production and support kidney function. These herbs can be enjoyed as teas or supplements, providing gentle support to your kidneys and assisting in their detoxification processes.

Monitoring your sodium intake is crucial for maintaining kidney health. Excessive sodium can put additional strain on your kidneys, so opting for low-sodium or salt-free options is wise. Flavoring your food with herbs and spices rather than salt can help reduce the workload on your kidneys and support their function.

Balancing your protein intake is another important factor in kidney health. While protein is essential, excessive consumption can stress the kidneys. Aim for moderate protein intake from sources like lean meats, beans, and legumes. This balance helps prevent kidney strain and supports long-term kidney health.

Incorporating these liver and kidney cleansing protocols into your daily routine doesn't have to be overwhelming. Begin by making small adjustments, such as drinking lemon water each morning or including kidney-friendly foods in your diet. Gradually add more practices as you become comfortable, always paying attention to your body's needs.

Herbal Detox Remedies for the Body

Detoxifying the body with herbs is a time-honored tradition that taps into the power of nature to support our health. Herbal remedies can help cleanse our systems, support vital organs, and promote overall well-being. Let's dive into some of the most effective herbal detox remedies that can help you feel revitalized and balanced.

Dandelion root is a fantastic herb for detoxifying the liver and supporting overall digestive health. Often found in teas and supplements, dandelion root acts as a natural diuretic, helping to flush out excess fluids and toxins from the body. It also stimulates bile production, which aids in the digestion of fats and supports liver function. Enjoy dandelion root tea to give your liver a gentle, natural boost and help keep your digestive system in check.

Milk thistle is renowned for its liver-supporting properties, thanks to a compound called silymarin. Silymarin has antioxidant and anti-inflammatory effects that help protect liver cells from damage and promote detoxification. Milk thistle can be found in various forms, including teas, capsules, and tinctures. Incorporating milk thistle into your detox regimen can help support liver health and enhance your body's natural detoxification processes.

Nettle leaf is a versatile herb that supports kidney health and helps with detoxification. It has natural diuretic properties, which means it can increase urine production and assist in flushing out toxins. Nettle leaf is also rich in vitamins and minerals, providing additional health benefits. You can enjoy nettle leaf as a tea or take it in supplement form to support kidney function and overall detoxification.

Cilantro, also known as coriander, is more than just a flavorful herb used in cooking. It has natural detoxifying properties that can help remove heavy metals from the body. Cilantro supports liver function and promotes the excretion of toxins, making it a great addition to your detox routine. Adding fresh cilantro to your meals or enjoying it as a tea can help boost your body's natural detoxification processes.

Ginger is a well-known herb with powerful detoxifying properties. It aids digestion, reduces inflammation, and helps eliminate toxins from the body. Ginger also has a stimulating effect on the digestive system, which can help with the breakdown and elimination of waste. You can enjoy ginger in various forms, such as fresh, dried, or as a tea. Incorporating ginger into your diet can help support your body's detox efforts and promote overall digestive health.

Turmeric is celebrated for its anti-inflammatory and antioxidant properties, making it a valuable herb for detoxification. The active compound in turmeric, curcumin, helps support liver function and enhances the body's ability to process and eliminate toxins. Turmeric can be added to your meals as a spice, taken as a supplement, or enjoyed in a soothing tea. Including turmeric in your detox regimen can help support your liver and overall health.

Parsley is a herb commonly used in cooking, but it also offers impressive detoxifying benefits. It acts as a natural diuretic, helping to flush out excess fluids and toxins from the body. Parsley is also rich in vitamins and antioxidants, supporting overall health and wellness. You can add fresh parsley to salads, soups, and smoothies or enjoy it as a herbal tea to benefit from its detoxifying properties.

Red clover is a gentle herb known for its detoxifying effects on the blood and lymphatic system. It supports the body's natural cleansing processes and can help improve skin health. Red clover is often consumed as a tea or in supplement form. Incorporating red clover into your detox routine can help promote a healthier, cleaner internal environment.

Incorporating these herbal remedies into your daily routine can be a simple and enjoyable way to support your body's natural detoxification processes. Start by choosing a few herbs that resonate with you and gradually add them to your diet or wellness routine. Whether you prefer herbal teas, fresh herbs in your meals, or supplements, each of these remedies offers unique benefits to help keep your body in balance.

The Role of Water in Detoxification

Water is often celebrated as one of the most fundamental elements of good health, and its role in detoxification is a prime example of this. Our bodies, composed of about 60% water, rely heavily on this vital fluid to maintain various physiological functions, including the critical process of detoxification. First and foremost, water is indispensable for the effective functioning of the kidneys, which are central to detoxification. The kidneys filter blood to remove waste and excess substances, which are then excreted through urine. Adequate water intake ensures that the kidneys can perform this filtration efficiently, helping to flush out toxins and prevent the buildup of waste products. Without enough water, the kidneys might struggle to filter out these impurities effectively, leading to potential health issues such as kidney stones or urinary tract infections.

Moreover, water plays a significant role in digestion and maintaining a healthy digestive system. It helps break down food so that nutrients can be absorbed by the intestines. Additionally, water aids in preventing constipation by softening stools and promoting regular bowel movements. This is crucial for detoxification, as a well-functioning digestive system can better eliminate waste and toxins from the body.

Water also facilitates the transport of nutrients to cells and helps carry away waste products. This transportation is essential for maintaining overall health and supporting the body's natural detoxification processes. Proper hydration ensures that nutrients are delivered efficiently and that waste products are effectively removed, contributing to a balanced and healthy internal environment.

To fully harness the benefits of water for detoxification, it is recommended to drink at least 8 glasses of water daily, though individual needs can vary based on factors such as activity level, climate, and overall health. Incorporating water-rich foods into your diet, such as fruits and vegetables, can also contribute to your hydration goals and enhance the detoxification process.

Detoxing Heavy Metals and Environmental Toxins

In today's world, our exposure to heavy metals and environmental toxins is almost unavoidable. From the air we breathe and the water we drink to the food we eat, these substances can accumulate in our bodies and potentially impact our health. While our bodies are equipped with natural detoxification mechanisms, they sometimes need a little extra support to handle the load effectively. Here's how you can help your body detox heavy metals and environmental toxins, so you can feel your best and maintain optimal health.

Understanding the sources of these toxins is the first step. Heavy metals like lead, mercury, and cadmium can enter our bodies through contaminated food, water, or air. Environmental toxins, including pesticides, industrial chemicals, and pollutants, can also be absorbed through our skin or ingested. These substances can interfere with our cellular functions and contribute to a range of health issues, from fatigue and digestive discomfort to more severe conditions like neurological disorders.

Supporting your body's natural detoxification processes is essential. One of the simplest and most effective ways to do this is by staying well-hydrated. Drinking plenty of water helps your kidneys filter out and eliminate waste products, including toxins. Aim for at least 8 glasses of water each day to ensure that your body can efficiently flush out these harmful substances. Adding lemon or cucumber slices to your water can not only enhance the flavor but also provide additional detoxifying benefits.

Your liver plays a crucial role in detoxification, processing and breaking down toxins so they can be eliminated from the body. Supporting liver health can help enhance this process. Incorporating foods rich in antioxidants and liver-friendly nutrients into your diet can make a significant difference. Leafy greens like spinach and kale, cruciferous vegetables such as broccoli and Brussels sprouts, and herbs like milk thistle and dandelion root are known for their liver-supportive properties.

Fiber also plays a vital role in detoxification. It helps bind toxins in the digestive tract and facilitates their removal from the body. Eating a diet high in fiber, with plenty of fruits, vegetables, whole grains, and legumes, can aid in this process and support regular bowel movements. This helps ensure that waste and toxins are efficiently expelled from your system.

Certain herbs have been traditionally used to support detoxification and help eliminate heavy metals. Cilantro, for example, is known for its potential to bind with heavy metals and assist in their removal from the body. Chlorella, a type of green algae, is another herb that may help with the elimination of heavy metals. If you're considering herbal remedies, it's a good idea to consult with a healthcare professional to ensure they're appropriate for your individual needs.

Adopting a healthy lifestyle can further enhance your detoxification efforts. Regular exercise helps improve circulation and supports the lymphatic system, which plays a role in removing toxins. Aim for at least 30 minutes of moderate exercise most days of the week. Reducing your exposure to environmental toxins is also important. Opt for organic foods when possible, use natural cleaning products, and minimize contact with harmful chemicals.

Quality sleep is another critical component of detoxification. During sleep, your body goes through restorative processes, including the removal of toxins. Aim for 7-9 hours of restful sleep each night to support overall health and effective detoxification.

Detoxing is a personal journey, and what works for one person might not work for another. Listen to your body and adjust your approach as needed. If you have specific health concerns or underlying conditions, consult with a healthcare provider to ensure that your detoxification strategies are safe and effective for you.

Supporting the Lymphatic System in Detox

Our lymphatic system might not get as much spotlight as the heart or the liver, but it's an unsung hero in our body's detoxification process. This intricate network of vessels, nodes, and organs plays a crucial role in keeping us healthy by removing waste, toxins, and other unwanted substances from our tissues. Here's a friendly guide on how you can support your lymphatic system to help it work its detoxifying magic.

The lymphatic system is essentially a fluid drainage system that helps clear out toxins and waste products from our cells. It's made up of lymph, a clear fluid that travels through lymphatic vessels, and lymph nodes, which act as filters to trap and destroy harmful substances. Proper functioning of this system is vital for maintaining overall health and boosting our body's natural detoxification capabilities.

One of the simplest ways to support your lymphatic system is to stay hydrated. Drinking plenty of water helps keep the lymph fluid flowing smoothly, which is crucial for effective detoxification. Aim to drink at least 8 glasses of water a day, and consider adding fresh lemon or cucumber slices for an extra boost of hydration and flavor.

Regular physical activity is another key player in lymphatic health. Unlike the circulatory system, which has the heart to pump blood, the lymphatic system relies on muscle contractions to help move lymph fluid through its vessels. Engaging in regular exercise, whether it's a brisk walk, a yoga session, or a swim, helps stimulate lymph flow and promotes efficient waste removal.

Dry brushing is a wonderful technique to support lymphatic function. Using a natural bristle brush, gently brush your skin in circular motions towards your heart. This not only exfoliates the skin but also stimulates lymphatic circulation and helps remove toxins from the surface of your skin.

Incorporating specific foods into your diet can also boost lymphatic health. Foods rich in antioxidants, like berries, leafy greens, and citrus fruits, can help protect lymphatic tissues from damage and support overall detoxification. Garlic and ginger, known for their anti-inflammatory properties, can also aid in maintaining a healthy lymphatic system.

Herbal teas can be another gentle way to support lymphatic detoxification. Herbs like cleavers, red clover, and dandelion root are traditionally used to promote lymphatic drainage and support detoxification processes. Drinking a cup of herbal tea daily can complement your efforts and provide additional support for your lymphatic system.

Adequate rest and relaxation are essential for maintaining lymphatic health. Stress and lack of sleep can negatively impact lymphatic function, so make sure to get plenty of restful sleep and incorporate stress-relief practices into your daily routine. This can include meditation, deep breathing exercises, or simply taking time to unwind and relax.

Lastly, be mindful of your overall lifestyle. Avoiding excessive alcohol consumption, reducing exposure to environmental toxins, and opting for a balanced diet can all contribute to a healthier lymphatic system. It's about creating a harmonious balance that supports your body's natural detoxification processes.

Colon Cleansing and Gut Health

When it comes to feeling vibrant and energetic, a healthy gut is essential. Your gut, including the colon, plays a vital role in digestion, nutrient absorption, and even immune function. Keeping this crucial part of your body in top shape can have a significant impact on your overall health. Here's a friendly guide to understanding colon cleansing and supporting your gut health.

The colon, or large intestine, is responsible for absorbing water and electrolytes from undigested food and forming waste products for elimination. A well-functioning colon is key to maintaining a healthy digestive system and ensuring that your body effectively gets rid of toxins and waste.

Colon cleansing is often discussed in the context of detoxifying the body and improving digestive health. The idea is to remove accumulated waste and toxins that can impact the colon's ability to function properly. While the colon is naturally capable of cleaning itself, some people find that a gentle cleanse can provide a refreshing boost to their digestive system.

One of the simplest ways to support colon health is to stay well-hydrated. Drinking plenty of water helps keep things moving through your digestive system and prevents constipation. Aim for at least 8 glasses of water a day, and consider adding hydrating foods like cucumbers and watermelon to your diet.

Fiber is another key player in maintaining a healthy colon. It helps bulk up stool, making it easier to pass and reducing the risk of constipation. Foods high in fiber, such as fruits, vegetables, whole grains, and legumes, can support regular bowel movements and contribute to a healthy digestive system.

If you're considering a colon cleanse, opt for gentle methods that complement your body's natural processes. Herbal teas, such as those made with ginger or peppermint, can help soothe the digestive tract and support digestion. You might also try incorporating foods known for their detoxifying properties, like leafy greens and citrus fruits.

In addition to dietary approaches, you might explore methods like colon hydrotherapy. This procedure involves flushing the colon with warm water to remove waste and toxins. If you choose this route, make sure to consult with a qualified practitioner to ensure it's done safely and effectively.

Probiotics are beneficial bacteria that help maintain a healthy balance in your gut. They support digestion, boost the immune system, and contribute to overall gut health. Including probiotic-rich foods in your diet, such as yogurt, kefir, sauerkraut, and kombucha, can be a great way to promote a healthy gut environment.

In addition to hydration, fiber, and probiotics, adopting healthy habits can enhance your gut health. Eating smaller, more frequent meals can ease the digestive process and reduce the burden on your colon. Avoiding excessive intake of processed foods, sugars, and unhealthy fats can also contribute to a healthier gut.

Managing stress is another important aspect of maintaining gut health. Stress can affect digestion and contribute to gastrointestinal issues. Incorporating stress-reducing practices, such as mindfulness, meditation, or gentle exercise, can help keep your digestive system functioning smoothly.

Everyone's digestive system is unique, so it's important to find what works best for you. If you're considering a colon cleanse or making significant changes to your diet, it's always a good idea to consult with a healthcare professional. They can provide personalized advice and ensure that your approach to colon health is safe and effective.

Book 29: Dr. Barbara Cookbook

Breakfast 20 recipes

Breakfast is often called the most important meal of the day, and for good reason! It's the first opportunity to fuel your body and set the tone for the day ahead. If you're looking for a variety of tasty and nutritious breakfast options, you've come to the right place. Here are 20 breakfast recipes that will help you start your day on a delicious and healthy note:

1. Avocado Toast with Poached Egg

Preparation Time: 10 minutes
Cooking Time: 10 minutes
Total Time: 20 minutes
Servings: 2
Ingredients:
- 2 ripe avocados
- 4 slices whole-grain bread
- 4 large eggs
- 1 tablespoon lemon juice
- 1 tablespoon olive oil
- Salt and pepper to taste
- Red pepper flakes (optional)
- Fresh herbs (such as cilantro or parsley, optional)

Directions:
1. Prepare the Avocados:
   - Cut the avocados in half, remove the pit, and scoop the flesh into a bowl.
   - Mash the avocado with a fork, then mix in the lemon juice, olive oil, salt, and pepper.
2. Toast the Bread:
   - Toast the whole-grain bread slices in a toaster or under a broiler until golden brown and crisp.
3. Poach the Eggs:
   - Fill a medium saucepan with water and bring to a gentle simmer. Add a splash of vinegar to help the eggs hold their shape.
   - Crack each egg into a small bowl, then gently slide it into the simmering water.
   - Cook for 3-4 minutes, until the whites are set but the yolks remain soft.
   - Use a slotted spoon to transfer the eggs to a plate lined with paper towels.
4. Assemble the Toast:
   - Spread the mashed avocado mixture evenly over the toasted bread slices.
   - Top each slice with a poached egg.
   - Season with additional salt, pepper, and red pepper flakes if desired.
   - Garnish with fresh herbs if using.

Nutrition Information (per serving):
Calories: 360
Protein: 14g
Carbohydrates: 32g
Dietary Fiber: 10g
Sugars: 3g
Fat: 22g
Saturated Fat: 3g

2. Greek Yogurt Parfait

Preparation Time: 10 minutes
Cooking Time: 0 minutes
Total Time: 10 minutes
Servings: 2
Ingredients:
- 2 cups Greek yogurt (plain or vanilla)
- 1 cup granola
- 1 cup mixed fresh berries (such as strawberries, blueberries, and raspberries)
- 2 tablespoons honey or maple syrup (optional)
- Fresh mint leaves for garnish (optional)

Directions:
1. Prepare the Ingredients:
   - Wash and pat dry the fresh berries.

2. Assemble the Parfait:
    - In serving glasses or bowls, layer 1/2 cup of Greek yogurt at the bottom.
    - Add 1/4 cup of granola on top of the yogurt.
    - Place 1/4 cup of mixed berries over the granola.
    - Repeat the layers until the glasses or bowls are filled.
3. Add Sweetener:
    - Drizzle honey or maple syrup over the top layer if desired.
4. Garnish:
    - Garnish with fresh mint leaves if using.

Nutrition Information (per serving):
Calories: 350
Protein: 15g
Carbohydrates: 40g
Dietary Fiber: 4g
Sugars: 20g
Fat: 12g
Saturated Fat: 2g

3. Oatmeal with Fresh Fruit

Preparation Time: 10 minutes
Cooking Time: 0 minutes
Total Time: 10 minutes
Servings: 2
Ingredients:
- 2 cups Greek yogurt (plain or vanilla)
- 1 cup granola
- 1 cup mixed fresh berries (such as strawberries, blueberries, and raspberries)
- 2 tablespoons honey or maple syrup (optional)
- Fresh mint leaves for garnish (optional)

Directions:
1. Prepare the Ingredients:
    - Wash and pat dry the fresh berries.
2. Assemble the Parfait:
    - In serving glasses or bowls, layer 1/2 cup of Greek yogurt at the bottom.
    - Add 1/4 cup of granola on top of the yogurt.
    - Place 1/4 cup of mixed berries over the granola.
    - Repeat the layers until the glasses or bowls are filled.
3. Add Sweetener:
    - Drizzle honey or maple syrup over the top layer if desired.
4. Garnish:
    - Garnish with fresh mint leaves if using.

Nutrition Information (per serving):
Calories: 350
Protein: 15g
Carbohydrates: 40g
Dietary Fiber: 4g
Sugars: 20g
Fat: 12g
Saturated Fat: 2g

4. Spinach and Feta Omelette

Preparation Time: 5 minutes
Cooking Time: 10 minutes
Total Time: 15 minutes
Servings: 2
Ingredients:
- 1 cup rolled oats
- 2 cups water or milk (or a mix of both)
- 1/2 teaspoon cinnamon
- 1 tablespoon honey or maple syrup (optional)
- 1 cup fresh fruit (such as sliced bananas, berries, or diced apples)
- 1 tablespoon chia seeds (optional)
- A pinch of salt

Directions:
1. Cook the Oats:
    - In a medium saucepan, bring the water or milk to a boil.
    - Stir in the rolled oats and a pinch of salt.
    - Reduce the heat to low and simmer for 5-7 minutes, stirring occasionally, until the oats are tender and have absorbed most of the liquid.
    - Stir in the cinnamon and sweetener if using.
2. Prepare the Fruit:
    - While the oats are cooking, wash and prepare the fresh fruit.
3. Assemble the Oatmeal:
    - Divide the cooked oatmeal between two bowls.
    - Top each serving with a portion of fresh fruit.
    - Sprinkle with chia seeds if desired.

Nutrition Information (per serving):
- Calories: 270
- Protein: 6g
- Carbohydrates: 45g
- Dietary Fiber: 5g
- Sugars: 12g
- Fat: 6g
- Saturated Fat: 1g

5. Smoothie Bowl

Preparation Time: 5 minutes
Cooking Time: 0 minutes
Total Time: 5 minutes
Servings: 2
Ingredients:
- 1 cup frozen berries (such as strawberries, blueberries, or raspberries)
- 1 banana, sliced
- 1/2 cup Greek yogurt (plain or vanilla)
- 1/2 cup milk or a dairy-free alternative
- 1 tablespoon honey or maple syrup (optional)
- Toppings: granola, fresh fruit slices, chia seeds, shredded coconut, nuts, or seeds

Directions:
1. Blend the Smoothie:
   - In a blender, combine the frozen berries, banana, Greek yogurt, and milk.
   - Blend until smooth and creamy. Add honey or maple syrup if desired for extra sweetness.
2. Assemble the Bowl:
   - Pour the smoothie into bowls.
   - Top with your choice of granola, fresh fruit slices, chia seeds, shredded coconut, nuts, or seeds.
3. Serve:
   - Serve immediately with a spoon.

Nutrition Information (per serving):
- Calories: 300
- Protein: 10g
- Carbohydrates: 45g
- Dietary Fiber: 7g
- Sugars: 20g
- Fat: 8g
- Saturated Fat: 3g

6. Chia Seed Pudding

Preparation Time: 5 minutes
Cooking Time: 0 minutes
Total Time: 5 minutes (plus chilling time)
Servings: 2
Ingredients:
- 1/4 cup chia seeds
- 1 cup milk or dairy-free alternative (such as almond milk or coconut milk)
- 1 tablespoon honey or maple syrup (optional)
- 1/2 teaspoon vanilla extract
- Fresh fruit or nuts for topping (optional)

Directions:
1. Mix Ingredients:
   - In a bowl or jar, combine the chia seeds, milk, honey or maple syrup (if using), and vanilla extract.
2. Stir and Chill:
   - Stir well to ensure the chia seeds are evenly distributed.
   - Cover and refrigerate for at least 2 hours or overnight to allow the chia seeds to absorb the liquid and thicken.
3. Serve:
   - Before serving, stir the pudding to break up any clumps.
   - Top with fresh fruit, nuts, or seeds if desired.

Nutrition Information (per serving):
- Calories: 200
- Protein: 5g
- Carbohydrates: 20g
- Dietary Fiber: 10g
- Sugars: 8g
- Fat: 12g
- Saturated Fat: 1g

7. Whole Wheat Banana Pancakes

Preparation Time: 10 minutes
Cooking Time: 15 minutes
Total Time: 25 minutes
Servings: 2
Ingredients:
- 1 cup whole wheat flour
- 1 tablespoon baking powder
- 1/4 teaspoon salt
- 1 cup milk
- 1 large egg
- 1 ripe banana, mashed

- 2 tablespoons honey or maple syrup
- 1 tablespoon olive oil or melted butter

Directions:
1. Prepare the Batter:
    - In a bowl, whisk together the whole wheat flour, baking powder, and salt.
    - In another bowl, mix the milk, egg, mashed banana, honey or maple syrup, and olive oil or melted butter.
    - Combine the wet and dry ingredients, stirring until just mixed. The batter may be slightly lumpy.
2. Cook the Pancakes:
    - Heat a non-stick skillet or griddle over medium heat and lightly grease with a bit of oil or butter.
    - Pour 1/4 cup of batter onto the skillet for each pancake.
    - Cook until bubbles form on the surface and the edges look set, about 2-3 minutes. Flip and cook for another 1-2 minutes, until golden brown.
3. Serve:
    - Serve the pancakes warm with your favorite toppings such as fresh fruit, yogurt, or a drizzle of honey or maple syrup.

Nutrition Information (per serving):
Calories: 320
Protein: 8g
Carbohydrates: 55g
Dietary Fiber: 6g
Sugars: 10g
Fat: 8g
Saturated Fat: 2g

8. Breakfast Burrito

Preparation Time: 10 minutes
Cooking Time: 10 minutes
Total Time: 20 minutes
Servings: 2
Ingredients:
- 2 large flour tortillas
- 4 large eggs
- 1/2 cup shredded cheddar cheese
- 1/2 cup cooked black beans (drained and rinsed)
- 1/2 cup cooked and crumbled breakfast sausage or bacon (optional)
- 1/2 cup diced bell peppers
- 1/4 cup diced onions
- 1 tablespoon olive oil
- Salt and pepper to taste
- Salsa or hot sauce for serving (optional)

Directions:
1. Prepare the Filling:
    - Heat olive oil in a skillet over medium heat.
    - Add the diced bell peppers and onions, and sauté until softened, about 3-4 minutes.
    - In a bowl, whisk the eggs with a pinch of salt and pepper. Pour the eggs into the skillet with the vegetables and cook, stirring occasionally, until scrambled and fully cooked.
    - Stir in the cooked black beans and breakfast sausage or bacon if using. Remove from heat.
2. Assemble the Burritos:
    - Warm the tortillas in a dry skillet or microwave until pliable.
    - Divide the egg mixture between the tortillas.
    - Sprinkle shredded cheddar cheese over the egg mixture.
3. Roll and Serve:
    - Fold in the sides of each tortilla and roll it up tightly to form a burrito.
    - Serve with salsa or hot sauce if desired.

Nutrition Information (per serving):
Calories: 450
Protein: 25g
Carbohydrates: 40g
Dietary Fiber: 6g
Sugars: 4g
Fat: 22g
Saturated Fat: 8g

9. Egg Muffins

Preparation Time: 10 minutes
Cooking Time: 20 minutes
Total Time: 30 minutes
Servings: 2

Ingredients:
- 6 large eggs
- 1/2 cup milk
- 1/2 cup shredded cheddar cheese
- 1/2 cup diced bell peppers
- 1/4 cup diced onions
- 1/2 cup cooked and crumbled breakfast sausage or bacon (optional)
- 1/2 cup fresh spinach, chopped
- Salt and pepper to taste
- Cooking spray or olive oil for greasing

Directions:
1. Prepare the Oven:
   - Preheat the oven to 375°F (190°C).
   - Lightly grease a muffin tin with cooking spray or olive oil.
2. Mix the Ingredients:
   - In a bowl, whisk together the eggs, milk, salt, and pepper.
   - Stir in the shredded cheddar cheese, diced bell peppers, diced onions, cooked sausage or bacon (if using), and chopped spinach.
3. Fill the Muffin Tin:
   - Pour the egg mixture evenly into the muffin cups, filling each about 3/4 full.
4. Bake:
   - Bake for 18-20 minutes, or until the egg muffins are set and slightly golden on top.
5. Cool and Serve:
   - Allow the muffins to cool slightly before removing them from the tin. Serve warm.

Nutrition Information (per muffin, assuming 6 muffins total):
- Calories: 120
- Protein: 8g
- Carbohydrates: 2g
- Dietary Fiber: 1g
- Sugars: 1g
- Fat: 9g
- Saturated Fat: 3g

10. Quinoa Breakfast Bowl

Preparation Time: 10 minutes
Cooking Time: 15 minutes
Total Time: 25 minutes
Servings: 2

Ingredients:
- 1/2 cup quinoa
- 1 cup water or milk (or a mix of both)
- 1/2 cup Greek yogurt
- 1/2 cup fresh fruit (such as berries, sliced banana, or diced apple)
- 1 tablespoon honey or maple syrup (optional)
- 2 tablespoons chopped nuts or seeds (such as almonds, walnuts, or chia seeds)
- 1/2 teaspoon cinnamon (optional)

Directions:
1. Cook the Quinoa:
   - Rinse the quinoa under cold water.
   - In a medium saucepan, bring the water or milk to a boil.
   - Stir in the quinoa, reduce the heat to low, cover, and simmer for 15 minutes, until the quinoa is tender and the liquid is absorbed. Let it sit covered for 5 minutes, then fluff with a fork.
2. Assemble the Bowl:
   - Divide the cooked quinoa between two bowls.
   - Top each bowl with Greek yogurt, fresh fruit, and chopped nuts or seeds.
   - Drizzle with honey or maple syrup if desired.
   - Sprinkle with cinnamon if using.
3. Serve:
   - Serve immediately, or store in the refrigerator for a quick breakfast later.

Nutrition Information (per serving):
Calories: 320
Protein: 12g
Carbohydrates: 45g
Dietary Fiber: 6g
Sugars: 15g
Fat: 12g
Saturated Fat: 2g

11. Berry Smoothie

Preparation Time: 5 minutes
Cooking Time: 0 minutes
Total Time: 5 minutes
Servings: 2
Ingredients:
- 1 cup frozen mixed berries (such as strawberries, blueberries, raspberries)

- 1 banana, sliced
- 1 cup Greek yogurt (plain or vanilla)
- 1/2 cup milk or a dairy-free alternative (such as almond milk)
- 1 tablespoon honey or maple syrup (optional)
- 1/2 teaspoon vanilla extract (optional)

Directions:
1. Blend the Ingredients:
    - In a blender, combine the frozen berries, banana, Greek yogurt, and milk.
    - Blend until smooth and creamy. Add honey or maple syrup and vanilla extract if desired.
2. Serve:
    - Pour the smoothie into glasses and serve immediately.

Nutrition Information (per serving):
Calories: 250
Protein: 10g
Carbohydrates: 45g
Dietary Fiber: 6g
Sugars: 25g
Fat: 3g
Saturated Fat: 1g

12. Cottage Cheese and Fruit

Preparation Time: 5 minutes
Cooking Time: 0 minutes
Total Time: 5 minutes
Servings: 2
Ingredients:
- 1 cup cottage cheese
- 1 cup fresh fruit (such as berries, diced apple, or sliced peaches)
- 1 tablespoon honey or maple syrup (optional)
- 1 tablespoon chopped nuts or seeds (optional)

Directions:
1. Prepare the Ingredients:
    - Wash and prepare the fresh fruit.
2. Assemble the Dish:
    - Divide the cottage cheese between two bowls.
    - Top each bowl with a portion of fresh fruit.
    - Drizzle with honey or maple syrup if desired.
    - Sprinkle with chopped nuts or seeds if using.
3. Serve:
    - Serve immediately or chill briefly before serving.

Nutrition Information (per serving):
Calories: 220
Protein: 15g
Carbohydrates: 20g
Dietary Fiber: 3g
Sugars: 15g
Fat: 10g
Saturated Fat: 5g

13. Sweet Potato Hash

Preparation Time: 10 minutes
Cooking Time: 15 minutes
Total Time: 25 minutes
Servings: 2
Ingredients:
- 2 medium sweet potatoes, peeled and diced
- 1 tablespoon olive oil
- 1/2 cup diced bell peppers
- 1/4 cup diced onions
- 1/2 teaspoon smoked paprika
- 1/4 teaspoon garlic powder
- Salt and pepper to taste
- Fresh herbs for garnish (optional)

Directions:
1. Cook the Sweet Potatoes:
    - Heat olive oil in a large skillet over medium heat.
    - Add the diced sweet potatoes and cook, stirring occasionally, for about 10 minutes, until they start to soften.
2. Add Vegetables and Seasonings:
    - Add the diced bell peppers and onions to the skillet.
    - Stir in the smoked paprika, garlic powder, salt, and pepper.
    - Continue to cook for an additional 5 minutes, or until the sweet potatoes are tender and slightly crispy.
3. Serve:
    - Garnish with fresh herbs if desired and serve hot.

Nutrition Information (per serving):
Calories: 220
Protein: 3g
Carbohydrates: 36g
Dietary Fiber: 5g

Sugars: 8g
Fat: 8g
Saturated Fat: 1g

14. Almond Butter and Banana Toast

Preparation Time: 5 minutes
Cooking Time: 0 minutes
Total Time: 5 minutes
Servings: 2
Ingredients:
- 2 slices whole grain or multigrain bread
- 2 tablespoons almond butter
- 1 ripe banana, sliced
- 1 teaspoon honey or maple syrup (optional)
- A pinch of cinnamon (optional)

Directions:
1. Toast the Bread:
    - Toast the slices of bread until golden brown.
2. Spread Almond Butter:
    - Spread 1 tablespoon of almond butter evenly on each slice of toast.
3. Add Banana Slices:
    - Top the almond butter with sliced banana.
4. Optional Toppings:
    - Drizzle with honey or maple syrup and sprinkle with a pinch of cinnamon if desired.
5. Serve:
    - Serve immediately.

Nutrition Information (per serving):
Calories: 250
Protein: 8g
Carbohydrates: 32g
Dietary Fiber: 5g
Sugars: 14g
Fat: 12g
Saturated Fat: 1g

15. Muesli with Almond Milk

Preparation Time: 5 minutes
Cooking Time: 0 minutes
Total Time: 5 minutes
Servings: 2
Ingredients:
- 1 cup muesli
- 1 cup almond milk (or other dairy-free milk)
- 1/2 cup fresh fruit (such as berries or sliced apple)
- 1 tablespoon honey or maple syrup (optional)
- 1 tablespoon chopped nuts or seeds (optional)

Directions:
1. Prepare the Muesli:
    - In a bowl, combine the muesli and almond milk.
2. Add Toppings:
    - Top with fresh fruit, and drizzle with honey or maple syrup if desired.
    - Sprinkle with chopped nuts or seeds if using.
3. Serve:
    - Serve immediately or let it sit for a few minutes to soften the muesli.

Nutrition Information (per serving):
Calories: 250
Protein: 6g
Carbohydrates: 40g
Dietary Fiber: 6g
Sugars: 12g
Fat: 8g
Saturated Fat: 1g

16. Egg and Veggie Breakfast Bowl

Preparation Time: 10 minutes
Cooking Time: 15 minutes
Total Time: 25 minutes
Servings: 2
Ingredients:
- 4 large eggs
- 1 cup cooked quinoa or brown rice
- 1/2 cup diced bell peppers
- 1/2 cup diced zucchini
- 1/4 cup diced onions
- 1 tablespoon olive oil
- Salt and pepper to taste
- 1/4 cup shredded cheese (optional)
- Fresh herbs for garnish (optional)

Directions:
1. Cook the Vegetables:
    - Heat olive oil in a skillet over medium heat.
    - Add the diced bell peppers, zucchini, and onions. Sauté for 5-7 minutes, until vegetables are tender. Season with salt and pepper.

2. Cook the Eggs:
    - In another skillet, scramble the eggs over medium heat until fully cooked.
3. Assemble the Bowl:
    - Divide the cooked quinoa or brown rice between two bowls.
    - Top with sautéed vegetables and scrambled eggs.
    - Sprinkle with shredded cheese if desired and garnish with fresh herbs.
4. Serve:
    - Serve warm.

Nutrition Information (per serving):
Calories: 350
Protein: 20g
Carbohydrates: 30g
Dietary Fiber: 6g
Sugars: 5g
Fat: 18g
Saturated Fat: 4g

17. Berry and Yogurt Smoothie

Preparation Time: 5 minutes
Cooking Time: 0 minutes
Total Time: 5 minutes
Servings: 2
Ingredients:
- 1 cup mixed berries (fresh or frozen)
- 1 cup Greek yogurt (plain or vanilla)
- 1/2 cup almond milk or other milk of choice
- 1 tablespoon honey or maple syrup (optional)
- 1/2 teaspoon vanilla extract (optional)

Directions:
1. Blend Ingredients:
    - In a blender, combine mixed berries, Greek yogurt, and almond milk.
    - Blend until smooth and creamy. Add honey or maple syrup and vanilla extract if desired.
2. Serve:
    - Pour into glasses and serve immediately.

Nutrition Information (per serving):
Calories: 220
Protein: 12g
Carbohydrates: 30g
Dietary Fiber: 4g
Sugars: 20g
Fat: 6g
Saturated Fat: 2g

18. Zucchini and Carrot Fritters

Preparation Time: 10 minutes
Cooking Time: 15 minutes
Total Time: 25 minutes
Servings: 2
Ingredients:
- 1 medium zucchini, grated
- 1 medium carrot, grated
- 1/4 cup all-purpose flour
- 1/4 cup grated Parmesan cheese
- 1 large egg
- 2 tablespoons chopped fresh parsley (optional)
- 1/4 teaspoon garlic powder
- Salt and pepper to taste
- 2 tablespoons olive oil

Directions:
1. Prepare Vegetables:
    - Place the grated zucchini and carrot in a clean kitchen towel or cheesecloth and squeeze out excess moisture.
2. Mix Ingredients:
    - In a bowl, combine the grated zucchini, carrot, flour, Parmesan cheese, egg, parsley (if using), garlic powder, salt, and pepper. Mix well.
3. Cook the Fritters:
    - Heat olive oil in a skillet over medium heat.
    - Drop spoonfuls of the mixture into the skillet, pressing them down slightly to form patties.
    - Cook for 3-4 minutes on each side, or until golden brown and crispy.
4. Serve:
    - Drain on paper towels if needed, and serve warm.

Nutrition Information (per serving, assuming 4 fritters per person):
Calories: 180
Protein: 8g
Carbohydrates: 16g
Dietary Fiber: 3g
Sugars: 5g
Fat: 10g

Saturated Fat: 3g

19. Nut and Seed Granola

Preparation Time: 10 minutes
Cooking Time: 20 minutes
Total Time: 30 minutes
Servings: 2
Ingredients:
- 1 cup rolled oats
- 1/2 cup mixed nuts (such as almonds, walnuts, or pecans), chopped
- 1/2 cup mixed seeds (such as sunflower, pumpkin, or chia seeds)
- 1/4 cup honey or maple syrup
- 1/4 cup coconut oil or olive oil
- 1/2 teaspoon vanilla extract
- 1/2 teaspoon ground cinnamon
- A pinch of salt

Directions:
1. Preheat Oven:
   - Preheat your oven to 350°F (175°C).
2. Mix Ingredients:
   - In a large bowl, combine the oats, nuts, and seeds.
   - In a small saucepan, heat the honey or maple syrup with the coconut oil until melted. Stir in the vanilla extract, cinnamon, and salt.
3. Combine and Bake:
   - Pour the liquid mixture over the oat mixture and stir until evenly coated.
   - Spread the mixture in a single layer on a baking sheet.
   - Bake for 15-20 minutes, stirring halfway through, until golden and crispy.
4. Cool and Store:
   - Allow the granola to cool completely before breaking into clusters.
   - Store in an airtight container at room temperature for up to 2 weeks.

Nutrition Information (per serving, assuming 2 servings total):
Calories: 300
Protein: 8g
Carbohydrates: 30g
Dietary Fiber: 5g
Sugars: 12g
Fat: 18g
Saturated Fat: 6g

20. Pumpkin Spice Overnight Oats

Preparation Time: 5 minutes
Cooking Time: 0 minutes
Total Time: 5 minutes (plus 4 hours chilling)
Servings: 2
Ingredients:
- 1 cup rolled oats
- 1/2 cup canned pumpkin (pure pumpkin, not pumpkin pie filling)
- 1/2 cup almond milk (or other milk of choice)
- 1/4 cup Greek yogurt (plain or vanilla)
- 2 tablespoons maple syrup or honey
- 1/2 teaspoon pumpkin pie spice
- 1/4 teaspoon vanilla extract
- A pinch of salt

Directions:
1. Combine Ingredients:
   - In a bowl, mix the rolled oats, canned pumpkin, almond milk, Greek yogurt, maple syrup, pumpkin pie spice, vanilla extract, and salt.
2. Refrigerate:
   - Cover the bowl and refrigerate for at least 4 hours or overnight to allow the oats to absorb the liquid and flavors.
3. Serve:
   - Stir the oats before serving. Add extra toppings like nuts, seeds, or fresh fruit if desired.

Nutrition Information (per serving):
Calories: 280
Protein: 10g
Carbohydrates: 40g
Dietary Fiber: 6g
Sugars: 15g
Fat: 8g
Saturated Fat: 1g

Lunch 20 recipes

When it comes to lunch, you want something that's not only delicious but also nourishing to get you through the rest of your day. Whether you're looking for something light and refreshing or hearty and filling, these 20 lunch recipes are here to offer a perfect blend of taste and nutrition. Here's a handy list of tasty ideas to inspire your midday meal:

1. Grilled Chicken Salad

Preparation Time: 10 minutes
Cooking Time: 10 minutes
Total Time: 20 minutes
Servings: 2
Ingredients:
- 2 boneless, skinless chicken breasts
- 1 tablespoon olive oil
- 1 teaspoon paprika
- 1/2 teaspoon garlic powder
- Salt and pepper to taste
- 4 cups mixed salad greens
- 1 cup cherry tomatoes, halved
- 1/2 cucumber, sliced
- 1/4 red onion, thinly sliced
- 1/4 cup crumbled feta cheese (optional)
- 2 tablespoons balsamic vinaigrette or dressing of choice

Directions:
1. Grill the Chicken:
   - Preheat the grill or a grill pan over medium-high heat.
   - Rub the chicken breasts with olive oil, paprika, garlic powder, salt, and pepper.
   - Grill the chicken for 5-7 minutes on each side, or until cooked through and juices run clear. Let the chicken rest for a few minutes before slicing.
2. Prepare the Salad:
   - In a large bowl, toss the mixed greens, cherry tomatoes, cucumber, and red onion.
3. Assemble the Salad:
   - Slice the grilled chicken and place it on top of the salad.
   - Sprinkle with feta cheese if using.
   - Drizzle with balsamic vinaigrette or your preferred dressing.
4. Serve:
   - Serve immediately.

Nutrition Information (per serving):
Calories: 300
Protein: 30g
Carbohydrates: 15g
Dietary Fiber: 4g
Sugars: 6g
Fat: 15g
Saturated Fat: 3g

2. Quinoa and Black Bean Bowl

Preparation Time: 10 minutes
Cooking Time: 15 minutes
Total Time: 25 minutes
Servings: 2
Ingredients:
- 1 cup quinoa
- 1 1/2 cups water or vegetable broth
- 1 can (15 oz) black beans, drained and rinsed
- 1 cup corn kernels (fresh, frozen, or canned)
- 1/2 red bell pepper, diced
- 1/2 cup cherry tomatoes, halved
- 1/4 cup chopped fresh cilantro
- 1 tablespoon olive oil
- Juice of 1 lime
- Salt and pepper to taste
- 1 avocado, sliced (optional)

Directions:
1. Cook Quinoa:
   - Rinse the quinoa under cold water.
   - In a medium saucepan, combine the quinoa and water (or broth). Bring to a boil, then reduce heat to low, cover, and simmer for 15 minutes or until quinoa is tender and water is absorbed. Fluff with a fork.
2. Prepare Vegetables:
   - While quinoa is cooking, heat olive oil in a skillet over medium heat. Add corn and red bell pepper, and cook for 5-7 minutes

until tender. Season with salt and pepper.
3. Combine Ingredients:
    - In a large bowl, combine the cooked quinoa, black beans, corn mixture, cherry tomatoes, and cilantro.
4. Season and Serve:
    - Drizzle with lime juice and toss to combine. Adjust seasoning with salt and pepper if needed.
    - Top with avocado slices if desired.

Nutrition Information (per serving):
Calories: 350
Protein: 12g
Carbohydrates: 50g
Dietary Fiber: 10g
Sugars: 6g
Fat: 12g
Saturated Fat: 2g

3. Turkey and Avocado Wrap

Preparation Time: 10 minutes
Cooking Time: 0 minutes
Total Time: 10 minutes
Servings: 2
Ingredients:
- 2 large whole wheat tortillas
- 4 ounces sliced turkey breast (deli or cooked)
- 1 ripe avocado, sliced
- 1/2 cup baby spinach or mixed greens
- 1/2 cup shredded cheese (such as cheddar or Swiss, optional)
- 2 tablespoons hummus or Greek yogurt (optional)
- Salt and pepper to taste

Directions:
1. Assemble the Wraps:
    - Lay out the tortillas on a flat surface.
    - Spread hummus or Greek yogurt on each tortilla if using.
    - Layer with sliced turkey, avocado, spinach, and shredded cheese if desired.
    - Season with salt and pepper to taste.
2. Wrap and Serve:
    - Roll up the tortillas tightly to enclose the fillings.
    - Slice in half and serve immediately or wrap in foil for a portable lunch.

Nutrition Information (per serving):
Calories: 350
Protein: 20g
Carbohydrates: 30g
Dietary Fiber: 8g
Sugars: 2g
Fat: 20g
Saturated Fat: 4g

4. Mediterranean Chickpea Salad

Preparation Time: 10 minutes
Cooking Time: 0 minutes
Total Time: 10 minutes
Servings: 2
Ingredients:
- 1 can (15 oz) chickpeas, drained and rinsed
- 1/2 cup cherry tomatoes, halved
- 1/2 cucumber, diced
- 1/4 cup red onion, finely chopped
- 1/4 cup Kalamata olives, sliced
- 1/4 cup crumbled feta cheese
- 2 tablespoons chopped fresh parsley
- 2 tablespoons olive oil
- 1 tablespoon red wine vinegar
- 1/2 teaspoon dried oregano
- Salt and pepper to taste

Directions:
1. Combine Ingredients:
    - In a large bowl, mix the chickpeas, cherry tomatoes, cucumber, red onion, olives, feta cheese, and parsley.
2. Make Dressing:
    - In a small bowl, whisk together olive oil, red wine vinegar, dried oregano, salt, and pepper.
3. Toss Salad:
    - Pour the dressing over the salad and toss gently to combine.
4. Serve:
    - Serve immediately or refrigerate for 30 minutes to allow flavors to meld.

Nutrition Information (per serving):
Calories: 280
Protein: 10g
Carbohydrates: 30g
Dietary Fiber: 8g
Sugars: 5g

Fat: 14g
Saturated Fat: 4g

5. Lentil Soup

Preparation Time: 10 minutes
Cooking Time: 30 minutes
Total Time: 40 minutes
Servings: 2
Ingredients:
- 1 cup dried green or brown lentils, rinsed
- 1 tablespoon olive oil
- 1 small onion, chopped
- 2 cloves garlic, minced
- 1 carrot, diced
- 1 celery stalk, diced
- 1 can (14.5 oz) diced tomatoes
- 4 cups vegetable or chicken broth
- 1 teaspoon ground cumin
- 1/2 teaspoon smoked paprika
- 1 bay leaf
- Salt and pepper to taste
- 1 cup chopped fresh spinach (optional)

Directions:
1. Sauté Vegetables:
   - Heat olive oil in a large pot over medium heat. Add onion and garlic, and cook until softened, about 5 minutes.
   - Add carrot and celery, and cook for another 5 minutes.
2. Cook Soup:
   - Stir in the lentils, diced tomatoes, broth, cumin, paprika, and bay leaf. Bring to a boil, then reduce heat and simmer for 25-30 minutes, or until lentils are tender.
   - Season with salt and pepper to taste.
3. Add Spinach (Optional):
   - If using, stir in the chopped spinach and cook for an additional 2-3 minutes until wilted.
4. Serve:
   - Remove bay leaf before serving. Enjoy hot.

Nutrition Information (per serving):
Calories: 250
Protein: 15g
Carbohydrates: 40g
Dietary Fiber: 15g
Sugars: 7g
Fat: 5g
Saturated Fat: 1g

6. Greek Chicken Pita

Preparation Time: 15 minutes
Cooking Time: 10 minutes
Total Time: 25 minutes
Servings: 2
Ingredients:
- 2 boneless, skinless chicken breasts
- 1 tablespoon olive oil
- 1 teaspoon dried oregano
- 1/2 teaspoon garlic powder
- 1/2 teaspoon paprika
- Salt and pepper to taste
- 2 whole wheat pita breads
- 1/2 cup Greek yogurt
- 1 tablespoon lemon juice
- 1 tablespoon chopped fresh dill (or 1 teaspoon dried dill)
- 1 cup shredded lettuce
- 1/2 cucumber, sliced
- 1/2 cup cherry tomatoes, halved
- 1/4 cup sliced red onion
- 1/4 cup Kalamata olives (optional)

Directions:
1. Cook the Chicken:
   - Preheat a grill or skillet over medium-high heat.
   - Rub the chicken breasts with olive oil, oregano, garlic powder, paprika, salt, and pepper.
   - Cook the chicken for 5-7 minutes on each side, or until cooked through and juices run clear. Let rest for a few minutes before slicing.
2. Prepare the Tzatziki Sauce:
   - In a small bowl, mix Greek yogurt, lemon juice, and dill. Season with salt and pepper to taste.
3. Assemble the Pitas:
   - Warm the pita breads if desired.
   - Spread a spoonful of tzatziki sauce inside each pita.
   - Layer with shredded lettuce, sliced cucumber, cherry tomatoes, red onion, and olives.
   - Top with sliced chicken.
4. Serve:
   - Serve immediately.

Nutrition Information (per serving):
- Calories: 350
- Protein: 30g
- Carbohydrates: 30g
- Dietary Fiber: 6g
- Sugars: 6g
- Fat: 15g
- Saturated Fat: 3g

7. Vegetable Stir-Fry

Preparation Time: 10 minutes
Cooking Time: 10 minutes
Total Time: 20 minutes
Servings: 2
Ingredients:
- 1 tablespoon olive oil
- 1 small onion, sliced
- 1 bell pepper, sliced
- 1 zucchini, sliced
- 1 cup broccoli florets
- 1 carrot, julienned
- 1/2 cup snow peas
- 2 tablespoons soy sauce (low sodium)
- 1 tablespoon sesame oil
- 1 teaspoon grated ginger
- 1 clove garlic, minced
- 1 tablespoon sesame seeds (optional)
- Cooked rice or noodles (optional for serving)

Directions:
1. Heat Oil and Sauté:
   - Heat olive oil in a large skillet or wok over medium-high heat.
   - Add onion, garlic, and ginger, and sauté for 1-2 minutes until fragrant.
2. Add Vegetables:
   - Add bell pepper, zucchini, broccoli, carrot, and snow peas.
   - Stir-fry for 5-7 minutes until vegetables are tender-crisp.
3. Season:
   - Add soy sauce and sesame oil to the stir-fry. Toss well to coat the vegetables.
4. Serve:
   - Garnish with sesame seeds if desired. Serve alone or over cooked rice or noodles.

Nutrition Information (per serving):
- Calories: 200
- Protein: 5g
- Carbohydrates: 25g
- Dietary Fiber: 6g
- Sugars: 8g
- Fat: 10g
- Saturated Fat: 1.5g

8. Sweet Potato and Black Bean Tacos

Preparation Time: 10 minutes
Cooking Time: 20 minutes
Total Time: 30 minutes
Servings: 2-4
Ingredients:
- 2 medium sweet potatoes, diced
- 1 tablespoon olive oil
- 1 teaspoon cumin
- 1/2 teaspoon paprika
- Salt and pepper to taste
- 1 can black beans, drained and rinsed
- 8 small corn tortillas
- 1/4 cup chopped cilantro
- 1/4 cup diced red onion
- 1 avocado, sliced
- Salsa (optional)

Directions:
1. Roast Sweet Potatoes:
   - Preheat oven to 400°F (200°C). Toss sweet potatoes with olive oil, cumin, paprika, salt, and pepper. Roast for 20 minutes, or until tender.
2. Warm Beans and Tortillas:
   - In a small saucepan, heat black beans over medium heat.
   - Warm tortillas in a dry skillet or microwave.
3. Assemble Tacos:
   - Fill tortillas with roasted sweet potatoes, black beans, cilantro, red onion, and avocado slices. Add salsa if desired.

Nutrition Information (per serving):
- Calories: 350
- Protein: 10g
- Carbohydrates: 58g
- Dietary Fiber: 14g
- Sugars: 7g
- Fat: 10g

9. Spinach and Feta Stuffed Chicken Breast

Preparation Time: 15 minutes
Cooking Time: 25 minutes
Total Time: 40 minutes
Servings: 2-4
Ingredients:
- 2 large chicken breasts
- 1 cup fresh spinach, chopped
- 1/4 cup feta cheese, crumbled
- 1 tablespoon olive oil
- 1 teaspoon garlic powder
- Salt and pepper to taste

Directions:
1. Prepare Chicken:
   - Preheat oven to 375°F (190°C). Slice a pocket into each chicken breast.
   - In a bowl, mix spinach, feta, garlic powder, salt, and pepper.
2. Stuff and Cook Chicken:
   - Stuff the spinach-feta mixture into each chicken breast.
   - Heat olive oil in a skillet over medium heat, sear the chicken for 3-4 minutes on each side, then transfer to the oven and bake for 20 minutes.
3. Serve:
   - Let rest for a few minutes before slicing and serving.

Nutrition Information (per serving):
Calories: 280
Protein: 34g
Carbohydrates: 2g
Dietary Fiber: 1g
Fat: 14g

10. Salmon and Avocado Sushi Rolls

Preparation Time: 15 minutes
Cooking Time: 10 minutes
Total Time: 25 minutes
Servings: 2-4
Ingredients:
- 1 cup sushi rice, cooked
- 2 tablespoons rice vinegar
- 4 sheets nori (seaweed)
- 4 oz fresh salmon, sliced thin
- 1 avocado, sliced
- Soy sauce for serving

Directions:
1. Prepare Sushi Rice:
   - Cook sushi rice according to package instructions. Mix rice with vinegar and let cool.
2. Assemble Rolls:
   - Place a nori sheet on a bamboo mat. Spread a thin layer of rice on the nori, leaving 1 inch at the top.
   - Lay slices of salmon and avocado in the center. Roll the sushi tightly, sealing with water.
3. Slice and Serve:
   - Slice into bite-sized pieces and serve with soy sauce.

Nutrition Information (per serving):
Calories: 300
Protein: 18g
Carbohydrates: 36g
Dietary Fiber: 5g
Fat: 10g

11. Butternut Squash Soup

Preparation Time: 10 minutes
Cooking Time: 25 minutes
Total Time: 35 minutes
Servings: 2-4
Ingredients:
- 1 medium butternut squash, peeled and cubed
- 1 onion, chopped
- 2 cloves garlic, minced
- 4 cups vegetable broth
- 1/2 teaspoon ground nutmeg
- Salt and pepper to taste
- 1 tablespoon olive oil

Directions:
1. Sauté Vegetables:
   - Heat olive oil in a large pot. Add onion and garlic, sauté until soft.
2. Cook Squash:
   - Add cubed squash and broth. Bring to a boil, reduce heat, and simmer for 20 minutes until squash is tender.
3. Blend and Serve:
   - Puree soup with a blender until smooth. Season with nutmeg, salt, and pepper. Serve warm.

Nutrition Information (per serving):
Calories: 120
Protein: 2g
Carbohydrates: 28g
Dietary Fiber: 6g

Fat: 4g

12. Caesar Salad with Grilled Shrimp

Preparation Time: 10 minutes
Cooking Time: 10 minutes
Total Time: 20 minutes
Servings: 2-4
Ingredients:
- 12 shrimp, peeled and deveined
- 4 cups romaine lettuce, chopped
- 1/4 cup grated Parmesan cheese
- 1/4 cup Caesar dressing
- 1 tablespoon olive oil
- Salt and pepper to taste

Directions:
1. Grill Shrimp:
    - Season shrimp with salt and pepper. Grill over medium heat for 2-3 minutes per side, until pink and cooked through.
2. Assemble Salad:
    - Toss romaine lettuce with Caesar dressing, top with grilled shrimp and Parmesan cheese.

Nutrition Information (per serving):
Calories: 220
Protein: 18g
Carbohydrates: 6g
Dietary Fiber: 2g
Fat: 14g

13. Chicken and Vegetable Skewers

Preparation Time: 15 minutes
Cooking Time: 15 minutes
Total Time: 30 minutes
Servings: 2-4
Ingredients:
- 2 chicken breasts, cubed
- 1 red bell pepper, cubed
- 1 zucchini, sliced
- 1 red onion, cubed
- 2 tablespoons olive oil
- 1 teaspoon paprika
- Salt and pepper to taste

Directions:
1. Prepare Skewers:
    - Thread chicken, bell pepper, zucchini, and onion onto skewers. Brush with olive oil and season with paprika, salt, and pepper.
2. Grill Skewers:
    - Grill over medium heat for 10-15 minutes, turning occasionally, until chicken is cooked through.

Nutrition Information (per serving):
Calories: 250
Protein: 30g
Carbohydrates: 8g
Dietary Fiber: 2g
Fat: 10g

14. Hummus and Veggie Wrap

Preparation Time: 10 minutes
Total Time: 10 minutes
Servings: 2-4
Ingredients:
- 4 whole wheat tortillas
- 1 cup hummus
- 1 cucumber, sliced
- 1 red bell pepper, sliced
- 1/2 cup shredded carrots
- 1/4 cup spinach leaves

Directions:
1. Assemble Wraps:
    - Spread hummus evenly over each tortilla. Layer with cucumber, bell pepper, carrots, and spinach. Roll tightly and slice in half.

Nutrition Information (per serving):
Calories: 220
Protein: 6g
Carbohydrates: 30g
Dietary Fiber: 7g
Fat: 8g

15. Bulgur Wheat Salad

Preparation Time: 10 minutes
Cooking Time: 15 minutes
Total Time: 25 minutes
Servings: 2-4
Ingredients:
- 1 cup bulgur wheat
- 2 cups water
- 1 cucumber, diced
- 1 tomato, diced
- 1/4 cup parsley, chopped
- 2 tablespoons lemon juice
- 2 tablespoons olive oil
- Salt and pepper to taste

Directions:
1. Cook Bulgur:
    - Boil water and pour over bulgur in a bowl. Cover and let sit for 15 minutes until absorbed. Fluff with a fork.
2. Mix Salad:
    - Combine cooked bulgur with cucumber, tomato, parsley, lemon juice, olive oil, salt, and pepper.

Nutrition Information (per serving):
Calories: 180
Protein: 5g
Carbohydrates: 30g
Dietary Fiber: 6g
Fat: 6g

16. Stuffed Bell Peppers

Preparation Time: 15 minutes
Cooking Time: 40 minutes
Total Time: 55 minutes
Servings: 2-4
Ingredients:
- 4 bell peppers, tops removed and seeds cleaned out
- 1/2 lb ground beef or turkey
- 1 cup cooked quinoa or rice
- 1 small onion, chopped
- 1 can diced tomatoes (14 oz)
- 1/2 cup shredded mozzarella cheese
- 1 teaspoon garlic powder
- 1 teaspoon paprika
- Salt and pepper to taste
- 2 tablespoons olive oil

Directions:
1. Preheat Oven:
   Preheat the oven to 375°F (190°C).
2. Cook Filling:
   Heat olive oil in a skillet over medium heat. Add onion and cook until translucent. Add ground beef or turkey, cook until browned. Stir in cooked quinoa or rice, diced tomatoes, garlic powder, paprika, salt, and pepper. Cook for 5-7 minutes.
3. Stuff Peppers:
   Stuff each bell pepper with the filling mixture. Place them upright in a baking dish.
4. Bake:
   Cover with foil and bake for 30 minutes. Remove foil, sprinkle with mozzarella cheese, and bake for another 10 minutes until the cheese is melted and bubbly.

Nutrition Information (per serving):
Calories: 280
Protein: 18g
Carbohydrates: 18g
Dietary Fiber: 4g
Fat: 15g

17. Thai Peanut Noodle Salad

Preparation Time: 20 minutes
Total Time: 20 minutes
Servings: 2-4
Ingredients:
- 8 oz rice noodles, cooked
- 1/2 cup shredded carrots
- 1/2 cup red bell pepper, sliced thin
- 1/2 cucumber, julienned
- 1/4 cup chopped peanuts
- 2 tablespoons cilantro, chopped

For Peanut Sauce:
- 1/4 cup peanut butter
- 2 tablespoons soy sauce
- 1 tablespoon sesame oil
- 1 tablespoon honey or maple syrup
- 1 tablespoon lime juice
- 1 clove garlic, minced
- 1 teaspoon grated ginger

Directions:
1. Make Peanut Sauce:
   In a small bowl, whisk together peanut butter, soy sauce, sesame oil, honey, lime juice, garlic, and ginger until smooth.
2. Toss Salad:
   In a large bowl, combine cooked noodles, shredded carrots, bell pepper, cucumber, and cilantro. Pour peanut sauce over the salad and toss to coat evenly.
3. Garnish and Serve:
   Sprinkle chopped peanuts on top and serve immediately.

Nutrition Information (per serving):
Calories: 350
Protein: 10g
Carbohydrates: 48g
Dietary Fiber: 5g
Fat: 14g

18. Eggplant Parmesan

Preparation Time: 20 minutes
Cooking Time: 45 minutes
Total Time: 65 minutes
Servings: 2-4
Ingredients:
- 1 large eggplant, sliced into 1/2-inch rounds
- 1 cup breadcrumbs
- 1/2 cup grated Parmesan cheese
- 1/2 cup flour
- 2 eggs, beaten
- 1 1/2 cups marinara sauce
- 1 cup shredded mozzarella cheese
- 1/4 cup fresh basil, chopped
- Olive oil for frying

Directions:
1. Prepare Eggplant:
   Salt the eggplant slices and let them sit for 15 minutes to draw out moisture. Pat them dry with paper towels.
2. Coat Eggplant:
   Dredge the eggplant slices in flour, dip into beaten eggs, and coat with a mixture of breadcrumbs and Parmesan cheese.
3. Fry Eggplant:
   Heat olive oil in a large skillet. Fry eggplant slices for 2-3 minutes on each side until golden brown. Drain on paper towels.
4. Bake:
   Preheat oven to 375°F (190°C). In a baking dish, layer fried eggplant slices, marinara sauce, and mozzarella cheese. Repeat layers and finish with mozzarella cheese on top.
5. Bake and Serve:
   Bake for 25 minutes until cheese is bubbly and golden. Garnish with fresh basil before serving.

Nutrition Information (per serving):
Calories: 400
Protein: 17g
Carbohydrates: 45g
Dietary Fiber: 9g
Fat: 18g

19. Chicken Caesar Wrap

Preparation Time: 10 minutes
Total Time: 10 minutes
Servings: 2-4
Ingredients:
- 2 cups cooked, shredded chicken breast
- 1/4 cup Caesar dressing
- 2 cups romaine lettuce, chopped
- 1/4 cup grated Parmesan cheese
- 4 whole wheat tortillas
- Salt and pepper to taste

Directions:
1. Prepare Chicken:
   In a bowl, combine shredded chicken with Caesar dressing, tossing to coat evenly. Add salt and pepper to taste.
2. Assemble Wraps:
   Place a layer of romaine lettuce on each tortilla, top with chicken mixture, and sprinkle with Parmesan cheese.
3. Wrap and Serve:
   Roll up the tortillas and slice in half. Serve immediately.

Nutrition Information (per serving):
Calories: 290
Protein: 24g
Carbohydrates: 20g
Dietary Fiber: 3g
Fat: 12g

20. Roasted Vegetable Quiche

Preparation Time: 15 minutes
Cooking Time: 35 minutes
Total Time: 50 minutes
Servings: 2-4
Ingredients:
- 1 pre-made pie crust
- 1 cup roasted vegetables (zucchini, bell pepper, onion)
- 4 large eggs
- 1/2 cup milk or cream
- 1/2 cup shredded cheddar cheese
- Salt and pepper to taste
- 1 tablespoon olive oil

Directions:
1. Preheat Oven:
   Preheat oven to 375°F (190°C).
2. Roast Vegetables:
   Toss vegetables in olive oil, spread on a baking sheet, and roast for 20 minutes until tender.
3. Prepare Filling:
   In a bowl, whisk together eggs, milk, salt, and pepper. Stir in roasted vegetables and cheddar cheese.
4. Bake Quiche:
   Pour the egg mixture into the pie crust.

Bake for 30-35 minutes until the quiche is set and the top is golden.
Nutrition Information (per serving):
Calories: 320
Protein: 14g
Carbohydrates: 20g
Dietary Fiber: 3g
Fat: 22g

Dinner 20 recipes

When it comes to dinner, you want something that's not only tasty but also comforting and fulfilling. Here's a collection of 20 dinner recipes that will make your evening meals delightful and satisfying. From hearty dishes to lighter options, these recipes cater to a variety of tastes and preferences. Here's your go-to list for a fantastic dinner:

1. Baked Salmon with Lemon and Dill

Preparation Time: 10 minutes
Cooking Time: 20 minutes
Total Time: 30 minutes
Servings: 2-4
Ingredients:
- 2 salmon fillets
- 1 lemon, sliced
- 2 tablespoons fresh dill, chopped
- 2 tablespoons olive oil
- Salt and pepper to taste

Directions:
1. Preheat Oven:
   Preheat the oven to 400°F (200°C).
2. Prepare Salmon:
   Place salmon fillets on a baking sheet lined with parchment paper. Drizzle with olive oil and season with salt and pepper.
3. Add Lemon and Dill:
   Place lemon slices on top of the salmon and sprinkle with fresh dill.
4. Bake:
   Bake for 15-20 minutes, or until the salmon is cooked through and flakes easily with a fork.

Nutrition Information (per serving):
Calories: 290
Protein: 28g
Carbohydrates: 2g
Dietary Fiber: 1g
Fat: 18g

2. Chicken Alfredo Pasta

Preparation Time: 15 minutes
Cooking Time: 20 minutes
Total Time: 35 minutes
Servings: 2-4
Ingredients:
- 8 oz fettuccine pasta
- 2 boneless chicken breasts, cooked and sliced
- 1 cup heavy cream
- 1/2 cup Parmesan cheese, grated
- 2 cloves garlic, minced
- 2 tablespoons butter
- Salt and pepper to taste
- Fresh parsley for garnish

Directions:
1. Cook Pasta:
   Cook fettuccine according to package instructions. Drain and set aside.
2. Prepare Alfredo Sauce:
   In a large skillet, melt butter over medium heat. Add minced garlic and sauté until fragrant. Stir in heavy cream and bring to a simmer. Gradually add Parmesan cheese, whisking until the sauce is smooth.
3. Combine Ingredients:
   Add cooked chicken to the sauce and toss to coat. Stir in the cooked pasta until everything is well combined. Season with salt and pepper.
4. Garnish and Serve:
   Garnish with fresh parsley and serve immediately.

Nutrition Information (per serving):
Calories: 580
Protein: 35g
Carbohydrates: 45g
Dietary Fiber: 3g
Fat: 28g

3. Vegetable Stir-Fry with Tofu

Preparation Time: 15 minutes
Cooking Time: 15 minutes
Total Time: 30 minutes
Servings: 2-4

Ingredients:
- 1 block firm tofu, cubed
- 2 cups mixed vegetables (broccoli, bell peppers, carrots)
- 2 tablespoons soy sauce
- 1 tablespoon sesame oil
- 2 cloves garlic, minced
- 1 tablespoon ginger, grated
- 1 tablespoon cornstarch (optional, for tofu crisping)

Directions:
1. Cook Tofu:
   Heat sesame oil in a skillet over medium heat. If desired, toss tofu in cornstarch before adding to the pan. Cook tofu until golden and crispy, about 5-7 minutes. Remove from the pan and set aside.
2. Sauté Vegetables:
   In the same pan, add garlic and ginger. Sauté for 1-2 minutes, then add the mixed vegetables. Stir-fry until tender-crisp, about 5 minutes.
3. Add Tofu and Sauce:
   Return the tofu to the pan and drizzle with soy sauce. Toss to coat and cook for another 2 minutes.
4. Serve:
   Serve hot, optionally with rice or noodles.

Nutrition Information (per serving):
Calories: 280
Protein: 15g
Carbohydrates: 18g
Dietary Fiber: 5g
Fat: 15g

4. Stuffed Bell Peppers

Preparation Time: 15 minutes
Cooking Time: 40 minutes
Total Time: 55 minutes
Servings: 2-4
Ingredients:
- 4 bell peppers, tops removed and seeds cleaned out
- 1/2 lb ground beef or turkey
- 1 cup cooked quinoa or rice
- 1 small onion, chopped
- 1 can diced tomatoes (14 oz)
- 1/2 cup shredded mozzarella cheese
- 1 teaspoon garlic powder
- Salt and pepper to taste
- 2 tablespoons olive oil

Directions:
1. Preheat Oven:
   Preheat the oven to 375°F (190°C).
2. Cook Filling:
   Heat olive oil in a skillet over medium heat. Add onion and cook until soft. Add ground meat and cook until browned. Stir in cooked quinoa or rice, diced tomatoes, garlic powder, salt, and pepper.
3. Stuff Peppers:
   Stuff each bell pepper with the filling mixture and place them upright in a baking dish.
4. Bake:
   Cover with foil and bake for 30 minutes. Remove foil, top with mozzarella cheese, and bake for an additional 10 minutes until cheese is melted.

Nutrition Information (per serving):
Calories: 320
Protein: 25g
Carbohydrates: 20g
Dietary Fiber: 5g
Fat: 15g

5. Beef and Broccoli Stir-Fry

Preparation Time: 15 minutes
Cooking Time: 10 minutes
Total Time: 25 minutes
Servings: 2-4
Ingredients:
- 1/2 lb beef sirloin, sliced thin
- 2 cups broccoli florets
- 2 tablespoons soy sauce
- 1 tablespoon oyster sauce
- 1 tablespoon sesame oil
- 2 cloves garlic, minced
- 1 tablespoon cornstarch (optional, for sauce thickening)

Directions:
1. Cook Beef:
   Heat sesame oil in a large skillet or wok. Add the beef slices and cook for 2-3 minutes until browned. Remove and set aside.
2. Stir-Fry Broccoli:
   In the same pan, add broccoli and garlic. Stir-fry for 3-4 minutes until tender but still crisp.
3. Add Beef and Sauce:
   Return beef to the pan and add soy sauce and oyster sauce. Toss to coat and cook

for an additional 2 minutes. If desired, mix cornstarch with 1 tablespoon water and stir into the sauce to thicken.
4. Serve:
   Serve hot with rice or noodles.

Nutrition Information (per serving):
   Calories: 350
   Protein: 30g
   Carbohydrates: 12g
   Dietary Fiber: 4g
   Fat: 20g

6. Spinach and Ricotta Stuffed Chicken

Preparation Time: 20 minutes
Cooking Time: 25 minutes
Total Time: 45 minutes
Servings: 2-4
Ingredients:
- 2 boneless, skinless chicken breasts
- 1 cup fresh spinach, chopped
- 1/2 cup ricotta cheese
- 1/4 cup grated Parmesan cheese
- 1 clove garlic, minced
- Salt and pepper to taste
- 2 tablespoons olive oil

Directions:
1. Preheat Oven:
   Preheat oven to 375°F (190°C).
2. Prepare Filling:
   In a bowl, mix together chopped spinach, ricotta, Parmesan, garlic, salt, and pepper.
3. Stuff Chicken:
   Cut a slit into each chicken breast to form a pocket. Stuff the chicken with the spinach-ricotta mixture.
4. Cook Chicken:
   Heat olive oil in a skillet over medium heat. Sear the chicken on both sides until golden, about 3 minutes per side. Transfer the chicken to a baking dish and bake for 20-25 minutes until cooked through.

Nutrition Information (per serving):
   Calories: 380
   Protein: 35g
   Carbohydrates: 5g
   Dietary Fiber: 1g
   Fat: 24g

7. Sweet Potato and Black Bean Chili

Preparation Time: 15 minutes
Cooking Time: 30 minutes
Total Time: 45 minutes
Servings: 2-4
Ingredients:
- 2 medium sweet potatoes, diced
- 1 can black beans, drained and rinsed
- 1 can diced tomatoes (14 oz)
- 1 small onion, chopped
- 2 cloves garlic, minced
- 1 tablespoon chili powder
- 1 teaspoon cumin
- 2 cups vegetable broth
- Salt and pepper to taste

Directions:
1. Cook Aromatics:
   Heat a large pot over medium heat. Add onion and garlic and sauté until soft.
2. Add Vegetables and Spices:
   Stir in diced sweet potatoes, chili powder, and cumin. Cook for 5 minutes.
3. Simmer:
   Add diced tomatoes, black beans, and vegetable broth. Bring to a simmer and cook for 25-30 minutes, or until sweet potatoes are tender.
4. Serve:
   Season with salt and pepper and serve hot.

Nutrition Information (per serving):
   Calories: 280
   Protein: 8g
   Carbohydrates: 52g
   Dietary Fiber: 12g
   Fat: 4g

8. Lemon Garlic Shrimp with Zucchini Noodles

Preparation Time: 10 minutes
Cooking Time: 10 minutes
Total Time: 20 minutes
Servings: 2-4
Ingredients:
- 1 lb shrimp, peeled and deveined
- 2 zucchinis, spiralized
- 3 cloves garlic, minced
- 2 tablespoons olive oil
- Juice of 1 lemon
- Salt and pepper to taste
- Fresh parsley for garnish

Directions:
1. Sauté Shrimp:
   Heat olive oil in a large skillet over medium heat. Add garlic and sauté until fragrant. Add shrimp, season with salt and pepper, and cook for 3-4 minutes, or until pink and opaque.
2. Add Lemon:
   Stir in lemon juice and cook for 1 minute.
3. Prepare Zucchini Noodles:
   In the same skillet, toss in zucchini noodles and cook for 2-3 minutes, until tender but crisp.
4. Serve:
   Plate the shrimp over zucchini noodles and garnish with fresh parsley.

Nutrition Information (per serving):
Calories: 250
Protein: 28g
Carbohydrates: 7g
Dietary Fiber: 2g
Fat: 12g

9. Quinoa and Vegetable Stuffed Acorn Squash

Preparation Time: 15 minutes
Cooking Time: 45 minutes
Total Time: 1 hour
Servings: 2-4
Ingredients:
- 2 acorn squash, halved and seeds removed
- 1 cup quinoa, cooked
- 1/2 cup bell peppers, diced
- 1/4 cup red onion, diced
- 1/4 cup dried cranberries
- 2 tablespoons olive oil
- Salt and pepper to taste
- Fresh thyme for garnish

Directions:
1. Roast Squash:
   Preheat oven to 400°F (200°C). Drizzle acorn squash halves with olive oil, season with salt and pepper, and place cut side down on a baking sheet. Roast for 35-40 minutes until tender.
2. Prepare Quinoa Filling:
   In a bowl, combine cooked quinoa, bell peppers, red onion, dried cranberries, and olive oil. Season with salt and pepper.
3. Stuff Squash:
   Once the squash is roasted, fill each half with the quinoa mixture.
4. Serve:
   Garnish with fresh thyme and serve warm.

Nutrition Information (per serving):
Calories: 320
Protein: 7g
Carbohydrates: 58g
Dietary Fiber: 8g
Fat: 10g

10. Chicken and Mushroom Skillet

Preparation Time: 10 minutes
Cooking Time: 20 minutes
Total Time: 30 minutes
Servings: 2-4
Ingredients:
- 2 boneless, skinless chicken breasts
- 1 cup mushrooms, sliced
- 2 cloves garlic, minced
- 1 tablespoon olive oil
- 1/2 cup chicken broth
- 1/4 cup heavy cream
- 1 tablespoon fresh thyme
- Salt and pepper to taste

Directions:
1. Cook Chicken:
   Heat olive oil in a skillet over medium heat. Season chicken with salt and pepper and cook for 5-7 minutes per side until golden and cooked through. Remove from skillet and set aside.
2. Sauté Mushrooms:
   In the same skillet, add garlic and mushrooms. Cook until the mushrooms are golden, about 5 minutes.
3. Add Sauce:
   Pour in chicken broth and heavy cream, stirring to combine. Return the chicken to the skillet, simmer for 5 minutes until the sauce thickens.
4. Serve:
   Garnish with fresh thyme and serve.

Nutrition Information (per serving):
Calories: 340
Protein: 30g
Carbohydrates: 5g
Dietary Fiber: 1g
Fat: 20g

11. Eggplant Parmesan

Preparation Time: 15 minutes
Cooking Time: 40 minutes
Total Time: 55 minutes
Servings: 2-4
Ingredients:
- 2 medium eggplants, sliced
- 1 cup marinara sauce
- 1 cup mozzarella cheese, shredded
- 1/2 cup Parmesan cheese, grated
- 1/2 cup breadcrumbs
- 1 egg, beaten
- Salt and pepper to taste
- Fresh basil for garnish

Directions:
1. Prepare Eggplant:
   Preheat oven to 375°F (190°C). Dip eggplant slices in the beaten egg, then coat with breadcrumbs.
2. Bake:
   Place the eggplant slices on a baking sheet and bake for 20 minutes until golden.
3. Layer:
   In a baking dish, layer eggplant slices, marinara sauce, mozzarella, and Parmesan. Repeat until all ingredients are used.
4. Bake Again:
   Bake for another 20 minutes until the cheese is bubbly and golden. Garnish with fresh basil.

Nutrition Information (per serving):
Calories: 320
Protein: 15g
Carbohydrates: 28g
Fat: 18g

12. Turkey Meatballs with Marinara Sauce

Preparation Time: 15 minutes
Cooking Time: 25 minutes
Total Time: 40 minutes
Servings: 2-4
Ingredients:
- 1 lb ground turkey
- 1/2 cup breadcrumbs
- 1 egg
- 1/4 cup Parmesan cheese, grated
- 2 cloves garlic, minced
- 1 cup marinara sauce
- Salt and pepper to taste
- Fresh parsley for garnish

Directions:
1. Prepare Meatballs:
   In a bowl, mix ground turkey, breadcrumbs, egg, Parmesan, and garlic. Form into small meatballs.
2. Cook:
   Heat a skillet over medium heat and cook meatballs for 10 minutes, turning occasionally.
3. Add Sauce:
   Pour marinara sauce over the meatballs and simmer for 10 minutes until fully cooked. Garnish with parsley.

Nutrition Information (per serving):
Calories: 280
Protein: 28g
Carbohydrates: 12g
Fat: 14g

13. Butternut Squash and Sage Risotto

Preparation Time: 10 minutes
Cooking Time: 40 minutes
Total Time: 50 minutes
Servings: 2-4
Ingredients:
- 1 cup Arborio rice
- 1/2 butternut squash, cubed
- 4 cups vegetable broth
- 1/4 cup Parmesan cheese, grated
- 2 tablespoons butter
- 1 tablespoon fresh sage, chopped
- Salt and pepper to taste

Directions:
1. Cook Squash:
   In a skillet, cook butternut squash in butter until tender, about 10 minutes.
2. Make Risotto:
   In another pot, heat the vegetable broth. Add rice to the skillet with squash and cook, stirring, while adding broth gradually until rice is tender, about 20 minutes.
3. Finish:
   Stir in Parmesan, sage, salt, and pepper. Serve warm.

Nutrition Information (per serving):
Calories: 320
Protein: 8g
Carbohydrates: 50g
Fat: 10g

14. BBQ Chicken Pizza

Preparation Time: 15 minutes
Cooking Time: 20 minutes
Total Time: 35 minutes
Servings: 2-4
Ingredients:
- 1 pre-made pizza crust
- 1/2 cup BBQ sauce
- 1 cup cooked chicken, shredded
- 1/2 cup mozzarella cheese, shredded
- 1/4 cup red onion, sliced
- Fresh cilantro for garnish

Directions:
1. Prepare Pizza:
   Preheat oven to 400°F (200°C). Spread BBQ sauce over pizza crust, add chicken, onion, and top with mozzarella.
2. Bake:
   Bake for 15-20 minutes until the cheese is melted and bubbly.
3. Serve:
   Garnish with fresh cilantro and serve.

Nutrition Information (per serving):
Calories: 350
Protein: 25g
Carbohydrates: 38g
Fat: 10g

15. Stuffed Portobello Mushrooms

Preparation Time: 10 minutes
Cooking Time: 25 minutes
Total Time: 35 minutes
Servings: 2-4
Ingredients:
- 4 large portobello mushrooms
- 1/2 cup spinach, chopped
- 1/4 cup feta cheese, crumbled
- 1/4 cup breadcrumbs
- 2 tablespoons olive oil
- Salt and pepper to taste

Directions:
1. Prepare Mushrooms:
   Preheat oven to 375°F (190°C). Remove stems from mushrooms and brush with olive oil.
2. Stuff:
   Mix spinach, feta, and breadcrumbs. Stuff each mushroom with the mixture.
3. Bake:
   Bake for 20-25 minutes until the mushrooms are tender.

Nutrition Information (per serving):
Calories: 200
Protein: 7g
Carbohydrates: 15g
Fat: 12g

16. Balsamic Glazed Pork Tenderloin

Preparation Time: 10 minutes
Cooking Time: 30 minutes
Total Time: 40 minutes
Servings: 2-4
Ingredients:
- 1 lb pork tenderloin
- 1/4 cup balsamic vinegar
- 2 tablespoons honey
- 2 cloves garlic, minced
- Salt and pepper to taste

Directions:
1. Prepare Glaze:
   In a small bowl, mix balsamic vinegar, honey, and garlic.
2. Cook Pork:
   Preheat oven to 375°F (190°C). Season pork with salt and pepper, then roast for 25-30 minutes, basting with the glaze.
3. Serve:
   Slice and serve with remaining glaze.

Nutrition Information (per serving):
Calories: 320
Protein: 30g
Carbohydrates: 12g
Fat: 14g

17. Lentil and Vegetable Stew

Preparation Time: 10 minutes
Cooking Time: 35 minutes
Total Time: 45 minutes
Servings: 2-4
Ingredients:
- 1 cup lentils
- 1 carrot, diced
- 1 celery stalk, diced
- 1 onion, chopped
- 2 cups vegetable broth
- 2 cloves garlic, minced
- Salt and pepper to taste

Directions:
1. Cook Vegetables:
   In a large pot, sauté onion, garlic, carrot, and celery until tender.

2. Simmer Stew:
      Add lentils and vegetable broth. Bring to a boil, then reduce heat and simmer for 30 minutes.
   3. Serve:
      Season with salt and pepper and serve warm.

Nutrition Information (per serving):
Calories: 250
Protein: 12g
Carbohydrates: 40g
Fat: 5g

18. Chicken Curry with Cauliflower Rice

Preparation Time: 15 minutes
Cooking Time: 25 minutes
Total Time: 40 minutes
Servings: 2-4
Ingredients:
- 2 chicken breasts, diced
- 1/2 cup coconut milk
- 2 tablespoons curry powder
- 1 onion, chopped
- 2 cups cauliflower rice
- Salt and pepper to taste

Directions:
   1. Cook Chicken:
      Sauté chicken and onion in a skillet until chicken is cooked through.
   2. Add Curry:
      Stir in curry powder and coconut milk. Simmer for 15 minutes.
   3. Serve:
      Serve over cauliflower rice.

Nutrition Information (per serving):
Calories: 320
Protein: 28g
Carbohydrates: 12g
Fat: 18g

19. Seafood Paella

Preparation Time: 20 minutes
Cooking Time: 30 minutes
Total Time: 50 minutes
Servings: 2-4
Ingredients:
- 1/2 lb shrimp
- 1/2 lb mussels
- 1 cup Arborio rice
- 2 cups chicken broth
- 1/4 cup peas
- 1/2 red bell pepper, chopped
- 1/2 teaspoon saffron
- Salt and pepper to taste

Directions:
   1. Cook Rice:
      Sauté rice with saffron and bell pepper in a large skillet, then add broth and simmer for 20 minutes.
   2. Add Seafood:
      Add shrimp, mussels, and peas. Cook until seafood is done, about 10 minutes.
   3. Serve:
      Season with salt and pepper.

Nutrition Information (per serving):
Calories: 340
Protein: 25g
Carbohydrates: 45g
Fat: 8g

20. Vegetarian Enchiladas

Preparation Time: 15 minutes
Cooking Time: 25 minutes
Total Time: 40 minutes
Servings: 2-4
Ingredients:
- 6 corn tortillas
- 1 cup black beans, cooked
- 1/2 cup corn kernels
- 1/4 cup enchilada sauce
- 1/2 cup cheddar cheese, shredded
- 1/2 onion, chopped
- Salt and pepper to taste

Directions:
   1. Prepare Filling:
      Sauté onion, black beans, and corn in a skillet. Season with salt and pepper.
   2. Assemble Enchiladas:
      Spoon filling into tortillas, roll up, and place in a baking dish. Cover with enchilada sauce and cheese.
   3. Bake:
      Bake at 375°F (190°C) for 20-25 minutes until bubbly.

Nutrition Information (per serving):
Calories: 300
Protein: 14g
Carbohydrates: 45g
Fat: 10g

Snacks 20 recipes

Snacks are the perfect way to satisfy your hunger between meals or to add a little joy to your day. Whether you're in the mood for something crunchy, sweet, or savory, this list of 20 snack recipes has you covered. Each recipe is designed to be both tasty and nutritious, making them ideal for any time of day. Here's a roundup of delightful snack ideas to enjoy:

1. Homemade Granola Bars

Preparation Time: 10 minutes
Cooking Time: 15 minutes
Total Time: 25 minutes
Servings: 2-4
Ingredients:
- 1 1/2 cups rolled oats
- 1/4 cup honey
- 1/4 cup peanut butter
- 1/4 cup mixed nuts, chopped
- 1/4 cup dried fruits, chopped
- 1/2 teaspoon vanilla extract

Directions:
1. Mix Ingredients:
   Combine oats, honey, peanut butter, nuts, dried fruits, and vanilla.
2. Bake:
   Press mixture into a greased pan. Bake at 350°F (175°C) for 15 minutes. Let cool, then cut into bars.

Nutrition Information (per serving):
   Calories: 220
   Protein: 6g
   Carbohydrates: 30g
   Fat: 10g

2. Baked Sweet Potato Chips

Preparation Time: 5 minutes
Cooking Time: 20 minutes
Total Time: 25 minutes
Servings: 2-4
Ingredients:
- 2 medium sweet potatoes, thinly sliced
- 1 tablespoon olive oil
- Salt to taste

Directions:
1. Prepare Potatoes:
   Toss sweet potato slices in olive oil and salt.
2. Bake:
   Arrange on a baking sheet and bake at 375°F (190°C) for 20 minutes, flipping halfway.

Nutrition Information (per serving):
   Calories: 130
   Protein: 2g
   Carbohydrates: 24g
   Fat: 4g

3. Stuffed Mini Bell Peppers

Preparation Time: 10 minutes
Cooking Time: N/A
Total Time: 10 minutes
Servings: 2-4
Ingredients:
- 8 mini bell peppers
- 1/2 cup cream cheese
- 1/4 cup feta cheese, crumbled
- 1 tablespoon fresh herbs (parsley or dill)

Directions:
1. Prepare Peppers:
   Slice peppers in half and remove seeds.
2. Stuff:
   Mix cream cheese, feta, and herbs. Fill pepper halves with the mixture.

Nutrition Information (per serving):
   Calories: 120
   Protein: 4g
   Carbohydrates: 8g
   Fat: 9g

4. Greek Yogurt and Honey Parfait

Preparation Time: 5 minutes
Cooking Time: N/A
Total Time: 5 minutes
Servings: 2-4
Ingredients:
- 1 cup Greek yogurt
- 2 tablespoons honey
- 1/4 cup granola
- 1/4 cup fresh berries

Directions:
1. Layer:
   In a glass, layer yogurt, honey, granola, and berries.

Nutrition Information (per serving):
  Calories: 150
  Protein: 8g
  Carbohydrates: 25g
  Fat: 4g

5. Roasted Chickpeas

Preparation Time: 5 minutes
Cooking Time: 30 minutes
Total Time: 35 minutes
Servings: 2-4
Ingredients:
- 1 can chickpeas, drained and rinsed
- 1 tablespoon olive oil
- 1 teaspoon paprika
- Salt to taste

Directions:
1. Toss Chickpeas:
   Mix chickpeas with olive oil, paprika, and salt.
2. Roast:
   Roast at 400°F (200°C) for 30 minutes, stirring occasionally.

Nutrition Information (per serving):
  Calories: 180
  Protein: 7g
  Carbohydrates: 25g
  Fat: 5g

6. Apple Slices with Almond Butter

Preparation Time: 5 minutes
Cooking Time: N/A
Total Time: 5 minutes
Servings: 2-4
Ingredients:
- 2 apples, sliced
- 1/4 cup almond butter

Directions:
1. Serve:
   Dip apple slices in almond butter and serve.

Nutrition Information (per serving):
  Calories: 180
  Protein: 3g
  Carbohydrates: 26g
  Fat: 8g

7. Veggie Sticks with Hummus

Preparation Time: 5 minutes
Cooking Time: N/A
Total Time: 5 minutes
Servings: 2-4
Ingredients:
- 1 carrot, cut into sticks
- 1 cucumber, cut into sticks
- 1/2 cup hummus

Directions:
1. Serve:
   Arrange veggie sticks and serve with hummus for dipping.

Nutrition Information (per serving):
  Calories: 100
  Protein: 3g
  Carbohydrates: 12g
  Fat: 6g

8. Energy Balls

Preparation Time: 10 minutes
Cooking Time: N/A
Total Time: 10 minutes
Servings: 2-4
Ingredients:
- 1 cup rolled oats
- 1/4 cup peanut butter
- 1/4 cup honey
- 1/4 cup dark chocolate chips
- 1/4 cup flaxseeds

Directions:
1. Mix and Shape:
   Mix all ingredients in a bowl. Form into small balls.
2. Chill:
   Refrigerate for 30 minutes before serving.

Nutrition Information (per serving):
  Calories: 150
  Protein: 4g
  Carbohydrates: 18g
  Fat: 7g

9. Spicy Roasted Almonds

Preparation Time: 5 minutes
Cooking Time: 15 minutes
Total Time: 20 minutes
Servings: 2-4
Ingredients:
- 1 cup raw almonds
- 1 tablespoon olive oil

- 1 teaspoon chili powder
- Salt to taste

Directions:
1. Toss Almonds:
   Mix almonds with olive oil, chili powder, and salt.
2. Roast:
   Bake at 350°F (175°C) for 15 minutes, stirring occasionally.

Nutrition Information (per serving):
Calories: 200
Protein: 6g
Carbohydrates: 6g
Fat: 18g

10. Cucumber and Avocado Sandwiches

Preparation Time: 10 minutes
Cooking Time: N/A
Total Time: 10 minutes
Servings: 2-4
Ingredients:
- 1 cucumber, sliced
- 1 avocado, mashed
- 4 slices whole-grain bread
- Salt and pepper to taste

Directions:
1. Assemble Sandwiches:
   Spread mashed avocado on bread slices, top with cucumber slices, and season with salt and pepper.

Nutrition Information (per serving):
Calories: 200
Protein: 6g
Carbohydrates: 28g
Fat: 10g

11. Chia Seed Pudding

Preparation Time: 5 minutes
Chill Time: 2 hours
Total Time: 2 hours 5 minutes
Servings: 2-4
Ingredients:
- 1/4 cup chia seeds
- 1 cup almond milk
- 1 tablespoon honey
- 1/4 teaspoon vanilla extract

Directions:
1. Mix Ingredients:
   Stir chia seeds, almond milk, honey, and vanilla together in a bowl.
2. Chill:
   Refrigerate for 2 hours until thickened.

Nutrition Information (per serving):
Calories: 120
Protein: 3g
Carbohydrates: 12g
Fat: 7g

12. Homemade Popcorn

Preparation Time: 2 minutes
Cooking Time: 5 minutes
Total Time: 7 minutes
Servings: 2-4
Ingredients:
- 1/4 cup popcorn kernels
- 1 tablespoon olive oil
- Salt to taste

Directions:
1. Pop Corn:
   Heat oil in a pot over medium heat. Add popcorn kernels, cover, and shake until popped.
2. Season:
   Sprinkle with salt and serve.

Nutrition Information (per serving):
Calories: 120
Protein: 3g
Carbohydrates: 18g
Fat: 5g

13. Fruit and Nut Energy Balls

Preparation Time: 10 minutes
Cooking Time: N/A
Total Time: 10 minutes
Servings: 2-4
Ingredients:
- 1/2 cup dried fruits (such as raisins or apricots)
- 1/4 cup mixed nuts (such as almonds and walnuts)
- 1 tablespoon honey
- 1/4 cup rolled oats

Directions:
1. Blend Ingredients:
   In a food processor, pulse dried fruits, nuts, and oats. Add honey and blend until combined.
2. Form Balls:
   Roll mixture into small balls. Chill before serving.

Nutrition Information (per serving):
Calories: 150
Protein: 4g
Carbohydrates: 20g
Fat: 8g

14. Baked Zucchini Fries

Preparation Time: 10 minutes
Cooking Time: 20 minutes
Total Time: 30 minutes
Servings: 2-4
Ingredients:
- 2 medium zucchinis, cut into fries
- 1/2 cup breadcrumbs
- 1/4 cup Parmesan cheese, grated
- 1 egg
- Salt and pepper to taste

Directions:
1. Prepare Coatings:
   Mix breadcrumbs, Parmesan, salt, and pepper. Dip zucchini fries in egg, then coat with the breadcrumb mixture.
2. Bake:
   Bake at 400°F (200°C) for 20 minutes or until crispy.

Nutrition Information (per serving):
Calories: 150
Protein: 6g
Carbohydrates: 18g
Fat: 7g

15. Cheese and Whole Grain Crackers

Preparation Time: 5 minutes
Cooking Time: N/A
Total Time: 5 minutes
Servings: 2-4
Ingredients:
- 4 whole grain crackers
- 4 slices cheese (cheddar or Swiss)

Directions:
1. Assemble:
   Top each cracker with a slice of cheese.

Nutrition Information (per serving):
Calories: 180
Protein: 8g
Carbohydrates: 18g
Fat: 10g

16. Yogurt and Berry Smoothie

Preparation Time: 5 minutes
Cooking Time: N/A
Total Time: 5 minutes
Servings: 2-4
Ingredients:
- 1 cup Greek yogurt
- 1/2 cup mixed berries
- 1/4 cup honey
- 1/4 cup milk

Directions:
1. Blend:
   Blend Greek yogurt, berries, honey, and milk until smooth.

Nutrition Information (per serving):
Calories: 150
Protein: 8g
Carbohydrates: 24g
Fat: 3g

17. Stuffed Dates

Preparation Time: 10 minutes
Cooking Time: N/A
Total Time: 10 minutes
Servings: 2-4
Ingredients:
- 12 dates, pitted
- 1/4 cup almond butter
- 1/4 cup chopped nuts (optional)

Directions:
1. Stuff Dates:
   Fill each date with almond butter. Optionally, top with chopped nuts.

Nutrition Information (per serving):
Calories: 180
Protein: 5g
Carbohydrates: 22g
Fat: 10g

18. Homemade Trail Mix

Preparation Time: 5 minutes
Cooking Time: N/A
Total Time: 5 minutes
Servings: 2-4
Ingredients:
- 1/2 cup almonds
- 1/2 cup walnuts
- 1/2 cup dried cranberries
- 1/4 cup dark chocolate chips

Directions:
1. Mix Ingredients:
   Combine all ingredients in a bowl.

Nutrition Information (per serving):
Calories: 200
Protein: 6g
Carbohydrates: 22g
Fat: 12g

19. Spiced Roasted Pumpkin Seeds

Preparation Time: 5 minutes
Cooking Time: 15 minutes
Total Time: 20 minutes
Servings: 2-4
Ingredients:
- 1 cup pumpkin seeds
- 1 tablespoon olive oil
- 1 teaspoon smoked paprika
- Salt to taste

Directions:
1. Season Seeds:
   Toss pumpkin seeds with olive oil, smoked paprika, and salt.
2. Roast:
   Roast at 350°F (175°C) for 15 minutes, stirring occasionally.

Nutrition Information (per serving):
Calories: 150
Protein: 7g
Carbohydrates: 10g
Fat: 10g

20. Avocado Toast

Preparation Time: 5 minutes
Cooking Time: N/A
Total Time: 5 minutes
Servings: 2-4
Ingredients:
- 2 slices whole grain bread, toasted
- 1 avocado, mashed
- Salt and pepper to taste
- 1/2 lemon, juiced

Directions:
1. Prepare Toast:
   Spread mashed avocado on toasted bread. Season with salt, pepper, and lemon juice.

Nutrition Information (per serving):
Calories: 200
Protein: 5g
Carbohydrates: 24g
Fat: 10g

Desserts 20 recipes

Everyone deserves a little sweetness in their life, and these 20 dessert recipes offer a delightful array of options. From rich and creamy to light and refreshing, each recipe is crafted to bring joy to your taste buds. Here's a tempting list of desserts to try:

1. Chocolate Avocado Mousse

Preparation Time: 10 minutes
Cooking Time: N/A
Total Time: 10 minutes
Servings: 2-4
Ingredients:
- 1 ripe avocado
- 1/4 cup cocoa powder
- 1/4 cup honey or maple syrup
- 1/2 teaspoon vanilla extract

Directions:
1. Blend Ingredients:
   Blend avocado, cocoa powder, honey, and vanilla extract until smooth. Chill before serving.

Nutrition Information (per serving):
Calories: 150
Protein: 2g
Carbohydrates: 18g
Fat: 8g

2. Berry Chia Seed Pudding

Preparation Time: 5 minutes
Cooking Time: N/A
Total Time: 5 minutes plus chilling
Servings: 2-4
Ingredients:
- 1/4 cup chia seeds
- 1 cup almond milk
- 1 tablespoon maple syrup
- 1/2 cup mixed berries

Directions:
1. Mix Ingredients:
   Combine chia seeds, almond milk, and maple syrup. Refrigerate for at least 4 hours. Top with berries before serving.

Nutrition Information (per serving):
Calories: 180
Protein: 5g
Carbohydrates: 24g
Fat: 8g

3. Coconut Milk Ice Cream

Preparation Time: 10 minutes
Cooking Time: N/A
Total Time: 10 minutes plus freezing
Servings: 2-4
Ingredients:
- 1 can full-fat coconut milk
- 1/4 cup honey or maple syrup
- 1 teaspoon vanilla extract

Directions:
1. Mix Ingredients:
   Combine coconut milk, honey, and vanilla extract. Pour into an ice cream maker and churn according to manufacturer instructions. Freeze until firm.

Nutrition Information (per serving):
Calories: 200
Protein: 2g
Carbohydrates: 18g
Fat: 14g

4. Baked Apples with Cinnamon

Preparation Time: 10 minutes
Cooking Time: 20 minutes
Total Time: 30 minutes
Servings: 2-4
Ingredients:
- 4 apples, cored
- 2 tablespoons honey
- 1 teaspoon cinnamon

Directions:
1. Prepare Apples:
   Stuff apples with honey and cinnamon. Bake at 350°F (175°C) for 20 minutes.

Nutrition Information (per serving):
Calories: 120
Protein: 0g
Carbohydrates: 32g
Fat: 0g

5. Almond Flour Brownies

Preparation Time: 10 minutes
Cooking Time: 20 minutes
Total Time: 30 minutes
Servings: 2-4
Ingredients:
- 1 cup almond flour
- 1/4 cup cocoa powder
- 1/4 cup honey
- 2 eggs
- 1/4 cup coconut oil

Directions:
1. Mix Ingredients:
   Combine all ingredients. Pour into a baking dish and bake at 350°F (175°C) for 20 minutes.

Nutrition Information (per serving):
Calories: 180
Protein: 6g
Carbohydrates: 14g
Fat: 12g

6. Frozen Banana Bites

Preparation Time: 10 minutes
Cooking Time: N/A
Total Time: 10 minutes plus freezing
Servings: 2-4
Ingredients:
- 2 bananas, sliced
- 1/4 cup dark chocolate chips
- 1 tablespoon coconut oil

Directions:
1. Prepare Bites:
   Melt chocolate chips with coconut oil. Dip banana slices in chocolate and freeze until firm.

Nutrition Information (per serving):
Calories: 120
Protein: 1g
Carbohydrates: 20g
Fat: 6g

7. Fruit Sorbet

Preparation Time: 10 minutes
Cooking Time: N/A
Total Time: 10 minutes plus freezing
Servings: 2-4
Ingredients:
- 2 cups fruit (such as berries or mango), frozen

- 1/4 cup honey or agave syrup
- 1/2 cup lemon juice

Directions:
1. Blend Ingredients:
   Blend frozen fruit, honey, and lemon juice until smooth. Freeze until firm.

Nutrition Information (per serving):
Calories: 100
Protein: 1g
Carbohydrates: 25g
Fat: 0g

8. Pumpkin Spice Muffins

Preparation Time: 10 minutes
Cooking Time: 20 minutes
Total Time: 30 minutes
Servings: 2-4
Ingredients:
- 1 cup pumpkin puree
- 1/4 cup honey
- 1/2 cup almond flour
- 1 teaspoon pumpkin pie spice
- 2 eggs

Directions:
1. Prepare Muffins:
   Mix all ingredients. Pour into muffin tins and bake at 350°F (175°C) for 20 minutes.

Nutrition Information (per serving):
Calories: 150
Protein: 4g
Carbohydrates: 18g
Fat: 7g

9. Coconut Energy Balls

Preparation Time: 10 minutes
Cooking Time: N/A
Total Time: 10 minutes plus chilling
Servings: 2-4
Ingredients:
- 1 cup shredded coconut
- 1/2 cup almond butter
- 1/4 cup honey

Directions:
1. Mix Ingredients:
   Combine coconut, almond butter, and honey. Roll into balls and chill before serving.

Nutrition Information (per serving):
Calories: 160
Protein: 4g
Carbohydrates: 16g
Fat: 10g

10. Homemade Apple Pie

Preparation Time: 20 minutes
Cooking Time: 45 minutes
Total Time: 1 hour 5 minutes
Servings: 2-4
Ingredients:
- 2 cups apples, peeled and sliced
- 1/4 cup honey
- 1 tablespoon cinnamon
- 1 pie crust

Directions:
1. Prepare Pie:
   Mix apples, honey, and cinnamon. Place in pie crust and bake at 375°F (190°C) for 45 minutes.

Nutrition Information (per serving):
Calories: 250
Protein: 2g
Carbohydrates: 35g
Fat: 12g

11. Chocolate Almond Clusters

Preparation Time: 10 minutes
Cooking Time: N/A
Total Time: 10 minutes plus chilling
Servings: 2-4
Ingredients:
- 1 cup almonds
- 1/2 cup dark chocolate chips
- 1 tablespoon coconut oil

Directions:
1. Prepare Clusters:
   Melt chocolate chips with coconut oil. Stir in almonds and drop spoonfuls onto parchment paper. Chill until set.

Nutrition Information (per serving):
Calories: 180
Protein: 4g
Carbohydrates: 15g
Fat: 12g

12. Peach Crisp

Preparation Time: 15 minutes
Cooking Time: 30 minutes
Total Time: 45 minutes
Servings: 2-4
Ingredients:
- 2 cups peaches, sliced

- 1/4 cup oats
- 1/4 cup almond flour
- 2 tablespoons honey
- 1/4 cup melted coconut oil

Directions:
1. Prepare Crisp:
   Mix peaches with honey. Combine oats, almond flour, and coconut oil. Sprinkle over peaches and bake at 350°F (175°C) for 30 minutes.

Nutrition Information (per serving):
- Calories: 200
- Protein: 3g
- Carbohydrates: 30g
- Fat: 8g

13. Lemon Bars

Preparation Time: 15 minutes
Cooking Time: 25 minutes
Total Time: 40 minutes
Servings: 2-4
Ingredients:
- 1 cup almond flour
- 1/4 cup honey
- 2 eggs
- 1/2 cup lemon juice

Directions:
1. Prepare Bars:
   Mix almond flour and honey for crust. Press into a pan. Combine eggs and lemon juice for filling and pour over crust. Bake at 350°F (175°C) for 25 minutes.

Nutrition Information (per serving):
- Calories: 180
- Protein: 4g
- Carbohydrates: 15g
- Fat: 12g

14. Berry Compote

Preparation Time: 10 minutes
Cooking Time: 15 minutes
Total Time: 25 minutes
Servings: 2-4
Ingredients:
- 2 cups mixed berries
- 1/4 cup honey
- 1 tablespoon lemon juice

Directions:
1. Cook Compote:
   Simmer berries, honey, and lemon juice until thickened. Cool before serving.

Nutrition Information (per serving):
Calories: 100
Protein: 1g
Carbohydrates: 25g
Fat: 0g

15. Date and Nut Truffles

Preparation Time: 10 minutes
Cooking Time: N/A
Total Time: 10 minutes plus chilling
Servings: 2-4
Ingredients:
- 1 cup dates, pitted
- 1/2 cup mixed nuts
- 1 tablespoon cocoa powder

Directions:
1. Blend and Roll:
   Blend dates, nuts, and cocoa powder until smooth. Roll into balls and chill.

Nutrition Information (per serving):
Calories: 150
Protein: 4g
Carbohydrates: 24g
Fat: 7g

16. Greek Yogurt Cheesecake

Preparation Time: 15 minutes
Cooking Time: 30 minutes
Total Time: 45 minutes plus chilling
Servings: 2-4
Ingredients:
- 1 cup Greek yogurt
- 1/2 cup honey
- 2 eggs
- 1 teaspoon vanilla extract

Directions:
1. Prepare Cheesecake:
   Mix all ingredients. Pour into a baking dish and bake at 325°F (160°C) for 30 minutes. Chill before serving.

Nutrition Information (per serving):
Calories: 180
Protein: 12g
Carbohydrates: 18g
Fat: 8g

17. Chocolate Chip Cookies

Preparation Time: 15 minutes
Cooking Time: 12 minutes
Total Time: 27 minutes
Servings: 2-4
Ingredients:
- 1 cup almond flour
- 1/4 cup coconut oil
- 1/4 cup honey
- 1/2 cup chocolate chips
- 1 egg

Directions:
1. Prepare Cookies:
   Mix all ingredients. Drop spoonfuls onto a baking sheet and bake at 350°F (175°C) for 12 minutes.

Nutrition Information (per serving):
Calories: 180
Protein: 4g
Carbohydrates: 15g
Fat: 12g

18. No-Bake Cheesecake

Preparation Time: 15 minutes
Cooking Time: N/A
Total Time: 15 minutes plus chilling
Servings: 2-4
Ingredients:
- 1 cup Greek yogurt
- 1/4 cup honey
- 1/2 cup graham cracker crumbs
- 1/4 cup melted butter

Directions:
1. Prepare Cheesecake:
   Mix Greek yogurt and honey. Press graham cracker crumbs mixed with melted butter into a pan. Top with yogurt mixture and chill.

Nutrition Information (per serving):
Calories: 160
Protein: 8g
Carbohydrates: 20g
Fat: 6g

19. Coconut Macaroons

Preparation Time: 10 minutes
Cooking Time: 20 minutes
Total Time: 30 minutes
Servings: 2-4
Ingredients:
- 2 cups shredded coconut
- 1/2 cup egg whites
- 1/4 cup honey

Directions:
1. Prepare Macaroons:
   Mix all ingredients. Drop spoonfuls onto a baking sheet and bake at 350°F (175°C) for 20 minutes.

Nutrition Information (per serving):
Calories: 150
Protein: 2g
Carbohydrates: 16g
Fat: 8g

20. Homemade Fruit Leather

Preparation Time: 15 minutes
Cooking Time: 6-8 hours
Total Time: 6-8 hours 15 minutes
Servings: 2-4
Ingredients:
- 2 cups fruit puree (such as apples or berries)
- 1/4 cup honey

Directions:
1. Prepare Leather:
   Mix fruit puree with honey. Spread on a baking sheet and dry in a low oven (140°F or 60°C) for 6-8 hours.

Nutrition Information (per serving):
Calories: 100
Protein: 1g
Carbohydrates: 25g
Fat: 0g

Book 30: Natural Remedies for Chronic Fatigue

Understanding Chronic Fatigue and Its Causes

Chronic fatigue is more than just a result of overworking or a late night; it's a persistent, overwhelming exhaustion that doesn't seem to lift, even with plenty of rest. Imagine waking up each day feeling as though you haven't slept at all, and no matter what you do, that heavy, draining feeling doesn't go away. It's like living with a constant cloud of fatigue hanging over you.

So, what exactly is chronic fatigue? Officially known as Chronic Fatigue Syndrome (CFS), this condition is characterized by extreme tiredness that lasts for six months or more. This fatigue doesn't improve with rest and isn't explained by any other medical condition. It's as though your energy reserves are perpetually low, no matter how much you try to recharge.

The exact cause of chronic fatigue isn't fully understood, but several factors are believed to contribute to it. One possibility is that the immune system may be malfunctioning. If your body's defenses aren't working properly, you might feel perpetually drained. Similarly, chronic fatigue can sometimes follow an illness or infection, like a viral infection. Even when the infection has cleared, your body might still be in recovery mode, leaving you feeling worn out.

Hormonal imbalances might also play a role. Hormones like thyroid hormones and cortisol are crucial for regulating energy levels, and any imbalance can lead to feelings of constant fatigue. Stress is another significant factor. Both emotional and physical stress can exhaust you over time, leading to a persistent sense of tiredness.

Sleep disorders are also a common cause of chronic fatigue. Conditions like sleep apnea can disrupt your sleep quality, so even if you spend enough time in bed, you might still wake up feeling exhausted. It's akin to trying to refill a tank that has a leak.

Mental health issues, such as depression or anxiety, can manifest as chronic fatigue. The emotional and mental strain from these conditions can significantly drain your energy. Additionally, nutritional deficiencies might be a contributing factor. If your diet lacks essential vitamins and minerals, it can affect your energy levels, leaving you feeling depleted.

Herbal Remedies for Energy Boosting

When you're feeling perpetually exhausted, natural remedies can offer a refreshing boost to your energy levels. Many herbs have been celebrated for their ability to invigorate and sustain vitality. Let's explore some herbal options that might help lift your energy and enhance your overall well-being.

Ginseng is a well-known herb used for centuries to combat fatigue and boost energy. It's revered for its ability to enhance physical stamina and mental clarity. Panax ginseng, in particular, is famous for its energizing effects. You can enjoy its benefits in various forms, such as teas, capsules, or extracts.

Rhodiola is another fantastic herb with adaptogenic properties, meaning it helps your body adapt to stress and reduce fatigue. It's often used to support physical endurance and mental performance.

Adding Rhodiola to your daily routine might help you better manage stress and maintain higher energy levels throughout your day.

Ashwagandha, another adaptogen, is known for its ability to restore balance and vitality. It helps the body cope with stress and improves overall stamina. Incorporating Ashwagandha into your regimen can help balance your energy levels and support a sense of well-being, especially if you're feeling consistently tired.

Maca root, a traditional Peruvian herb, is celebrated for its energizing and stamina-enhancing properties. It's used to boost energy, improve mood, and support endurance. You can add Maca to smoothies, oatmeal, or take it as a supplement to invigorate your day.
Peppermint is not only refreshing but also has stimulating properties that can help you feel more awake and energized. Sipping on peppermint tea or inhaling peppermint essential oil can refresh your senses and help combat fatigue.

Ginger, known for its digestive benefits, also has energizing effects. It can improve circulation and reduce feelings of sluggishness. Incorporating fresh ginger into your meals or enjoying a cup of ginger tea can give you a natural lift.
Yerba mate, a traditional South American herb, is packed with caffeine and other compounds that enhance alertness and energy. It's a great alternative to coffee and can provide a steady boost without the jitters that sometimes come with caffeine.

Green tea is another excellent option for a natural energy boost. It contains a modest amount of caffeine and L-theanine, which promotes alertness while helping to reduce stress. Green tea can help maintain steady energy levels throughout the day.

Nutritional Support for Fighting Fatigue

When you're battling chronic fatigue, the right nutrition can be a powerful ally in restoring your energy levels. Eating a balanced diet rich in specific nutrients can help keep your energy up and fight off that relentless sense of tiredness. Let's explore some key dietary strategies and foods that can give you the boost you need.

First off, incorporating complex carbohydrates into your diet is essential. Unlike simple sugars, complex carbs provide a steady release of energy. Think whole grains like oats, quinoa, and brown rice. These foods help maintain stable blood sugar levels, which can prevent those annoying energy crashes.

Protein is another vital component for combating fatigue. It helps build and repair tissues and keeps you feeling full and energized. Including lean proteins like chicken, turkey, tofu, and beans in your meals can keep your energy levels steady throughout the day.
Don't forget about healthy fats, which are crucial for maintaining energy. Nuts, seeds, avocados, and olive oil are excellent sources of healthy fats. They provide long-lasting energy and help your body absorb essential vitamins.

Vitamins and minerals play a significant role in your overall energy levels. Iron is especially important because it helps transport oxygen throughout your body. Foods like spinach, lentils, and lean meats are great sources of iron. Vitamin B12 and folate are also key players in energy production. You can find B12 in animal products like meat, eggs, and dairy, while folate is abundant in leafy greens, beans, and fortified cereals.

Magnesium is another mineral that supports energy production and muscle function. Include magnesium-rich foods such as nuts, seeds, and leafy green vegetables in your diet. These can help alleviate fatigue and promote better sleep.

Hydration is often overlooked but is just as important. Dehydration can lead to feelings of tiredness and low energy. Aim to drink plenty of water throughout the day. Herbal teas like peppermint or ginger can also be a refreshing way to stay hydrated and energized.

Incorporating a variety of fruits and vegetables into your meals ensures you get a range of vitamins, minerals, and antioxidants that support overall health and energy levels. Aim for a colorful plate with a mix of different fruits and veggies to maximize your nutrient intake.

Finally, consider moderating your caffeine and sugar intake. While these can provide a quick boost, they often lead to crashes later on. Instead, focus on stable sources of energy from your meals and snacks.

Managing Adrenal Fatigue Naturally

Adrenal fatigue can leave you feeling drained and overwhelmed, as if your body is running on empty. Your adrenal glands, which are responsible for producing hormones that help regulate your stress response, can become overworked and sluggish when you're under prolonged stress. But don't worry—there are natural ways to support and rejuvenate your adrenal glands. Let's explore some gentle, holistic approaches to managing adrenal fatigue.

First and foremost, it's important to focus on reducing stress. Chronic stress can seriously tax your adrenal glands, so finding ways to manage stress is crucial. Activities like deep breathing exercises, meditation, or yoga can help calm your mind and body. Even short daily practices can make a significant difference in how you feel.

Getting enough quality sleep is another key factor. Your body needs restful sleep to recover and recharge, so aim for 7-9 hours each night. Establishing a consistent sleep routine, avoiding screens before bed, and creating a relaxing bedtime ritual can all contribute to better sleep.

Incorporating adaptogenic herbs into your routine can be incredibly beneficial for adrenal support. Adaptogens are natural substances that help your body adapt to stress and restore balance. Herbs like ashwagandha, rhodiola, and holy basil are popular choices for supporting adrenal health. You can find these herbs in teas, capsules, or tinctures.

Eating a balanced diet is equally important. Focus on whole, nutrient-dense foods to provide your body with the vitamins and minerals it needs to function optimally. Include plenty of fresh fruits and vegetables, lean proteins, and healthy fats in your meals. Foods rich in vitamin C, B vitamins, and magnesium, like citrus fruits, leafy greens, and nuts, can be particularly supportive of adrenal function.

Regular physical activity is also beneficial. While you might not have the energy for intense workouts, even moderate exercise like walking, swimming, or gentle stretching can help improve your energy levels and overall well-being. Just be sure not to overdo it—listen to your body and find a balance that feels right for you.

Stay hydrated by drinking plenty of water throughout the day. Proper hydration supports every function in your body, including adrenal health. Herbal teas like chamomile or peppermint can also be soothing and help with relaxation.

Lastly, consider reducing your caffeine intake. While caffeine can provide a temporary boost, it can also strain your adrenal glands if consumed in excess. Opt for herbal teas or decaffeinated beverages if you're looking for a gentler alternative.

The Role of Detoxification in Fatigue Recovery

Feeling constantly exhausted can often be linked to the buildup of toxins in your body. Detoxification, or the process of removing these harmful substances, can play a significant role in helping you recover from fatigue. Let's dive into how detoxification can aid in boosting your energy levels and improving your overall well-being.

First, it's helpful to understand what detoxification involves. Your body naturally has systems in place, like the liver, kidneys, and lymphatic system, that work to filter out toxins and waste. However, factors such as stress, poor diet, and environmental pollutants can overwhelm these systems. Detoxification helps support and enhance your body's natural ability to cleanse itself.

One of the most effective ways to support detoxification is through your diet. Eating plenty of fresh fruits and vegetables can provide your body with essential nutrients and antioxidants that help fight off oxidative stress and support liver function. Cruciferous vegetables like broccoli, cauliflower, and Brussels sprouts are particularly good at boosting detoxification processes.
Drinking plenty of water is also crucial. Staying hydrated helps flush out toxins through your kidneys and urine. Aim for at least eight glasses of water a day, and consider adding herbal teas such as dandelion or green tea, which are known for their detoxifying properties.

Incorporating foods that promote liver health can further support detoxification. The liver plays a central role in breaking down and eliminating toxins. Foods like garlic, ginger, and turmeric can help stimulate liver function and enhance its ability to process and remove harmful substances. Including these in your meals can give your liver a helping hand.
Another useful practice is to engage in regular physical activity. Exercise encourages sweating, which is another way your body can eliminate toxins. Activities like brisk walking, jogging, or yoga can boost circulation and lymphatic flow, aiding in the detoxification process.

Consider periodic detox programs, such as juice cleanses or short-term elimination diets. These can help give your digestive system a break and reduce your intake of processed foods and chemicals. However, it's important to approach these programs carefully and ideally under the guidance of a healthcare professional to ensure they're safe and appropriate for you.

Lastly, reducing your exposure to environmental toxins can make a big difference. Simple changes like using natural cleaning products, avoiding excessive use of plastics, and choosing organic foods when possible can help minimize the amount of toxins your body has to deal with.

Restoring Sleep and Energy Levels Naturally

When chronic fatigue takes hold, it often disrupts your sleep, creating a frustrating cycle where poor sleep leads to lower energy levels, which in turn makes getting good rest even harder. Fortunately, there are several natural strategies you can use to restore your sleep quality and boost your energy levels. Here's how you can gently guide your body back to feeling refreshed and revitalized.

Creating a relaxing sleep environment is a great place to start. Your bedroom should be a tranquil space dedicated to rest. Aim for a cool, dark, and quiet environment to promote better sleep. Consider using blackout curtains, a white noise machine, or a fan to block out disturbances. A comfortable mattress and supportive pillows are also essential, so make sure your sleep setup is cozy and inviting.

Establishing a consistent sleep schedule can greatly benefit your sleep quality. Try to go to bed and wake up at the same time every day, even on weekends. This helps regulate your internal clock and makes it easier for your body to fall asleep and wake up naturally. Consistency reinforces your body's natural sleep-wake cycle, making restful sleep more attainable.

Developing a calming bedtime routine can signal to your body that it's time to wind down. Engaging in soothing activities like reading a book, taking a warm bath, or practicing gentle yoga can help prepare your mind and body for sleep. It's best to avoid stimulating activities, such as watching TV or using electronic devices, as the blue light from screens can interfere with your ability to fall asleep.

Managing stress and anxiety is crucial for improving both sleep and energy levels. Incorporating stress-reducing practices into your daily routine can make a big difference. Techniques like mindfulness meditation, deep breathing exercises, or simply talking about your worries with a trusted friend can help calm your mind before bedtime.

Herbal remedies can also support better sleep. Chamomile tea, known for its calming effects, can help you relax and fall asleep more easily. Valerian root is another herb traditionally used to improve sleep quality. You can find these herbs in various forms, including teas, capsules, or tinctures.

Regular physical activity can enhance both sleep quality and energy levels. Aim for at least 30 minutes of moderate exercise most days of the week. Activities such as walking, cycling, or swimming can boost your overall energy and contribute to deeper, more restorative sleep. However, avoid exercising too close to bedtime, as it might make it harder to fall asleep.

Nutrition plays a key role in how well you sleep and how energetic you feel. Avoid heavy or rich meals close to bedtime, as they can cause discomfort and disrupt sleep. Instead, opt for a light snack that includes sleep-supportive nutrients, such as a small bowl of yogurt or a banana with a bit of nut butter. Foods rich in magnesium, like nuts and leafy greens, can help relax your muscles and improve sleep quality. Keeping your blood sugar levels steady throughout the day with balanced meals can also help prevent energy crashes.

Staying hydrated is important, but be mindful of your fluid intake before bed to avoid waking up during the night. Drink enough water throughout the day to stay hydrated, but try to limit large amounts of fluids right before bedtime.

Avoiding stimulants like caffeine and nicotine, especially in the afternoon and evening, can help you fall asleep more easily. Opt for caffeine-free beverages or herbal teas instead.

Exposure to natural light during the day can help regulate your body's internal clock and improve sleep quality. Try to spend some time outside each day, particularly in the morning. If natural light is limited, especially during winter months, consider using a light therapy box to simulate sunlight.

Book 31: Healing Infections with Natural Remedies

The Body's Natural Defense Against Infections

Our bodies are incredible machines, constantly working behind the scenes to keep us healthy and protect us from infections. Understanding how your body defends itself can help you appreciate the complex processes involved and support your immune system naturally. Here's a friendly guide to how your body naturally defends against infections and how you can support these processes.

The Immune System at Work: The immune system is your body's primary defense mechanism against infections. It's made up of a network of cells, tissues, and organs, including the bone marrow, thymus, spleen, and lymph nodes. These components work together to detect and destroy harmful invaders like bacteria, viruses, and fungi. Think of it as an intricate security system, constantly on the lookout for threats.

White Blood Cells: The Frontline Defenders: White blood cells (or leukocytes) are your immune system's front-line soldiers. They patrol your body, identifying and attacking pathogens. There are different types of white blood cells, each with a specific role. For example, neutrophils quickly respond to bacterial infections, while lymphocytes, such as T-cells and B-cells, are crucial for recognizing and remembering specific pathogens.

The Role of Antibodies: Antibodies are special proteins produced by B-cells that specifically target and neutralize pathogens. Once your body has encountered a pathogen, it creates antibodies tailored to fight it. This means that if the same pathogen tries to invade again, your body can respond more rapidly and effectively, thanks to this "memory" of previous infections.

The Importance of Inflammation: Inflammation is a natural response to infection or injury. It involves the increased production of white blood cells and other substances that help fight off invaders. While inflammation can cause symptoms like redness and swelling, it's a crucial part of the healing process. However, chronic inflammation can be harmful, so it's important to support your body in managing inflammation effectively.

Fever as a Defense Mechanism: When your body detects an infection, it may raise your temperature to create an environment less favorable for pathogens. This is why fevers are often a sign that your immune system is working hard to fight off an infection. While fever can be uncomfortable, it's usually a sign that your body is doing its job.

Mucosal Defenses: Your body has protective barriers to keep pathogens from entering. The skin acts as a physical barrier, while mucous membranes in the respiratory and digestive tracts trap and expel invaders. Mucus, along with other substances like saliva and stomach acid, helps neutralize and flush out harmful organisms before they can cause an infection.

Gut Health and Immunity: Your digestive system plays a crucial role in immune function. A significant portion of your immune system resides in your gut, where beneficial bacteria help keep harmful pathogens in check. Maintaining a healthy gut microbiome through a balanced diet rich in fiber, probiotics, and prebiotics can support your body's natural defenses.

Supporting Natural Defenses with Nutrition: What you eat can impact how well your body can defend itself. Nutrient-rich foods, such as fruits, vegetables, nuts, seeds, and lean proteins, provide essential vitamins and minerals that support immune function. Vitamins like C and D, zinc, and antioxidants help enhance your body's ability to fight off infections and heal effectively.

Hydration and Healing: Staying well-hydrated is essential for overall health and can support your body's natural defenses. Water helps maintain optimal body function, supports circulation, and aids in the removal of toxins. Drinking enough fluids can help your immune system work efficiently and support your body's healing processes.

Rest and Recovery: Your body needs adequate rest to keep your immune system functioning at its best. When you're well-rested, your body can produce more white blood cells and other immune system components to combat infections. Aim for 7-9 hours of sleep each night and listen to your body when it needs rest.

Herbal Antibiotics and Antivirals

Nature provides us with a rich selection of herbs that can act as natural antibiotics and antivirals, offering a supportive boost to our immune system and helping to fight off infections. Here's a closer look at how these herbal remedies work and how you might use them to enhance your health.

Herbal antibiotics are plants that have natural properties capable of combating bacteria. Garlic is one such powerful herb, celebrated for its ability to fight a variety of bacteria thanks to a compound called allicin. Incorporating fresh garlic into your meals or taking it in supplement form can help bolster your defenses against bacterial infections.

Another effective herbal antibiotic is Echinacea. This herb is often used to support the immune system by stimulating the production of white blood cells, which are essential for fighting infections. Echinacea is particularly known for its effectiveness against upper respiratory infections such as colds and flu.

Goldenseal is another herb that is commonly used for its antimicrobial properties. It contains a compound known as berberine, which has been shown to combat various bacterial infections, especially those affecting the digestive and respiratory systems. Goldenseal can be taken as a tincture or in capsule form.

Oregano oil is also a notable herbal antibiotic. It contains carvacrol and thymol, compounds with strong antibacterial properties. Oregano oil can be used in cooking or taken as a supplement to help fight off bacterial infections and support respiratory health.

When it comes to antiviral properties, certain herbs excel in inhibiting the replication of viruses, thereby reducing the severity and duration of infections. Elderberry is a prime example. Elderberry is known for its antiviral effects, particularly against influenza viruses. The berries contain anthocyanins that help inhibit viral replication and reduce inflammation. Elderberry syrup or supplements can be taken at the onset of symptoms to boost your immune response.

Licorice root is another herb with strong antiviral and immune-boosting properties. It contains glycyrrhizin, which can help to inhibit viral activity and manage inflammation. Licorice root can be consumed as a tea or taken in supplement form to support your body during viral infections.

Astragalus is also valued for its ability to fight off viruses and enhance immune function. Traditionally used to prevent and treat colds and flu, Astragalus helps to boost the immune system and can be taken as a tea or in capsule form.

Sage, known for its antiviral and antibacterial properties, can be particularly helpful for soothing sore throats and reducing symptoms of respiratory infections. Sage tea or tincture can offer relief and support your immune system.

Incorporating these herbal remedies into your routine can be both enjoyable and beneficial. You might add garlic and oregano to your cooking for their antimicrobial benefits while sipping herbal teas like elderberry and sage for soothing relief. Supplements and tinctures are also available for a more concentrated dose of these herbs.

Supporting the Immune System During Infections

When your body is battling an infection, giving your immune system a helping hand can make all the difference in how quickly and effectively you recover. The immune system is your body's natural defense mechanism, working tirelessly to fight off harmful pathogens. By supporting it with the right practices and nutrients, you can boost its ability to fend off infections and speed up your recovery. Here's how you can help support your immune system during an infection.

Prioritize Rest and Recovery: Rest is crucial when your body is fighting an infection. Your immune system needs extra energy to combat pathogens, and getting plenty of sleep helps it function at its best. Aim for 7-9 hours of sleep each night, and listen to your body's signals to rest when needed. Adequate rest allows your immune system to produce more white blood cells and other immune components, enhancing its ability to fight off infections.

Stay Hydrated: Hydration plays a vital role in supporting your immune system. Water helps to maintain optimal bodily functions, including the production of immune cells and the removal of toxins. Drinking plenty of fluids like water, herbal teas, and clear broths helps keep your body hydrated, supports overall health, and can ease symptoms such as congestion.

Eat a Nutrient-Rich Diet: Your diet has a significant impact on your immune system. Focus on consuming a variety of nutrient-dense foods that support immune health. Fruits and vegetables are rich in vitamins and minerals, such as vitamin C, vitamin A, and zinc, which play essential roles in immune function. Foods like citrus fruits, bell peppers, carrots, and leafy greens can provide these vital nutrients.

Incorporate Immune-Boosting Herbs: Certain herbs can provide additional support to your immune system. Echinacea and elderberry, for instance, are well-known for their immune-boosting properties. Drinking teas made from these herbs or taking them in supplement form can help enhance your body's ability to fight off infections. Similarly, herbs like ginger and garlic have antimicrobial properties that can further support your immune system.

Maintain a Balanced Lifestyle: A balanced lifestyle supports overall immune function. Regular physical activity helps keep your immune system strong, while reducing stress through practices like meditation, deep breathing, or yoga can prevent the immune system from being compromised. Avoiding excessive alcohol and smoking is also important, as these can weaken your immune defenses.

Support Gut Health: A significant portion of your immune system is located in the gut, so maintaining a healthy digestive system is crucial. Eating probiotic-rich foods like yogurt, kefir, and fermented vegetables can help promote a healthy gut microbiome. This, in turn, supports your body's immune response.

Practice Good Hygiene: During an infection, practicing good hygiene can prevent the spread of pathogens and help your immune system focus on fighting the infection. Regular handwashing, using tissues when coughing or sneezing, and avoiding close contact with others can help reduce the risk of transmitting or acquiring additional infections.

Consider Supplements Wisely: While a well-balanced diet should provide most of the nutrients needed for immune support, some people may benefit from supplements. Vitamin C, vitamin D, and zinc supplements can be helpful in boosting immune function. However, it's essential to consult with a healthcare provider before starting any new supplements to ensure they are appropriate for your specific needs.

Stay Positive and Manage Stress: Stress can negatively impact your immune system, making it harder for your body to recover from infections. Engaging in activities that bring you joy, practicing relaxation techniques, and maintaining a positive outlook can help manage stress levels and support immune function.

Managing Bacterial and Fungal Infections Naturally

Dealing with bacterial and fungal infections can be challenging, but nature offers a range of remedies that can help support your body's healing process. By incorporating natural approaches into your care routine, you can complement conventional treatments and potentially enhance your recovery. Here's a friendly guide on managing bacterial and fungal infections naturally.

Embrace the Power of Garlic: Garlic isn't just for flavoring your meals; it's also a natural powerhouse against infections. Garlic contains allicin, a compound with potent antibacterial and antifungal properties. To harness its benefits, try incorporating fresh garlic into your diet or consider taking garlic supplements. Just be sure to use it as part of a balanced approach to managing your infection.

Tea Tree Oil for Fungal Infections: Tea tree oil is a well-known natural remedy for fungal infections, especially those affecting the skin and nails. It has strong antifungal properties and can be applied topically to the affected area. Dilute tea tree oil with a carrier oil (like coconut oil) before applying to avoid irritation. It's important to use this remedy consistently and monitor for any adverse reactions.

Aloe Vera for Skin Infections: Aloe vera is not only soothing but also has antimicrobial properties that can aid in healing skin infections. Apply pure aloe vera gel directly to the affected area to reduce inflammation and promote healing. It's a gentle and natural way to support your skin's recovery.

Use Honey for Wound Healing: Honey has been used for centuries as a natural remedy for wounds and infections. Its antibacterial properties can help prevent infection and speed up the healing process. Apply raw honey to minor wounds or cuts and cover with a sterile bandage. Honey's natural enzymes and sugars create an environment that supports healing.

Incorporate Probiotics: Probiotics are beneficial bacteria that support a healthy gut microbiome, which plays a crucial role in overall immune function. When dealing with bacterial infections, taking probiotic supplements or consuming probiotic-rich foods (like yogurt and kefir) can help balance your gut flora and enhance your body's ability to fight off harmful bacteria.

Turmeric for Its Anti-Inflammatory Effects: Turmeric contains curcumin, a compound with strong anti-inflammatory and antimicrobial properties. Adding turmeric to your diet or taking it as a supplement can help reduce inflammation and support your body's natural defenses against infections. It can be especially useful for managing symptoms and supporting recovery.

Consider Apple Cider Vinegar: Apple cider vinegar is known for its antibacterial and antifungal properties. It can be used as a natural remedy for various infections. For a sore throat, dilute apple cider vinegar in water and use it as a gargle. For skin infections, dilute it with water and apply to the affected area. Always ensure proper dilution to avoid irritation.

Maintain Good Hygiene Practices: Good hygiene is key to preventing and managing infections. Regularly wash your hands, avoid sharing personal items, and keep affected areas clean and dry. For fungal infections, such as athlete's foot, keeping your feet dry and changing socks frequently can help prevent the spread of the infection.

Stay Hydrated and Eat Well: Proper hydration and nutrition play an essential role in supporting your body's ability to fight infections. Drink plenty of water, eat a balanced diet rich in fruits, vegetables, and whole grains, and ensure you're getting the necessary vitamins and minerals to support your immune system.

Consult with a Healthcare Professional: While natural remedies can be effective, it's important to consult with a healthcare provider, especially if you have a severe or persistent infection. They can help guide you on the best course of treatment and ensure that your natural remedies are used safely and effectively in conjunction with conventional care.

Detoxifying After Infections

Once you've overcome an infection, giving your body a little extra care can help you bounce back fully and restore your overall well-being. Detoxifying after an infection is about supporting your body's natural ability to cleanse and heal, ensuring you feel your best as you recover. Here's a friendly guide on how to detoxify naturally and rejuvenate after an infection.

Rehydrate and Replenish: After an infection, your body can be dehydrated from fever and sweating. Start by drinking plenty of water to help flush out any remaining toxins and rehydrate your system. Herbal teas like chamomile or peppermint can also be soothing and supportive, aiding digestion and providing additional antioxidants.

Focus on Nutrient-Dense Foods: Eating a diet rich in fruits, vegetables, and whole grains supports your body's detoxification processes. These foods are packed with vitamins, minerals, and antioxidants that help repair tissues, boost your immune system, and eliminate toxins. Incorporate a variety of colorful vegetables and fruits to ensure you're getting a broad range of nutrients.

Add Detoxifying Herbs and Spices: Certain herbs and spices can aid in detoxification and support your body's natural cleansing processes. Ginger and turmeric are excellent choices; they have anti-inflammatory and detoxifying properties that can help soothe your digestive system and promote overall health. Adding these to your meals or enjoying them as teas can be beneficial.

Support Your Liver: The liver plays a crucial role in detoxifying the body. To support liver health, consider incorporating liver-friendly foods like leafy greens, beets, and artichokes into your diet. These foods help boost liver function and support the body's natural detoxification processes.

Maintain Regular Bowel Movements: A healthy digestive system is key to effective detoxification. Ensure you're getting enough fiber from fruits, vegetables, and whole grains to keep your digestive system moving smoothly. Regular bowel movements help eliminate toxins and waste products from your body.

Engage in Gentle Exercise: Light to moderate exercise can support your body's detoxification efforts by promoting circulation and helping your body eliminate toxins through sweat. Activities like walking, yoga, or swimming can be beneficial. Just be sure to listen to your body and start slowly, especially if you're still recovering from an infection.

Get Plenty of Rest: Rest is essential for recovery and detoxification. Ensure you're getting enough sleep each night to allow your body to repair and rejuvenate. A well-rested body is more effective at cleansing and healing.

Practice Stress Management: Stress can impact your body's ability to detoxify effectively. Incorporate stress-reducing practices into your routine, such as meditation, deep breathing exercises, or spending time in nature. Managing stress helps support overall health and well-being.

Avoid Toxins: After an infection, it's a good idea to avoid exposure to additional toxins. This means cutting back on processed foods, reducing alcohol intake, and avoiding smoking. Opt for natural, whole foods and a clean, healthy environment to support your body's detoxification efforts.

Consider Gentle Detoxification Practices: Gentle detox practices like saunas or steam baths can support your body's natural detoxification processes. These practices help to sweat out toxins and promote relaxation. Just be sure to stay hydrated and consult with a healthcare provider if you have any concerns.

Listen to Your Body: Pay attention to how you're feeling as you go through the detoxification process. Everyone's body responds differently, so it's important to listen to your own needs and adjust your approach as needed. If you have any specific concerns or symptoms, don't hesitate to reach out to a healthcare professional for personalized advice.

Probiotics and Gut Health During Infections

When you're fighting off an infection, your gut health plays a surprisingly important role in how well you recover. Your gut is home to a vast community of microorganisms, known as the microbiome, which are crucial for supporting your immune system and overall health. One way to support this balance is by incorporating probiotics into your routine. Let's dive into how probiotics and gut health can make a difference during infections.

Understanding the Gut-Immune Connection: Your gut and immune system are closely linked. About 70% of your immune system resides in your gut, so maintaining a healthy microbiome can significantly influence how effectively your body responds to infections.

A balanced gut microbiome helps regulate inflammation and supports the production of immune cells, which are essential for fighting off pathogens.

What Are Probiotics? Probiotics are beneficial bacteria that help maintain a healthy balance of microorganisms in your gut. They can be found in fermented foods like yogurt, kefir, sauerkraut, and kimchi, or taken as dietary supplements. These friendly bacteria help crowd out harmful bacteria, support digestion, and promote a strong immune response.

How Probiotics Support Infection Recovery: During an infection, your gut flora can be disrupted, especially if you've been on antibiotics. Antibiotics, while necessary to treat bacterial infections, can also kill off beneficial bacteria along with harmful ones. Probiotics help replenish these beneficial bacteria, restoring balance to your gut microbiome and supporting your body's natural healing processes.

Choose the Right Probiotics: Not all probiotics are created equal, so it's important to select strains that are known for their health benefits. Common strains like Lactobacillus acidophilus and Bifidobacterium bifidum have been studied for their positive effects on gut health and immune function. Look for supplements with a variety of strains to support a diverse microbiome.

Incorporate Probiotic-Rich Foods: Adding probiotic-rich foods to your diet can be a delicious way to support gut health. Greek yogurt, kefir, miso, and fermented vegetables are excellent choices. These foods provide live cultures that help to repopulate your gut with beneficial bacteria.

Prebiotics Are Just as Important: While probiotics are beneficial bacteria, prebiotics are the nutrients that feed these good bacteria. Foods high in prebiotics, like bananas, onions, garlic, and asparagus, provide the fuel necessary for probiotics to thrive and support a healthy gut environment.

Timing and Dosage: For the best results, try to incorporate probiotics regularly into your diet, rather than just during illness. For those taking supplements, follow the recommended dosage on the label or consult with a healthcare provider for personalized advice. Consistency is key to maintaining a balanced gut microbiome.

Listen to Your Body: Everyone's gut is unique, and it's important to pay attention to how your body responds to probiotics. If you experience any discomfort or digestive changes, it's a good idea to adjust your intake or consult with a healthcare provider to ensure you're choosing the right approach for your needs.

Maintain a Balanced Diet: Probiotics are most effective when combined with a balanced diet. Eating a variety of whole, unprocessed foods supports overall gut health and complements the benefits of probiotics. Focus on a diet rich in fiber, fruits, vegetables, and lean proteins.

Consider Your Overall Health: If you have underlying health conditions or are on specific medications, such as immunosuppressants, discuss with your healthcare provider before starting probiotics. They can help determine the best approach based on your individual health needs.

Preventing Future Infections with Lifestyle Changes

Once you've recovered from an infection, it's natural to want to take steps to reduce the risk of future illnesses. Adopting a few lifestyle changes can significantly bolster your immune system and help keep infections at bay. Here's a friendly guide to making some practical adjustments that can help you stay healthy and strong.

Prioritize Hand Hygiene: One of the simplest yet most effective ways to prevent infections is by practicing good hand hygiene. Regularly washing your hands with soap and water for at least 20 seconds can help remove germs and reduce the spread of infections. Make it a habit to wash your hands before meals, after using the restroom, and when you've been in public places.

Boost Your Immune System: A strong immune system is your best defense against infections. Eating a balanced diet rich in fruits, vegetables, whole grains, and lean proteins can provide your body with the nutrients it needs to stay resilient. Vitamins and minerals like vitamin C, zinc, and vitamin D are particularly important for immune health.

Stay Active: Regular physical activity has numerous health benefits, including supporting a robust immune system. Aim for at least 150 minutes of moderate exercise or 75 minutes of vigorous activity per week. Activities like walking, jogging, or yoga can help keep your body in shape and improve your overall well-being.

Get Quality Sleep: Never underestimate the power of a good night's sleep. Your body needs adequate rest to repair itself and maintain a healthy immune system. Strive for 7-9 hours of quality sleep each night, and establish a regular sleep schedule to support your body's natural rhythms.

Manage Stress: Chronic stress can weaken your immune system and make you more susceptible to infections. Finding healthy ways to manage stress is crucial for maintaining good health. Consider incorporating relaxation techniques such as meditation, deep breathing exercises, or engaging in hobbies you enjoy.

Stay Hydrated: Proper hydration is essential for overall health and helps your body function optimally. Drinking enough water throughout the day supports your immune system, aids digestion, and helps flush out toxins. Aim for about 8 glasses of water daily, or more if you're active or live in a hot climate.

Practice Safe Food Handling: Preventing foodborne illnesses is another important aspect of avoiding infections. Practice safe food handling by washing fruits and vegetables thoroughly, cooking meats to the proper temperature, and avoiding cross-contamination between raw and cooked foods.

Maintain a Clean Environment: Keeping your living space clean can help reduce the presence of germs and bacteria. Regularly disinfect commonly touched surfaces like doorknobs, light switches, and countertops. Ensure good ventilation in your home to help prevent the buildup of indoor pollutants.

Avoid Smoking and Limit Alcohol Consumption: Smoking can impair your immune system and increase your risk of infections. If you smoke, seek support to quit. Additionally, excessive alcohol consumption can weaken your immune defenses, so it's best to drink in moderation or avoid alcohol altogether.

Get Vaccinated: Vaccinations play a crucial role in preventing infections by helping your body build immunity against specific pathogens. Stay up-to-date with recommended vaccinations for diseases like influenza, pneumonia, and other preventable infections. Consult with your healthcare provider for guidance on which vaccines are appropriate for you.

Foster Social Connections: Positive social interactions and maintaining relationships can have a beneficial impact on your overall health. Social support can help reduce stress, promote emotional well-being, and encourage healthy lifestyle choices.

Regular Health Check-ups: Regular visits to your healthcare provider can help catch any potential health issues early and ensure you're on track with preventive measures. Discuss any concerns you have about infections or your overall health to get personalized advice and recommendations.

Book 32: Encyclopedia of Healing Herbs

Introduction to Herbal Medicine

Welcome to the fascinating world of herbal medicine! This time-tested practice harnesses the power of plants to promote health and healing. Whether you're new to herbal remedies or looking to deepen your understanding, this guide will give you a warm and friendly introduction to the basics of herbal medicine.

Herbal medicine, also known as phytotherapy, is the use of plant-based substances to treat ailments, support health, and improve well-being. It involves using various parts of plants—such as leaves, roots, flowers, and seeds—to create remedies. These remedies can be found in many forms, including teas, tinctures, capsules, and extracts.

Herbal medicine has been around for thousands of years, with evidence of its use in ancient civilizations like Egypt, China, and Greece. Ancient texts and traditional practices reveal how cultures have relied on herbs for healing and health maintenance. Today, herbal medicine continues to be a cornerstone of healthcare in many parts of the world and is gaining recognition in modern medicine.

Herbs contain a complex mix of active compounds, such as alkaloids, flavonoids, and essential oils, that interact with our bodies to promote health. These compounds can have a variety of effects, from reducing inflammation to boosting the immune system. Herbal medicine works by supporting the body's natural processes and helping it to restore balance.

One of the great things about herbal medicine is its holistic approach. Rather than just addressing symptoms, it aims to treat the whole person—mind, body, and spirit. Herbal remedies can be gentle and supportive, often with fewer side effects compared to pharmaceutical drugs. Many people find that herbs offer a natural way to enhance their well-being and address chronic conditions.

Selecting the right herbs involves understanding what each herb does and how it can benefit you. For example, ginger is known for its digestive support, while lavender is often used for relaxation. It's important to match the herb to your specific needs and health goals. Consulting with a qualified herbalist or healthcare provider can help you make informed choices.

Herbal remedies come in various forms, each with its own benefits. Teas are great for gentle, daily use, while tinctures (alcohol extracts) are more concentrated and can offer quicker effects. Capsules and tablets provide convenience, and topical applications, like salves and oils, can be used for external issues. Understanding these forms helps you choose the one that best fits your needs.

Not all herbal products are created equal, so it's essential to ensure you're using high-quality herbs from reputable sources. Look for products that are well-tested and free from contaminants. As with any medicine, proper dosage and usage are key to safety. If you're unsure, seek guidance from a knowledgeable herbalist or healthcare provider.

Incorporating herbal medicine into your daily routine can be a wonderful way to support your health. Whether you're sipping a calming chamomile tea before bed or using an echinacea tincture to boost your immune system, herbs can be a beneficial addition to your wellness practices. Start with simple remedies and observe how they work for you.

Herbal medicine is experiencing a resurgence as more people seek natural and holistic approaches to health. Modern research continues to explore and validate the benefits of many herbs, blending traditional knowledge with contemporary science. This ongoing exploration promises exciting developments in how we understand and use herbal remedies.

Embrace the Journey

Exploring herbal medicine is a journey of discovery and learning. It invites you to connect with nature and embrace a holistic approach to health. As you begin this journey, remember to approach it with curiosity and respect for the plants that have been cherished for generations.

100 Healing Herbs

Welcome to the wonderful world of healing herbs! Here's a friendly guide to 100 herbs that have been cherished for their therapeutic properties. Whether you're new to herbal remedies or a seasoned enthusiast, this list will give you a great starting point for exploring the diverse and fascinating realm of herbal medicine.

1. Aloe Vera: Known for its soothing gel, aloe vera is a popular remedy for minor burns, cuts, and skin irritations. It also has moisturizing properties that are beneficial for dry skin.

2. Echinacea: Often used to boost the immune system, echinacea is a go-to herb for preventing and treating colds and infections.

3. Lavender: Lavender isn't just lovely; it's also great for calming the mind and easing anxiety. It's often used in aromatherapy and as a gentle sleep aid.

4. Peppermint: Peppermint is fantastic for soothing digestive issues, such as bloating and indigestion. It also has a refreshing and invigorating scent.

5. Ginger: Ginger is well-known for its anti-nausea and anti-inflammatory properties. It's excellent for digestive health and can help ease motion sickness.

6. Chamomile: Chamomile is a calming herb that's often enjoyed as a tea before bed to promote relaxation and improve sleep quality.

7. Turmeric: Turmeric contains curcumin, a powerful anti-inflammatory compound. It's commonly used to support joint health and reduce inflammation.

8. Ginseng: Ginseng is prized for its energy-boosting and stress-reducing properties. It's often used to enhance overall vitality and mental clarity.

9. Rosemary: Rosemary is more than a flavorful herb for cooking; it also has antioxidant properties and can support cognitive function.

10. Thyme: Thyme is known for its antimicrobial properties, making it useful for respiratory health and as a natural remedy for coughs.

11. Sage: Sage is traditionally used for its digestive benefits and to support respiratory health. It also has antimicrobial properties.

12. Lemon Balm: Lemon balm has a lemony scent and is used to ease stress and anxiety, as well as to promote relaxation and improve sleep.

13. Valerian Root: Valerian root is a popular herb for promoting restful sleep and managing anxiety. It's often used in sleep aids and calming teas.

14. Dandelion: Dandelion is more than a weed—it's a powerhouse herb for liver health, digestion, and detoxification.

15. St. John's Wort: St. John's Wort is well-known for its mood-enhancing properties and is often used to support mental well-being.

16. Holy Basil (Tulsi) : Holy basil, or tulsi, is revered in Ayurvedic medicine for its stress-relieving and immune-boosting properties.

17. Milk Thistle: Milk thistle supports liver health and detoxification. Its active compound, silymarin, helps protect liver cells from damage.

18. Calendula: Calendula is a wonderful herb for soothing skin irritations, including minor cuts, bruises, and rashes.

19. Nettles: Nettle leaves are rich in nutrients and are used to support urinary health and reduce inflammation.

20. Yarrow: Yarrow is traditionally used for its wound-healing properties and to support digestive and respiratory health.

21. Hawthorn: Hawthorn is known for supporting cardiovascular health and improving circulation. It's often used to strengthen the heart.

22. Peppermint: Peppermint is great for digestive issues and can also help relieve headaches with its cooling effect.

23. Eucalyptus: Eucalyptus oil is known for its respiratory benefits, helping to clear congestion and ease coughs.

24. Fennel: Fennel seeds support digestion and can help relieve bloating and gas.

25. Ginger: Ginger is great for nausea and digestive issues and can also help reduce inflammation.

26. Garlic: Garlic has powerful antibacterial and antiviral properties and supports immune health.

27. Anise: Anise seeds are used to support digestion and can help alleviate symptoms like bloating and gas.

28. Burdock Root: Burdock root is often used to support liver health and improve skin conditions.

29. Catnip: Catnip is known for its calming effects, particularly for easing anxiety and promoting relaxation.

30. Astragalus: Astragalus is used to boost the immune system and support overall vitality.

31. Gotu Kola: Gotu kola is traditionally used for enhancing cognitive function and promoting wound healing.

32. Juniper Berries: Juniper berries support urinary health and have diuretic properties.

33. Licorice Root: Licorice root is soothing for the digestive tract and supports respiratory health.

34. Coriander: Coriander seeds aid in digestion and have anti-inflammatory properties.

35. Passionflower: Passionflower is used to relieve anxiety and improve sleep quality.

36. Red Clover: Red clover supports hormonal balance and is often used for menopausal symptoms.

37. Slippery Elm: Slippery elm is known for its soothing properties, particularly for the digestive tract and sore throats.

38. Ginger: Ginger helps with nausea, digestive issues, and inflammation.

39. Wormwood: Wormwood is used to support digestive health and manage parasitic infections.

40. Cumin: Cumin seeds are used for digestive support and have antioxidant properties.

41. Moringa: Moringa is packed with nutrients and is used to support overall health and energy levels.

42. Chaga: Chaga mushroom is known for its immune-boosting and antioxidant properties.

43. Reishi: Reishi mushroom supports the immune system and helps with stress management.

44. Shiitake: Shiitake mushrooms have immune-boosting properties and support overall vitality.

45. Ginkgo Biloba: Ginkgo biloba supports cognitive function and improves circulation.

46. Mullein: Mullein is used to soothe respiratory issues and support lung health.

47. Holy Basil (Tulsi) : Holy basil helps with stress and supports the immune system.

48. Marshmallow Root: Marshmallow root soothes mucous membranes and supports digestive health.

49. Red Raspberry Leaf: Red raspberry leaf is often used to support women's reproductive health.

50. Sage: Sage supports digestive health and has antimicrobial properties.

51. Thyme: Thyme supports respiratory health and has antimicrobial properties.

52. Anise: Anise seeds aid digestion and alleviate bloating.

53. Bay Leaf: Bay leaves support digestion and have antioxidant properties.

54. Chervil: Chervil is used for its digestive benefits and mild diuretic effect.

55. Dill: Dill supports digestive health and has anti-inflammatory properties.

56. Echinacea: Echinacea boosts the immune system and helps with infections.

57. Elderberry: Elderberry supports the immune system and helps with colds and flu.

58. Flaxseed: Flaxseeds support heart health and digestion.

59. Goji Berry: Goji berries are rich in antioxidants and support overall health.

60. Jujube: Jujube is used to support digestion and reduce stress.

61. Linden Flower: Linden flowers support relaxation and help with anxiety.

62. Oregano: Oregano has antimicrobial properties and supports respiratory health.

63. Pomegranate: Pomegranate supports heart health and has antioxidant properties.

64. Rosemary: Rosemary supports cognitive function and has antioxidant properties.

65. Schisandra: Schisandra supports liver health and reduces stress.

66. Soursop: Soursop is used to support immune health and has anti-inflammatory properties.

67. Tarragon: Tarragon supports digestion and has mild diuretic properties.

68. Thyme: Thyme supports respiratory health and has antimicrobial properties.

69. Turmeric: Turmeric supports joint health and reduces inflammation.

70. Valerian Root: Valerian root promotes relaxation and improves sleep.

71. Yarrow: Yarrow supports wound healing and digestive health.

72. Aloe Vera: Aloe vera soothes skin and supports digestion.

73. Angelica Root: Angelica root supports digestive health and has mild diuretic properties.

74. Berberine: Berberine supports blood sugar levels and has antimicrobial properties.

75. Borage: Borage supports skin health and has anti-inflammatory properties.

76. Catuaba: Catuaba supports sexual health and has mood-enhancing properties.

77. Dong Quai: Dong quai supports menstrual health and has anti-inflammatory properties.

78. Eleuthero: Eleuthero, also known as Siberian ginseng, supports energy and stress resilience.

79. Ginger: Ginger aids in digestion and reduces nausea.

80. Gotu Kola: Gotu kola supports cognitive function and wound healing.

81. Holy Basil (Tulsi) : Holy basil helps with stress and immune support.

82. Kava: Kava promotes relaxation and reduces anxiety.

83. Lemon Balm: Lemon balm supports relaxation and aids digestion.

84. Maca Root: Maca root supports energy levels and hormone balance.

85. Marshmallow Root: Marshmallow root soothes mucous membranes and supports digestive health.

86. Milk Thistle: Milk thistle supports liver health and detoxification.

87. Nettle: Nettle supports urinary health and has anti-inflammatory properties.

88. Passionflower: Passionflower helps with anxiety and improves sleep.

89. Red Clover: Red clover supports hormonal balance and is used for menopausal symptoms.

90. Siberian Ginseng: Siberian ginseng supports energy and stress resilience.

91. Slippery Elm: Slippery elm soothes the digestive tract and helps with sore throats.

92. Sweet Wormwood: Sweet wormwood supports digestive health and manages parasitic infections.

93. Usnea: Usnea has antimicrobial properties and supports immune health.

94. White Willow Bark: White willow bark supports pain relief and has anti-inflammatory properties.

95. Wormwood: Wormwood supports digestive health and has antimicrobial properties.

96. Yarrow: Yarrow supports wound healing and digestive health.

97. Astragalus: Astragalus boosts the immune system and supports overall vitality.

98. Burdock Root: Burdock root supports liver health and detoxification.

99. Dandelion: Dandelion supports liver health and aids digestion.

100. Echinacea: Echinacea boosts the immune system and helps with infections.

Book 33: Natural Pain Management Strategies

Understanding Chronic Pain and Its Causes

Chronic pain is a persistent, often debilitating condition that affects many people around the world. Unlike acute pain, which typically arises from a specific injury or illness and fades as the underlying issue heals, chronic pain lasts for more than three to six months and can continue even after the initial cause has been resolved.

The nature of chronic pain is multifaceted. It can be caused by a range of factors, sometimes occurring in combination. For some, it begins after an injury or surgery, but the pain persists long after the physical damage has healed. This lingering discomfort can result from nerves becoming overly sensitive, continuing to send pain signals even in the absence of ongoing injury.

Inflammatory conditions are another common cause of chronic pain. Diseases like arthritis, fibromyalgia, and lupus involve ongoing inflammation, which can contribute to persistent pain. When the body's immune system is in a constant state of activity, it can lead to sustained discomfort in various parts of the body.

Nerve damage is another factor that can lead to chronic pain. Conditions such as diabetes or shingles can cause neuropathy, where damaged nerves send pain signals to the brain without a clear external cause. Similarly, issues with muscles, bones, or joints, such as chronic back pain or repetitive strain injuries, can result in ongoing pain.

In some cases, the pain system itself becomes overly active, a phenomenon known as central sensitization. In these situations, the central nervous system, including the brain and spinal cord, becomes hypersensitive, amplifying pain signals and leading to chronic pain even in the absence of a physical injury.

Psychological factors also play a significant role in chronic pain. Stress, anxiety, and depression can not only worsen the perception of pain but also contribute to its persistence. Emotional and mental well-being are closely intertwined with physical pain, making it crucial to address both aspects in managing chronic pain.

The impact of chronic pain extends beyond physical discomfort. It can significantly affect emotional well-being, leading to frustration, depression, or anxiety. The ongoing nature of the pain can interfere with daily activities, reduce social interactions, and affect one's ability to perform work or household tasks. Moreover, chronic pain often disrupts sleep, leading to fatigue and further diminishing quality of life.

Managing chronic pain requires a comprehensive approach that considers both physical and emotional factors. This may include medical treatments such as medications and physical therapy, along with lifestyle changes like regular exercise, a healthy diet, and good sleep hygiene. Mind-body techniques, such as mindfulness and relaxation exercises, can also be beneficial in addressing the emotional aspects of pain. Additionally, support from healthcare providers, therapists, and support groups can provide valuable resources and encouragement.

Herbal Pain Relievers for Common Conditions

When it comes to managing pain naturally, herbal remedies can offer a gentle yet effective alternative to traditional pain relief methods. Many herbs have been used for centuries to alleviate various types of pain, and they come with the added benefit of being generally safe when used appropriately. Let's explore some herbal options for managing pain associated with common conditions.

Turmeric, with its active compound curcumin, is renowned for its anti-inflammatory properties. It's particularly beneficial for conditions like arthritis, where inflammation contributes to joint pain. Turmeric can be taken as a spice in your food, brewed into a tea, or used as a supplement. Its ability to reduce inflammation helps ease pain and improve joint function.

Ginger is another powerhouse herb with anti-inflammatory and analgesic (pain-relieving) properties. It's often used to soothe muscle soreness, including pain from overuse or exercise. You can enjoy ginger as a tea, add it to your meals, or take it in capsule form. Regular consumption can help alleviate discomfort and promote faster recovery.

Willow bark has been used historically as a natural remedy for pain relief, particularly for back pain and headaches. It contains salicin, which is similar to the active ingredient in aspirin. Willow bark can be taken as a tea or in supplement form to help reduce pain and inflammation.

Peppermint is known for its cooling and soothing effects, making it a great choice for relieving tension headaches. The menthol in peppermint helps relax muscles and improve circulation. You can apply diluted peppermint oil to your temples, drink peppermint tea, or inhale the steam from a peppermint-infused bowl of hot water for relief.

Arnica is a popular herb for treating bruises, sprains, and muscle aches. It's available as a topical cream or gel, which can be applied directly to the affected area. Arnica's anti-inflammatory and pain-relieving properties make it a go-to remedy for minor injuries and muscle soreness.

Chamomile is often associated with relaxation and sleep, but it also has mild analgesic properties that can help with general pain relief. Chamomile tea is a soothing way to alleviate minor aches and pains and promote overall well-being.

Lavender's calming and relaxing effects make it beneficial for stress-related pain, such as tension headaches or muscle tightness. You can use lavender essential oil in aromatherapy, add a few drops to a warm bath, or use it in a massage oil to ease pain and reduce stress.

Cayenne pepper contains capsaicin, which is known for its ability to reduce nerve pain. Capsaicin works by depleting substance P, a neurotransmitter involved in pain transmission. You can use cayenne pepper in topical creams or ointments for targeted relief of nerve pain and discomfort.

Eucalyptus has soothing properties that can help with respiratory issues and associated pain, such as chest discomfort from coughing or congestion. Eucalyptus oil can be added to a steam inhalation or used in a chest rub to relieve symptoms and support respiratory health.

Valerian root is well-known for its sedative effects, which can be helpful for relaxing muscles and easing spasms. It's commonly used as a tincture or tea to promote muscle relaxation and alleviate related pain.

The Role of Nutrition in Reducing Inflammation and Pain

When it comes to managing pain and inflammation, the foods you choose to eat can have a profound impact. Nutrition is a key player in either fueling inflammation or helping to soothe it. By making mindful food choices, you can support your body's natural ability to handle pain and promote overall health.

Inflammation is a natural response by your immune system to injury or infection, but when it becomes chronic, it can contribute to ongoing pain and a variety of health issues, such as arthritis and cardiovascular diseases. The right diet can help mitigate this inflammatory response and provide relief. Foods known for their anti-inflammatory properties can be particularly beneficial. Fruits and vegetables are at the top of the list, offering a wealth of antioxidants and vitamins that combat inflammation. For example, berries, oranges, tomatoes, and leafy greens like spinach and kale are rich in compounds that help reduce oxidative stress and inflammation.

Fatty fish such as salmon, mackerel, and sardines are also excellent choices. These fish are high in omega-3 fatty acids, which have been shown to lower the production of inflammatory compounds in the body, thereby reducing pain and inflammation.

Nuts and seeds like almonds, walnuts, chia seeds, and flaxseeds provide healthy fats and antioxidants that further help lower inflammation. Similarly, extra virgin olive oil, which contains oleocanthal, a compound with anti-inflammatory properties, can be a great alternative to other cooking oils.
Herbs and spices play an important role as well. Turmeric, with its active ingredient curcumin, and ginger are well-regarded for their anti-inflammatory effects. Turmeric can be used in various dishes, and ginger can be added to teas or meals to help alleviate pain and inflammation.

Conversely, there are certain foods that can exacerbate inflammation and should be consumed in moderation or avoided. Processed foods high in refined sugars, trans fats, and artificial additives can increase inflammation. This includes sugary snacks, fast foods, and processed snacks.
Red and processed meats are also known to contribute to inflammation. Opting for leaner proteins and plant-based alternatives can be beneficial. Additionally, refined carbohydrates, such as those found in white bread and pastries, can spike blood sugar levels and promote inflammation. Choosing whole grains instead offers more fiber and nutrients.

Excessive alcohol consumption can also promote inflammation and negatively affect overall health. Moderation is key if you choose to drink. Similarly, high-sodium foods can lead to inflammation and water retention, so cutting back on salty foods and opting for low-sodium alternatives can help.
By incorporating a variety of nutrient-rich foods into your daily meals and limiting inflammatory foods, you can create a balanced approach to managing pain and inflammation. Eating a diet rich in fruits, vegetables, lean proteins, and healthy fats supports your body's natural ability to reduce inflammation and handle pain more effectively.

Managing Joint and Muscle Pain Naturally

When dealing with joint and muscle pain, it's natural to seek relief that doesn't rely on medication. Fortunately, there are several natural strategies that can help manage and alleviate this type of pain. Let's explore some effective approaches to soothing joint and muscle discomfort without the need for pharmaceutical interventions.

Exercise is essential for maintaining joint and muscle health, but it's important to approach it wisely. Gentle activities like walking, swimming, and cycling can help keep your muscles and joints flexible without putting too much strain on them. Incorporating stretching exercises into your routine can also improve flexibility and reduce stiffness. Yoga and Pilates are excellent options as they focus on stretching, strengthening, and balancing muscles, which can be particularly beneficial for managing pain.

Applying heat or cold to painful areas can provide immediate relief. Heat therapy, such as a warm bath, hot water bottle, or heating pad, helps relax tight muscles and improve blood flow, which can ease pain. Cold therapy, using an ice pack or a cold compress, reduces inflammation and numbs the area, which can be especially helpful after a flare-up or injury. Alternating between hot and cold treatments can also be effective in managing chronic pain.

Incorporating anti-inflammatory foods into your diet can help reduce joint and muscle pain. Foods like fatty fish, nuts, seeds, and leafy greens are rich in anti-inflammatory compounds. Herbs such as turmeric and ginger are known for their pain-relieving properties. Turmeric contains curcumin, which helps reduce inflammation, while ginger can help alleviate muscle soreness. Adding these herbs to your meals or taking them as supplements can be beneficial.

Excess weight can put additional stress on your joints, particularly those in the lower body like the knees and hips. Maintaining a healthy weight through a balanced diet and regular exercise can reduce the strain on your joints and help manage pain more effectively. If weight loss is needed, focus on a combination of healthy eating and physical activity to achieve gradual and sustainable results.

Certain supplements may support joint and muscle health and alleviate pain. Glucosamine and chondroitin are popular for joint health, as they help maintain cartilage and improve joint function. Omega-3 fatty acids, found in fish oil supplements, have anti-inflammatory effects that can help reduce joint pain. Always consult with a healthcare provider before starting any new supplements to ensure they are appropriate for you.

Mind-body practices such as mindfulness meditation, deep breathing, and progressive muscle relaxation can help manage pain by reducing stress and improving your overall sense of well-being. These techniques can help you manage the emotional aspects of chronic pain and promote relaxation, which in turn can reduce muscle tension and discomfort.

Massage therapy can help relax tight muscles, improve circulation, and alleviate pain. A professional massage therapist can use various techniques to target specific areas of discomfort. Acupuncture, a traditional Chinese medicine practice, involves inserting thin needles into specific points on the body to relieve pain and promote healing. Both treatments have been shown to be effective in managing joint and muscle pain for many people.

Proper hydration is crucial for maintaining healthy muscles and joints. Drinking enough water helps keep tissues lubricated and can prevent muscle cramps and stiffness. Aim to drink plenty of water throughout the day, and consider including hydrating foods like fruits and vegetables in your diet.

Finally, it's important to listen to your body and avoid activities that worsen your pain. If you experience increased discomfort during or after certain activities, it's a sign to modify your approach or seek guidance from a healthcare professional. Taking a balanced and mindful approach to managing pain can help you maintain a better quality of life.

Detoxifying the Body to Alleviate Pain

Detoxifying your body can be a powerful way to manage and alleviate pain. By supporting your body's natural detoxification processes, you can help reduce inflammation, improve overall health, and potentially ease pain. Here's a friendly guide to understanding how detoxification can help and some simple ways to incorporate it into your daily routine.

Detoxification is the process by which your body removes toxins and waste products. This is primarily done through the liver, kidneys, and other organs like the skin and intestines. When these organs are overwhelmed or not functioning optimally, toxins can accumulate, potentially leading to inflammation and pain. By supporting these detoxifying organs, you can enhance your body's ability to eliminate harmful substances and reduce pain.

One of the simplest and most effective ways to support detoxification is by staying well-hydrated. Drinking plenty of water helps flush toxins out of your system through urine and sweat. Aim for at least 8 glasses of water a day, and consider adding a squeeze of lemon for an extra detoxifying boost. Lemon water can help stimulate digestion and enhance the liver's detoxification efforts.

Certain foods are known for their detoxifying properties and can help support your body's natural cleansing processes. Leafy greens like spinach and kale, cruciferous vegetables such as broccoli and Brussels sprouts, and fruits like berries and apples are all excellent choices. These foods are rich in vitamins, minerals, and antioxidants that help neutralize and eliminate toxins.

Herbal teas can be a soothing and effective way to support detoxification. Green tea is packed with antioxidants that help combat oxidative stress and support liver function. Dandelion root tea is known for its diuretic properties, which can help flush out excess fluids and toxins. Milk thistle tea supports liver health and enhances the liver's ability to detoxify.

Fiber plays a crucial role in detoxification by aiding digestion and helping your body eliminate waste. Foods rich in fiber, such as whole grains, legumes, fruits, and vegetables, help keep your digestive system moving smoothly and prevent the buildup of toxins. Aim to include a variety of fiber-rich foods in your diet to support regular bowel movements and effective detoxification.

Exercise is not only beneficial for overall health but also supports detoxification. Physical activity helps improve circulation, boost metabolism, and promote sweating, which can assist in the elimination of toxins through the skin. Whether it's a brisk walk, a yoga session, or a workout at the gym, regular exercise helps keep your body's detoxification systems functioning optimally.

Gentle detox methods, such as a short-term cleanse or detox diet, can help give your body a break from processed foods and excess toxins. A typical detox might involve focusing on whole, unprocessed foods and eliminating common allergens or irritants like caffeine, sugar, and alcohol for a period of time. Always consult with a healthcare provider before starting any new detox program, especially if you have underlying health conditions.

Your liver and kidneys are key players in detoxification. Supporting their health can enhance your body's ability to detoxify effectively. Eating foods known for their liver-supportive properties, such as beets, garlic, and turmeric, can help. Similarly, maintaining kidney health through proper hydration and a balanced diet is essential for effective detoxification.

Sleep is an important aspect of the detoxification process. During sleep, your body focuses on repair and recovery, including the elimination of waste products. Aim for 7-9 hours of quality sleep each night to support your body's natural detoxification processes and overall well-being.

Finally, it's important to listen to your body and pay attention to how you feel during the detoxification process. If you experience any discomfort or adverse effects, it's a sign to adjust your approach or seek guidance from a healthcare professional.

Mind-Body Techniques for Pain Management

When it comes to managing pain, your mind plays a powerful role. Mind-body techniques harness the connection between mental and physical well-being to help alleviate pain and improve your quality of life. Here's a friendly guide to some effective mind-body techniques that can help you manage pain naturally.

Mindfulness meditation involves focusing on the present moment without judgment. By practicing mindfulness, you can learn to observe your pain without becoming overwhelmed by it. This technique helps reduce stress and can alter the way you perceive pain. Simple mindfulness exercises, such as paying attention to your breath or body sensations, can help you develop a more accepting and less reactive attitude toward pain.

Deep breathing exercises can help calm the nervous system and reduce pain perception. Try taking slow, deep breaths through your nose, allowing your abdomen to rise, and then exhaling fully through your mouth. This practice helps relax tense muscles, lowers stress levels, and can create a soothing effect that eases discomfort.

Progressive muscle relaxation involves systematically tensing and then relaxing different muscle groups in your body. This technique helps reduce muscle tension and stress, which can contribute to pain. Start by tensing the muscles in your feet for a few seconds, then release and relax. Gradually work your way up through each muscle group, from your legs to your head, focusing on the sensation of relaxation.

Visualization and guided imagery involve imagining a peaceful, relaxing scene or using mental imagery to alter your pain experience. You might picture yourself in a serene place, like a beach or forest, and focus on the sensory details of that scene. Guided imagery can also involve listening to recorded scripts that lead you through relaxation techniques and positive imagery, helping shift your focus away from pain.

Yoga and Tai Chi combine gentle movement, stretching, and mindfulness to help manage pain. Both practices focus on balancing the body and mind, improving flexibility, and reducing stress. Yoga offers various poses and breathing techniques that can help release muscle tension and enhance relaxation. Tai Chi involves slow, flowing movements that improve balance and promote a sense of calm.

Biofeedback is a technique that teaches you to control physiological functions by providing real-time feedback on bodily processes like heart rate and muscle tension. Using biofeedback, you can learn to consciously regulate these functions, helping to reduce pain and improve relaxation. This technique often involves specialized equipment and guidance from a trained practitioner.

Emotional Freedom Techniques, also known as tapping, combines elements of cognitive therapy and acupressure. It involves tapping on specific points on the body while focusing on pain or discomfort. EFT helps address the emotional aspects of pain and can lead to a reduction in both physical and emotional symptoms.

Journaling and expressive writing allow you to process your thoughts and emotions related to pain. Writing about your experiences, feelings, and coping strategies can help you gain insight and release emotional tension. This practice can also provide a sense of control and empowerment, contributing to pain relief.

Focusing on gratitude and positive aspects of your life can shift your mindset and reduce the impact of pain. Keeping a gratitude journal or taking a few moments each day to reflect on things you're thankful for can enhance your overall well-being and help you manage pain more effectively.

Combining various mind-body techniques can offer even greater benefits. For example, you might practice mindfulness meditation along with yoga or deep breathing exercises. Experimenting with different approaches and finding what works best for you can enhance your ability to manage pain naturally.

Long-Term Strategies for Pain-Free Living

Achieving a pain-free life is a journey that often requires a combination of lifestyle changes, self-care practices, and a positive mindset. While it may not be possible to eliminate pain completely, there are effective long-term strategies that can help you manage pain better and improve your overall quality of life. Here's a friendly guide to some practical and sustainable approaches for long-term pain relief.

A nutritious diet plays a crucial role in managing pain and promoting overall health. Focus on eating a variety of whole foods, including fruits, vegetables, lean proteins, and whole grains. Foods rich in antioxidants, omega-3 fatty acids, and anti-inflammatory compounds—such as berries, fatty fish, and leafy greens—can help reduce inflammation and support joint health. Avoiding processed foods high in sugar and unhealthy fats can also contribute to reduced pain and improved well-being.

Regular physical activity is essential for managing pain and maintaining overall health. Engaging in low-impact exercises like walking, swimming, or cycling can help keep your body flexible, strengthen your muscles, and improve your mood. Activities such as yoga and stretching can enhance your flexibility and reduce muscle tension. Finding an exercise routine that you enjoy and can sustain over time is key to long-term pain management.

Quality sleep is vital for pain management and overall health. Establishing a regular sleep schedule and creating a relaxing bedtime routine can help improve your sleep quality. Aim for 7-9 hours of restful sleep each night, and create a sleep-friendly environment by keeping your bedroom dark, quiet, and cool. Good sleep supports your body's natural healing processes and can help you manage pain more effectively.

Chronic stress can exacerbate pain and contribute to various health issues. Incorporate stress-reducing practices into your daily routine to help manage pain and improve your overall well-being. Techniques such as mindfulness meditation, deep breathing exercises, and progressive muscle relaxation can help calm your mind and body. Finding healthy outlets for stress, such as hobbies, social activities, or creative pursuits, can also be beneficial.

Creating a comprehensive pain management plan with the help of healthcare professionals can help you address your pain more effectively. Work with your doctor or a pain specialist to develop a personalized plan that includes medication, physical therapy, and other treatments as needed. Regular check-ins with your healthcare team can help you adjust your plan and stay on track with your pain management goals.

Complementary therapies, such as acupuncture, chiropractic care, and massage therapy, can be effective in managing pain and improving your overall quality of life. These therapies can help address underlying issues, reduce muscle tension, and promote relaxation. Explore different complementary therapies and find those that resonate with you and complement your overall pain management strategy.

A positive mindset can have a significant impact on your experience of pain and your ability to manage it effectively. Focus on your strengths, set realistic goals, and celebrate your progress. Surround yourself with supportive friends and family, and seek out social connections that uplift and inspire you. A positive attitude can enhance your resilience and help you navigate the challenges of living with pain.

Staying informed about your condition and available treatments can empower you to make informed decisions about your pain management. Keep up with the latest research and developments in pain management, and communicate openly with your healthcare providers. Knowledge can help you better understand your condition and explore new strategies for managing pain.

Self-care is a vital component of long-term pain management. Make time for activities that bring you joy and relaxation, whether it's reading a book, taking a bath, or spending time in nature. Regular self-care helps recharge your mental and emotional energy, which can positively impact your experience of pain.

Setting realistic and achievable goals can help you stay motivated and focused on your pain management journey. Break larger goals into smaller, manageable steps and celebrate your accomplishments along the way. Setting goals that align with your values and interests can provide a sense of purpose and help you maintain a positive outlook.

Book 34: Enhancing Longevity with Natural Approaches

The Science of Longevity and Aging

Understanding the science behind longevity and aging can be both fascinating and empowering. It's a journey into how our bodies change over time and how we can influence these changes to lead longer, healthier lives. Here's a friendly look at the science of aging and what you can do to enhance your longevity.

Aging is a complex process involving gradual changes at the cellular, tissue, and organ levels. As we age, our cells undergo a series of alterations. These include a decrease in the efficiency of cellular repair processes, the accumulation of cellular damage, and changes in cellular function. On a broader scale, aging affects our body systems, contributing to decreased muscle mass, bone density, and cognitive function.

Our genetics play a significant role in determining how we age. Certain genes are associated with longevity and the risk of age-related diseases. However, genetics are just one part of the equation. Environmental factors, such as diet, physical activity, exposure to toxins, and lifestyle choices, also influence how we age. This means that while we can't change our genes, we can make choices that positively impact our health and longevity.

One of the key concepts in aging research is cellular aging, which is closely linked to telomeres. Telomeres are protective caps at the ends of our chromosomes that shorten as cells divide. When telomeres become too short, cells can no longer divide effectively and may become senescent or die. Maintaining telomere length through a healthy lifestyle is thought to play a role in longevity.

Oxidative stress is another important factor in aging. This occurs when there is an imbalance between free radicals (unstable molecules) and antioxidants (molecules that neutralize free radicals) in the body. Excessive free radicals can damage cells, proteins, and DNA, contributing to aging and disease. Eating a diet rich in antioxidants, such as fruits, vegetables, and nuts, can help counteract oxidative stress and support overall health.

Chronic inflammation is linked to many age-related conditions, including heart disease, diabetes, and arthritis. As we age, our bodies can experience increased levels of inflammation, often referred to as "inflammaging." Adopting anti-inflammatory practices, such as consuming omega-3 fatty acids from fish or flaxseeds, can help reduce inflammation and support healthy aging.

Aging brings about changes in hormone levels, which can impact various aspects of health. For example, levels of growth hormone and sex hormones like estrogen and testosterone typically decline with age, affecting muscle mass, bone density, and energy levels. Hormone replacement therapies and lifestyle changes can sometimes help manage these changes, but it's important to discuss options with a healthcare provider.

Your daily habits have a profound impact on how you age. Regular physical activity helps maintain muscle mass, bone density, and cardiovascular health. A balanced diet supports overall health and can help manage weight and reduce the risk of chronic diseases. Adequate sleep, stress management, and avoiding harmful habits like smoking also contribute to healthy aging.

Mental and social factors play a crucial role in longevity. Staying mentally active through activities like reading, puzzles, and learning new skills can help keep your brain sharp. Social connections are equally important; maintaining strong relationships and engaging in social activities can enhance emotional well-being and longevity.

Exciting developments in aging research continue to emerge, offering new insights into how we can promote longevity. Researchers are exploring areas like genetic modification, cellular therapies, and novel drugs that target the aging process. While many of these advancements are still in the experimental stage, they hold promise for the future of healthy aging.

Incorporating healthy habits into your daily routine can make a significant difference in your longevity and quality of life. Aim for a balanced diet, regular exercise, sufficient sleep, and stress management. Stay curious and engaged with new research on aging and consider consulting with healthcare professionals for personalized advice.

Anti-Aging Nutritional Strategies

Eating well is one of the best ways to support your body's ability to stay youthful and vibrant as you age. The right foods can boost your energy, enhance your skin's appearance, and help protect your body against age-related diseases. Let's explore some friendly and practical anti-aging nutritional strategies to help you feel and look your best!

Antioxidants are your body's best allies in the fight against aging. They help neutralize free radicals—unstable molecules that can cause damage to your cells and contribute to aging. Incorporate plenty of colorful fruits and vegetables into your diet, such as berries, oranges, spinach, and bell peppers. These foods are rich in antioxidants like vitamins C and E, which can help protect your skin and support overall health.

Omega-3 fatty acids are essential fats that have anti-inflammatory properties and can help maintain heart health. They also support brain function and skin health. To boost your intake, enjoy fatty fish like salmon, mackerel, and sardines. If you're vegetarian or vegan, consider adding flaxseeds, chia seeds, and walnuts to your meals, or use algae-based supplements to get your omega-3s.

Whole grains are packed with nutrients and fiber that support digestive health and keep you feeling full longer. They also help stabilize blood sugar levels, which is important for maintaining energy and reducing the risk of chronic diseases. Choose whole grains like quinoa, brown rice, oats, and whole wheat over refined grains. These provide essential vitamins, minerals, and antioxidants that support overall well-being.

Not all fats are created equal. Healthy fats, such as those found in avocados, nuts, seeds, and olive oil, can help improve your cholesterol levels, support brain health, and keep your skin supple. Incorporate these healthy fats into your diet in moderation, and try to reduce your intake of saturated and trans fats found in processed and fried foods.

Protein is vital for maintaining muscle mass and supporting your body's repair processes. Choose lean protein sources like chicken, turkey, tofu, legumes, and low-fat dairy products. Including a variety of protein sources in your diet can help ensure you get all the essential amino acids your body needs for optimal health.

Proper hydration is key to maintaining youthful skin and overall health. Water helps flush out toxins, supports digestion, and keeps your joints lubricated. Aim to drink plenty of water throughout the day, and consider including hydrating foods like cucumbers, watermelon, and herbal teas. Avoid excessive consumption of sugary or caffeinated beverages that can contribute to dehydration.

Fiber supports digestive health and helps regulate blood sugar levels. High-fiber foods also contribute to a feeling of fullness, which can be helpful for weight management. Include a variety of fiber-rich foods in your diet, such as fruits, vegetables, legumes, and whole grains. These foods not only aid digestion but also provide essential nutrients that support overall health.

Herbs and spices are not only flavorful but also packed with antioxidants and anti-inflammatory compounds. Turmeric, ginger, garlic, and cinnamon are excellent choices to include in your cooking. They can add delicious flavor to your meals while providing health benefits that support your body's natural defenses and reduce inflammation.

While it's important to focus on nutrient-dense foods, it's also essential to practice moderation. Enjoying a variety of foods in balanced portions can help you maintain a healthy weight and reduce the risk of chronic diseases. Allow yourself the occasional treat, and remember that overall dietary patterns are more important than individual foods.

Aim to create balanced meals that include a mix of vegetables, fruits, lean proteins, whole grains, and healthy fats. This approach ensures that you're getting a wide range of nutrients that support different aspects of your health. Meal planning and prepping in advance can help you stay on track and make healthy eating easier.

Herbs and Supplements for Healthy Aging

As we age, our bodies can benefit from a little extra support to maintain vitality and health. Herbs and supplements can play a helpful role in promoting longevity and enhancing well-being. Here's a friendly guide to some of the best herbs and supplements for healthy aging, and how they can be part of your daily routine.

Ginseng is a popular herb known for its ability to boost energy and improve overall vitality. It has adaptogenic properties, which means it helps your body adapt to stress and maintain balance. Ginseng can also support cognitive function and enhance mood. You can find ginseng in various forms, including teas, capsules, and extracts. It's best to use it as part of a balanced approach to health, rather than as a quick fix.

Turmeric is a golden spice renowned for its anti-inflammatory and antioxidant properties. The active compound in turmeric, curcumin, can help reduce inflammation in the body, which is beneficial for managing symptoms of arthritis and supporting joint health. To get the most out of turmeric, consider adding it to your meals or taking it as a supplement. Pair it with black pepper to enhance absorption.

Garlic is more than just a flavor enhancer—it's also a heart-healthy herb. It contains allicin, a compound that has been shown to support cardiovascular health by helping to reduce cholesterol levels and blood pressure. Including fresh garlic in your diet or taking garlic supplements can help maintain a healthy heart and overall well-being.

Ashwagandha is an adaptogenic herb known for its ability to help manage stress and support adrenal health. It can also improve sleep quality and boost overall energy levels. Ashwagandha supplements are available in various forms, including capsules and powders. If you're feeling overwhelmed or stressed, incorporating ashwagandha into your routine may offer some relief.

Ginkgo biloba is well-known for its potential to enhance cognitive function and improve memory. It works by increasing blood flow to the brain, which can help support mental clarity and focus. Ginkgo supplements are often used to help with age-related cognitive decline and to boost overall brain health.

Omega-3 fatty acids, found in fish oil and flaxseed oil, are essential for maintaining brain health and cardiovascular function. They help reduce inflammation, support cognitive function, and promote heart health. Including omega-3-rich foods in your diet, such as fatty fish, or taking a high-quality omega-3 supplement can offer significant benefits.

Vitamin D is crucial for maintaining bone health and supporting the immune system. As we age, our ability to produce vitamin D from sunlight decreases, making supplementation important. Vitamin D helps with calcium absorption, which is vital for bone strength. Consider taking a vitamin D supplement, especially if you have limited sun exposure or are at risk of deficiency.

Coenzyme Q10 (CoQ10) is a nutrient that plays a key role in cellular energy production. As we age, our natural levels of CoQ10 can decrease, which can impact energy levels and overall vitality. Supplementing with CoQ10 can help support cardiovascular health and improve energy levels. It's available in various forms, including capsules and soft gels.

Green tea is packed with antioxidants, particularly catechins, which can help protect cells from oxidative damage. Green tea extract supplements can provide a concentrated dose of these beneficial compounds, supporting overall health and longevity. Drinking green tea regularly or taking a green tea extract supplement can help enhance your antioxidant defenses.

Resveratrol is a powerful antioxidant found in red wine, grapes, and berries. It has been linked to various health benefits, including supporting cardiovascular health and promoting longevity. Resveratrol supplements can help provide these benefits in a more concentrated form, helping to combat the effects of aging and support overall well-being.

Detoxing for Longevity and Vitality

Detoxing might sound like a trend, but it's actually a time-honored practice that supports your body's natural ability to stay healthy and vibrant. By giving your body a little extra help in eliminating toxins and waste, you can enhance your overall well-being and promote longevity. Let's dive into some friendly and practical ways to detox for a longer, more energetic life.

Water is your body's natural detoxifier. It helps flush out toxins through urine and sweat, keeps your organs functioning optimally, and supports overall vitality. Make it a habit to drink plenty of water throughout the day.

Adding a splash of lemon or cucumber to your water can make it more refreshing and provide extra benefits. Staying hydrated is one of the simplest and most effective ways to support your body's natural detoxification processes.

Eating a variety of colorful fruits and vegetables is like giving your body a nutrient-packed boost. These foods are rich in antioxidants, vitamins, and minerals that help neutralize free radicals and support your detox organs, like the liver and kidneys. Aim to fill half your plate with vegetables and fruits at each meal. Dark leafy greens, berries, and cruciferous vegetables like broccoli and cauliflower are particularly beneficial.

Certain herbs and spices have natural detoxifying properties that can support your body's cleansing processes. Turmeric, ginger, and cilantro are great choices. Turmeric contains curcumin, which helps reduce inflammation and support liver health. Ginger aids digestion and can help with nausea. Cilantro is known for its ability to bind to heavy metals and help remove them from the body. Add these herbs and spices to your meals or enjoy them as teas for a detoxifying boost.

Physical activity is a powerful way to support your body's detoxification and longevity. Exercise helps stimulate circulation, promotes lymphatic drainage, and encourages sweating—all of which aid in the elimination of toxins. Aim for at least 30 minutes of moderate exercise most days of the week. Whether it's a brisk walk, a yoga session, or a fun dance class, find activities that you enjoy and make them a regular part of your routine.

Your liver is a key player in detoxification, so it's important to support it with the right foods. Incorporate foods that promote liver health, such as beets, garlic, and green tea. Beets contain betalains, which support liver function. Garlic has sulfur compounds that help detoxify and support liver enzymes. Green tea is rich in antioxidants and can help protect your liver from damage. A diet rich in these supportive foods can help keep your liver in top shape.

How you eat can be just as important as what you eat. Practice mindful eating by paying attention to your hunger cues and savoring each bite. Eating slowly and chewing your food thoroughly can aid digestion and support detoxification. Avoid overeating and try to limit processed and sugary foods, as they can burden your digestive system and contribute to toxin buildup.

A healthy gut is essential for effective detoxification. Probiotics are beneficial bacteria that support a balanced gut microbiome and aid in digestion. Foods like yogurt, kefir, sauerkraut, and kombucha are excellent sources of probiotics. By maintaining a healthy gut, you support your body's ability to eliminate waste and absorb nutrients more efficiently.

Your body's detoxification processes work best when you're well-rested. Quality sleep is crucial for overall health and longevity. During sleep, your body performs essential repair and detoxification functions. Aim for 7-9 hours of restful sleep each night and create a calming bedtime routine to improve your sleep quality. This will help ensure your body has the time it needs to rejuvenate and detoxify.

If you're looking for a more structured approach, consider trying a gentle detox program. These programs typically include a combination of dietary changes, herbal supplements, and lifestyle practices designed to support your body's natural detoxification processes. Look for programs that emphasize whole foods, hydration, and balanced nutrition. Always consult with a healthcare professional before starting any detox program to ensure it's right for you.

Finally, remember that detoxing should feel good, not overwhelming. Listen to your body's signals and adjust your approach as needed. If you experience any discomfort or have specific health concerns, it's important to consult with a healthcare professional to tailor your detox strategy to your individual needs.

Managing Stress for a Longer Life

Stress is a part of life, but managing it effectively can make a big difference in your overall health and longevity. Chronic stress can take a toll on your body and mind, leading to various health issues and potentially shortening your life. Luckily, there are plenty of natural and enjoyable ways to manage stress and support a longer, healthier life. Here's a friendly guide to keeping stress in check and boosting your well-being.

Finding ways to relax and unwind is essential for managing stress. Techniques like deep breathing, progressive muscle relaxation, and meditation can help calm your mind and reduce stress levels. Deep breathing exercises involve taking slow, deep breaths to help your body relax. Progressive muscle relaxation focuses on tensing and then relaxing different muscle groups to release tension. Meditation, even just for a few minutes a day, can help center your thoughts and promote a sense of peace.

Exercise is a fantastic stress-buster. Physical activity releases endorphins, which are natural mood lifters that help reduce stress and anxiety. Whether it's a brisk walk, a bike ride, a yoga class, or dancing to your favorite tunes, find activities that you enjoy and make them a regular part of your routine. Aim for at least 30 minutes of moderate exercise most days of the week. Not only will you feel better mentally, but regular exercise also supports overall health and longevity.

Social connections play a crucial role in stress management and overall well-being. Spending time with family and friends can provide emotional support, increase feelings of belonging, and offer a break from daily stressors. Make an effort to nurture your relationships and engage in meaningful social activities. Whether it's a phone call, a coffee date, or a family gathering, connecting with others can help alleviate stress and boost your mood.

Mindfulness involves staying present and fully engaging with the current moment, rather than worrying about the past or future. It can help reduce stress by shifting your focus away from anxious thoughts and promoting relaxation. Gratitude practices, like keeping a gratitude journal or simply reflecting on the positive aspects of your life, can also help improve your mood and reduce stress. Taking time each day to acknowledge what you're thankful for can make a big difference in how you feel.

Self-care is all about taking care of your physical, mental, and emotional needs. Set aside time each day for activities that you enjoy and that help you relax. This could include reading a book, taking a warm bath, practicing a hobby, or spending time in nature. Taking care of yourself isn't selfish—it's essential for maintaining your health and managing stress. Make self-care a regular part of your routine and listen to your body's needs.

What you eat can impact how you feel. A balanced diet rich in whole foods, including fruits, vegetables, lean proteins, and whole grains, can help stabilize your mood and energy levels. Avoid excessive caffeine and sugar, as they can contribute to anxiety and stress. Hydration is also key—drink plenty of water to support overall health and well-being. Eating a variety of nutritious foods can help your body cope better with stress and promote longevity.

Sleep is crucial for managing stress and maintaining overall health. Aim for 7-9 hours of quality sleep each night. Establish a relaxing bedtime routine and create a sleep-friendly environment by keeping your bedroom dark, quiet, and cool. Avoid screens and stimulating activities before bedtime, as they can interfere with your ability to fall asleep. Good sleep supports your body's stress response and helps you feel refreshed and ready to face the day.

Engaging in hobbies and activities you enjoy can be a great way to unwind and reduce stress. Whether it's gardening, painting, knitting, or playing an instrument, find activities that bring you joy and relaxation. Hobbies provide a break from daily pressures and give you a sense of accomplishment and satisfaction. Make time for these activities regularly to keep stress levels in check and enhance your overall quality of life.

Feeling overwhelmed by a long to-do list can increase stress levels. Set realistic goals for yourself and prioritize tasks based on importance and deadlines. Break large tasks into smaller, manageable steps and tackle them one at a time. Don't be afraid to delegate or ask for help when needed. Organizing and managing your responsibilities in a thoughtful way can reduce stress and improve productivity.

If stress becomes overwhelming or persistent, it's important to seek professional support. A therapist or counselor can help you develop coping strategies and provide guidance on managing stress. There's no shame in seeking help—mental health professionals are trained to support you and offer valuable tools for managing stress and enhancing your well-being.

The Role of Physical Activity in Aging Gracefully

Physical activity is like a magic elixir for aging gracefully. It not only helps keep our bodies strong and flexible but also has a range of benefits that contribute to a vibrant and fulfilling life as we age. Let's dive into why staying active is so important and how it can help us age with grace and vitality.

As we age, our muscles naturally lose strength and flexibility. Regular physical activity, especially strength training and stretching exercises, can help counteract this. Lifting weights, doing resistance exercises, and incorporating stretching into your routine can keep your muscles and joints healthy. This not only helps you maintain independence but also reduces the risk of falls and injuries. Imagine being able to enjoy everyday activities with ease—whether it's gardening, dancing, or playing with grandchildren.

Cardiovascular health becomes increasingly important as we age. Engaging in activities like walking, cycling, or swimming can help keep your heart strong and efficient. Regular aerobic exercise improves circulation, lowers blood pressure, and helps manage cholesterol levels. By keeping your cardiovascular system in good shape, you're setting yourself up for a longer and healthier life. Plus, staying active can boost your energy levels and overall mood, making daily life more enjoyable.

Physical activity isn't just good for your body; it's great for your brain too. Exercise has been shown to improve cognitive function and memory, helping to keep your mind sharp as you age. Activities that require coordination and balance, such as dancing or tai chi, can also be particularly beneficial. Regular exercise increases blood flow to the brain, supports the growth of new brain cells, and reduces the risk of cognitive decline. It's like giving your brain a workout, which can lead to clearer thinking and better mental health.

Staying active is a natural mood booster. Exercise triggers the release of endorphins, the body's feel-good chemicals, which can help reduce stress and anxiety. Physical activity also provides a sense of accomplishment and can improve your self-esteem. Whether it's taking a brisk walk in the park, joining a fitness class, or practicing yoga, finding activities that you enjoy can significantly enhance your emotional well-being. It's a great way to lift your spirits and feel more positive about life.

Physical activity can also be a wonderful way to connect with others. Joining a local sports team, attending group fitness classes, or participating in community walks can provide opportunities to socialize and make new friends. Social interactions are important for mental and emotional health, and they can add a fun and fulfilling dimension to your fitness routine. Engaging with a community of like-minded individuals can also help keep you motivated and committed to staying active.

Maintaining a healthy weight is crucial for overall health and longevity. Regular physical activity helps regulate body weight by burning calories and building muscle. A balanced exercise routine, combined with a nutritious diet, can help you achieve and maintain a healthy weight, which in turn reduces the risk of chronic conditions like diabetes and heart disease. It's all about finding a balance that works for you and supports your long-term health goals.

Getting enough quality sleep is essential for good health and well-being. Engaging in regular physical activity can help improve sleep patterns and promote more restful sleep. Exercise helps regulate your body's internal clock and reduces symptoms of insomnia. Just be sure to finish exercising a few hours before bedtime to allow your body to wind down. A good night's sleep contributes to overall health and can enhance your ability to handle daily stressors.

To truly reap the benefits of physical activity, it's important to make it a regular part of your life. Find activities that you enjoy and can stick with in the long term. It could be as simple as taking a daily walk, joining a local fitness group, or practicing yoga at home. The key is to set realistic goals and create a routine that fits your lifestyle. Consistency is more important than intensity, so focus on making exercise a fun and rewarding part of your daily life.

By incorporating regular physical activity into your routine, you're investing in your future health and well-being. It's a natural way to stay strong, vibrant, and engaged as you age. Embrace the joy of movement and enjoy the many benefits that come with staying active. Aging gracefully is all about taking care of yourself, and physical activity is a fantastic way to do just that. So lace up those sneakers, find your favorite activities, and celebrate the vitality that comes with staying active and healthy.

Preventing Age-Related Diseases Naturally

As we age, our bodies undergo various changes that can sometimes lead to age-related diseases. However, with a bit of proactive care, it's possible to maintain our health and well-being well into our later years. Embracing natural approaches to prevent these conditions can not only enhance your quality of life but also keep you feeling vibrant and energetic. Let's explore some effective natural strategies to prevent age-related diseases and support long-term health.

A well-balanced diet is fundamental to preventing age-related diseases. Focus on incorporating a variety of whole foods, including fresh fruits, vegetables, lean proteins, whole grains, and healthy fats. Foods rich in antioxidants, such as berries, nuts, and leafy greens, help combat oxidative stress and inflammation—two factors linked to many chronic diseases.

Don't forget to include sources of omega-3 fatty acids, like fatty fish and flaxseeds, which support heart health and cognitive function. Eating a rainbow of foods ensures you get a broad spectrum of nutrients to support your overall health.

Regular physical activity is one of the most effective ways to ward off age-related diseases. Exercise helps maintain a healthy weight, improves cardiovascular health, strengthens bones and muscles, and supports mental well-being. Aim for a mix of aerobic exercises, such as walking or swimming, and strength training exercises, like lifting weights or doing resistance band workouts. Incorporate flexibility and balance exercises, such as yoga or tai chi, to enhance your overall mobility and reduce the risk of falls. Finding activities you enjoy makes it easier to stick with a routine.

Mental and emotional well-being plays a crucial role in preventing age-related diseases. Chronic stress and mental health issues can negatively impact physical health, contributing to conditions like high blood pressure and heart disease. Practice stress management techniques such as mindfulness, meditation, or deep-breathing exercises. Engaging in hobbies, staying connected with loved ones, and seeking support when needed can also improve mental health. Keeping your mind active through puzzles, reading, or learning new skills helps support cognitive function as you age.

Adequate and restorative sleep is essential for maintaining health and preventing age-related diseases. Poor sleep can contribute to various health problems, including weakened immune function, increased risk of cardiovascular disease, and cognitive decline. Establish a regular sleep routine by going to bed and waking up at the same time each day. Create a relaxing bedtime routine and ensure your sleep environment is comfortable and free from distractions. Aim for 7-9 hours of quality sleep each night to support overall health and well-being.

Proper hydration is vital for maintaining health and preventing age-related issues. As we age, our sense of thirst can diminish, making it important to consciously drink enough fluids throughout the day. Water is the best choice, but herbal teas and water-rich foods like fruits and vegetables can also contribute to your daily intake. Staying hydrated supports digestive health, maintains skin elasticity, and helps regulate body temperature. Aim to drink at least 8 glasses of water a day, adjusting based on your activity level and climate.

Certain herbs and natural supplements can offer additional support in preventing age-related diseases. For instance, turmeric and ginger are known for their anti-inflammatory properties, while ginkgo biloba may support cognitive function. Omega-3 supplements can benefit heart health, and probiotics help maintain a healthy gut. Always consult with a healthcare provider before starting any new supplements to ensure they are appropriate for your individual needs and health conditions.

Steering clear of harmful habits is essential for long-term health. Smoking and excessive alcohol consumption can significantly increase the risk of age-related diseases, including cancer, heart disease, and liver damage. If you smoke, seek support to quit, and limit alcohol consumption to moderate levels. Adopting a healthy lifestyle helps reduce the risk of many chronic conditions and supports overall well-being.

Regular health check-ups and screenings are important for early detection and prevention of age-related diseases. Schedule routine visits with your healthcare provider to monitor key health indicators, such as blood pressure, cholesterol levels, and glucose levels. Staying on top of recommended screenings and vaccinations helps catch potential issues early and ensures you receive appropriate care.

Book 35: Natural Remedies for Cardiovascular Health

The Role of Nutrition in Heart Health

Taking care of your heart is one of the most important things you can do for your overall health, and a big part of maintaining heart health starts with what you put on your plate. By making thoughtful food choices, you can help keep your heart in great shape and reduce your risk of cardiovascular issues. Here's how nutrition plays a crucial role in heart health and some tips for eating your way to a healthier heart.

Not all fats are created equal, and some are better for your heart than others. Opt for healthy fats that can help improve your cholesterol levels and reduce inflammation. Sources of these heart-healthy fats include avocados, nuts, seeds, and olive oil. Fatty fish like salmon and mackerel are rich in omega-3 fatty acids, which are particularly beneficial for heart health. They can help lower blood pressure and reduce the risk of heart disease. On the other hand, try to limit saturated fats found in red meats and full-fat dairy products, and avoid trans fats, which are often present in processed and fried foods.

Whole grains are an excellent choice for maintaining heart health. They're packed with fiber, which helps lower LDL cholesterol (the "bad" cholesterol) and keeps your blood sugar levels stable. Foods like oats, brown rice, quinoa, and whole wheat products are great options. Fiber not only helps with cholesterol levels but also supports healthy digestion and helps you feel fuller for longer, which can aid in weight management—a key factor in heart health.

Fruits and vegetables are loaded with essential vitamins, minerals, and antioxidants that support heart health. These nutrients help reduce inflammation and oxidative stress, both of which can contribute to heart disease. Aim to fill half your plate with a colorful variety of fruits and veggies at each meal. Berries, leafy greens, oranges, and bell peppers are particularly rich in heart-friendly nutrients. The more variety you include, the more benefits you'll reap.

Excess sodium in your diet can lead to high blood pressure, which is a major risk factor for heart disease. Many processed and packaged foods contain hidden sodium, so it's important to read labels and choose lower-sodium options when possible. Instead of relying on salt to add flavor, try using herbs, spices, and lemon juice to enhance your dishes. Cooking at home allows you to control the amount of salt in your meals and makes it easier to stick to a heart-healthy diet.

Drinking plenty of water is essential for maintaining heart health. Proper hydration supports overall cardiovascular function, helps regulate blood pressure, and ensures that your body's systems are operating efficiently. Aim for at least 8 glasses of water a day, and remember that staying hydrated also involves consuming water-rich foods like fruits and vegetables.

When it comes to protein sources, choose lean options that are lower in saturated fats. Skinless poultry, beans, lentils, and tofu are excellent alternatives to red and processed meats. These lean proteins provide essential nutrients without the added fats that can negatively impact heart health. Additionally, plant-based proteins often come with extra fiber and beneficial nutrients.

Nuts and seeds are a fantastic addition to a heart-healthy diet. They're rich in healthy fats, fiber, and antioxidants. Almonds, walnuts, chia seeds, and flaxseeds are particularly good for heart health. They can help lower cholesterol levels and reduce inflammation. A small handful of nuts or a sprinkle of seeds on your salad or yogurt can provide a nutritious boost.

If you choose to drink alcohol, do so in moderation. Some studies suggest that moderate alcohol consumption, particularly red wine, may offer heart benefits due to its antioxidant content. However, excessive alcohol intake can lead to high blood pressure and other heart-related issues. Moderation is key, which generally means up to one drink per day for women and up to two drinks per day for men.

Herbal Remedies for Lowering Blood Pressure

Managing blood pressure is crucial for maintaining overall heart health, and herbal remedies can be a natural and effective way to support this process. Many herbs have been traditionally used to help keep blood pressure in check, thanks to their various beneficial properties. Let's explore some herbal allies that can assist in lowering blood pressure and supporting a heart-healthy lifestyle.

Garlic is a well-known herb with numerous health benefits, including its ability to help lower blood pressure. The active compound in garlic, allicin, has been shown to relax blood vessels and improve blood flow. Incorporating fresh garlic into your diet can enhance flavor and provide these heart-healthy benefits. You can also take garlic supplements, but it's best to consult with a healthcare provider before starting any new supplement regimen.

Hibiscus tea is not only refreshing but also a great option for managing blood pressure. Studies have shown that hibiscus can help lower both systolic and diastolic blood pressure. This vibrant red tea is rich in antioxidants, which help protect the blood vessels and promote cardiovascular health. Enjoy a cup of hibiscus tea daily as part of your routine to support healthy blood pressure levels.

Hawthorn has been used for centuries to support heart health, and it's particularly noted for its ability to help manage blood pressure. This herb works by improving blood flow and strengthening the heart muscle. Hawthorn can be taken in various forms, including teas, capsules, or tinctures. It's a good idea to consult with a healthcare professional to determine the appropriate dosage and form for your needs.

Ginger is another versatile herb that can aid in lowering blood pressure. It has anti-inflammatory and antioxidant properties that help relax the blood vessels and improve circulation. You can easily incorporate ginger into your diet by adding it to your meals, teas, or smoothies. Fresh ginger root or powdered ginger can both be effective, and they add a delightful zing to your dishes.

Celery seed is a lesser-known herb that has been traditionally used to support cardiovascular health. It contains compounds that may help relax blood vessels and promote a healthy blood pressure level. Celery seed supplements are available, but you can also use celery seeds in cooking to add flavor and benefit from their potential effects on blood pressure.

Green tea is packed with antioxidants, particularly catechins, which have been shown to help lower blood pressure. Drinking green tea regularly can provide a gentle boost to your cardiovascular health. In addition to its blood pressure-lowering effects, green tea supports overall wellness and can be a soothing addition to your daily routine.

Beetroot, while not an herb, deserves a mention for its impressive effects on blood pressure. It's rich in nitrates, which help relax and dilate blood vessels, leading to lower blood pressure. Drinking beetroot juice or incorporating beets into your meals can be a tasty way to support healthy blood pressure levels.

Dandelion is often considered a weed, but it's also a powerful herb with potential benefits for blood pressure. It acts as a diuretic, helping the body to get rid of excess fluid and sodium, which can reduce blood pressure. Dandelion tea or supplements can be a helpful addition to your regimen, especially if you're looking to support overall fluid balance.

Managing Cholesterol Naturally

Keeping cholesterol levels in check is essential for maintaining heart health and reducing the risk of cardiovascular disease. Fortunately, there are several natural strategies you can adopt to manage your cholesterol levels effectively. By focusing on lifestyle changes and incorporating certain foods and practices into your daily routine, you can support healthy cholesterol levels and promote overall cardiovascular wellness.

What you eat plays a significant role in managing cholesterol levels. Focus on including plenty of fruits, vegetables, whole grains, and legumes in your diet. These foods are rich in fiber, which helps lower LDL (bad) cholesterol and improve overall cholesterol balance. Foods like oats, beans, lentils, apples, and carrots are excellent choices for boosting your fiber intake.

Not all fats are bad for you. In fact, incorporating healthy fats into your diet can help improve your cholesterol levels. Opt for unsaturated fats found in foods like avocados, nuts, seeds, and olive oil. These fats can help lower LDL cholesterol while increasing HDL (good) cholesterol. Try to limit saturated fats, which are found in red meats and full-fat dairy products, as well as avoid trans fats present in many processed and fried foods.

Omega-3 fatty acids, found in fatty fish such as salmon, mackerel, and sardines, are known for their heart health benefits. They can help lower triglycerides and improve cholesterol levels. If you're not a fan of fish, consider omega-3 supplements derived from algae or flaxseeds, chia seeds, and walnuts as alternative sources.

Nuts and seeds are packed with healthy fats, fiber, and antioxidants that support heart health. Almonds, walnuts, flaxseeds, and chia seeds are particularly beneficial for managing cholesterol. A small handful of nuts or a sprinkle of seeds on your salads, yogurt, or oatmeal can provide a crunchy, heart-healthy boost.

Incorporating plant-based proteins like beans, lentils, and tofu into your diet can help manage cholesterol levels while providing essential nutrients. Fatty fish, rich in omega-3s, also supports heart health. Try to include a variety of these protein sources in your meals for a balanced approach.

Fiber is a key player in managing cholesterol. Soluble fiber, found in foods like oats, barley, and apples, helps lower LDL cholesterol by binding to it and removing it from the bloodstream. Including a variety of fiber-rich foods in your diet ensures you get the benefits of this essential nutrient.

Excessive sugar and processed foods can contribute to unhealthy cholesterol levels and overall poor heart health. Cut back on sugary beverages, snacks, and processed foods high in unhealthy fats. Instead, focus on whole, unprocessed foods that support heart health.

Drinking plenty of water is important for overall health, including maintaining healthy cholesterol levels. Proper hydration supports digestion, metabolism, and the elimination of waste products from the body. Aim to drink at least 8 glasses of water a day and choose water-rich foods like fruits and vegetables. Regular physical activity is crucial for managing cholesterol levels. Aim for at least 30 minutes of moderate exercise most days of the week. Activities like brisk walking, cycling, or swimming can help raise HDL (good) cholesterol while lowering LDL (bad) cholesterol and triglycerides.

Chronic stress can negatively impact cholesterol levels and heart health. Incorporate stress-management techniques such as deep breathing, meditation, yoga, or spending time in nature to help keep stress in check and support overall well-being.

Strengthening Blood Vessels with Natural Solutions

Maintaining healthy blood vessels is crucial for overall cardiovascular health. Strong, flexible blood vessels ensure that your blood flows efficiently throughout your body, supporting heart function and reducing the risk of cardiovascular issues. Fortunately, there are several natural solutions you can incorporate into your lifestyle to strengthen your blood vessels and support vascular health.

Antioxidants help protect your blood vessels from oxidative stress and inflammation. Foods high in antioxidants, such as berries (blueberries, strawberries, and raspberries), dark chocolate, and green tea, can support the health of your blood vessels. Adding these to your diet not only enhances flavor but also provides essential nutrients that help maintain the integrity of your blood vessel walls.

Omega-3 fatty acids are known for their cardiovascular benefits, including their ability to strengthen blood vessels. These healthy fats, found in fatty fish like salmon, mackerel, and sardines, as well as flaxseeds, chia seeds, and walnuts, can help reduce inflammation and improve blood vessel function. Aim to include these sources of omega-3s in your diet regularly.

Garlic is a powerhouse herb that supports vascular health by improving blood circulation and reducing inflammation. The active compounds in garlic, such as allicin, help relax blood vessels and promote healthy blood flow. Adding fresh garlic to your cooking or taking garlic supplements can be an effective way to boost your cardiovascular health.

Proper hydration is essential for maintaining healthy blood vessels. Water helps keep your blood volume and pressure at optimal levels, which supports overall vascular function. Aim to drink plenty of water throughout the day, and consider incorporating hydrating foods like cucumbers, melons, and oranges into your diet.

Beets are rich in nitrates, which can help relax blood vessels and improve circulation. Drinking beet juice or adding beets to salads, soups, or smoothies can provide a natural boost to your vascular health. Beets are also packed with essential nutrients and antioxidants that support overall cardiovascular wellness.

Green tea is packed with catechins, powerful antioxidants that support blood vessel health. Drinking green tea regularly can help improve blood flow and reduce inflammation. For added benefits, try incorporating a few cups of green tea into your daily routine.

Incorporate healthy fats, such as those found in avocados, nuts, and olive oil, into your diet. These fats support the flexibility of blood vessel walls and help reduce inflammation. Using olive oil in your cooking or snacking on a handful of nuts can be both delicious and heart-healthy.

Physical activity is key to maintaining strong blood vessels. Exercise helps improve circulation, reduce blood pressure, and enhance overall vascular function. Aim for at least 150 minutes of moderate-intensity exercise per week, such as brisk walking, cycling, or swimming, to support your vascular health.

Maintaining a healthy weight is important for cardiovascular health. Excess weight can put extra strain on your blood vessels and increase the risk of hypertension. Adopting a balanced diet and regular exercise routine can help you achieve and maintain a healthy weight, supporting the strength of your blood vessels.

Chronic stress can negatively impact blood vessel health. Incorporate stress-reducing activities such as mindfulness, meditation, or yoga into your routine to help keep your stress levels in check. Managing stress effectively can support overall vascular health and improve your well-being.

Detoxing for Heart Health

Taking care of your heart involves more than just eating well and exercising; it also means giving your body a chance to clear out toxins that could affect your cardiovascular health. Detoxing isn't just about drastic cleanses or fad diets; it's about supporting your body's natural processes to promote heart health and overall well-being. Here's how you can gently detoxify for a healthier heart:

Water is essential for flushing out toxins and supporting every function in your body, including your heart. Drinking plenty of water helps your kidneys filter waste products and supports healthy blood circulation. Aim for at least eight glasses of water a day, and consider starting your morning with a glass of warm lemon water to kickstart your detox.

Fiber helps sweep toxins out of your digestive system and supports healthy cholesterol levels. Include plenty of fruits, vegetables, whole grains, and legumes in your diet. Foods like apples, beans, and oats are particularly good at helping your body eliminate waste and support heart health.

Antioxidants fight oxidative stress and inflammation, which can contribute to heart disease. Foods like berries, leafy greens, nuts, and dark chocolate are packed with antioxidants. Adding these to your diet can help protect your heart and support overall detoxification.

Certain herbal teas can support detoxification and cardiovascular health. Green tea, for example, is rich in antioxidants and can help improve blood flow. Dandelion tea is another great choice, as it supports liver function and helps flush out toxins. Sip on these teas throughout the day to support your detox efforts.

Processed foods can be high in unhealthy fats, sugars, and sodium, all of which can negatively impact heart health. By reducing your intake of processed foods and focusing on whole, natural ingredients, you help your body reduce the toxic load it needs to process.

Healthy fats, such as those found in avocados, nuts, seeds, and olive oil, support heart health and help your body absorb essential nutrients. These fats can also aid in the detoxification process by supporting liver health, which is crucial for clearing toxins from the body.

Your liver is a key player in detoxification. Supporting its function can help your body effectively eliminate toxins. Foods like garlic, turmeric, and beets can help boost liver health. Garlic has compounds that support liver detoxification, while turmeric is known for its anti-inflammatory properties and support for liver function.

Regular exercise supports your body's natural detoxification processes by improving circulation and helping to eliminate toxins through sweat. Aim for at least 30 minutes of moderate exercise most days of the week. Activities like walking, cycling, or swimming can be particularly beneficial for cardiovascular health.

Chronic stress can negatively impact your heart and overall health. Incorporating stress-reducing activities like yoga, meditation, or deep-breathing exercises into your daily routine can help reduce stress levels and support your detox efforts.

Sleep is a crucial component of detoxification. During sleep, your body works to repair and rejuvenate itself, including clearing out toxins. Aim for 7-9 hours of quality sleep each night to support heart health and overall well-being.

Preventing Heart Disease with a Holistic Lifestyle

When it comes to heart health, a holistic approach can make a significant difference. Instead of focusing solely on isolated dietary changes or exercises, embracing a holistic lifestyle involves looking at the bigger picture—how various aspects of your life come together to support cardiovascular health. Here's how you can weave heart-healthy habits into your daily routine for long-term wellness:

A balanced diet is the cornerstone of heart health. Aim to fill your plate with a variety of nutrient-dense foods. Focus on whole grains, fruits, vegetables, lean proteins, and healthy fats. Foods rich in omega-3 fatty acids, like salmon, walnuts, and chia seeds, are particularly beneficial for heart health. Reducing your intake of processed foods, sugars, and unhealthy fats can help keep your cholesterol and blood pressure in check.

Exercise is a powerful tool for maintaining cardiovascular health. It helps strengthen your heart muscle, improve circulation, and manage weight. Find activities you enjoy—whether it's brisk walking, cycling, swimming, or dancing—and aim for at least 150 minutes of moderate exercise or 75 minutes of vigorous activity per week. Incorporating strength training exercises a few times a week can also benefit your heart.

Chronic stress can negatively impact your heart health by raising blood pressure and contributing to unhealthy habits. Incorporate stress-reducing techniques into your routine, such as mindfulness meditation, yoga, or deep-breathing exercises. Finding activities that bring you joy and relaxation can also help you manage stress more effectively.

Adequate sleep is essential for overall health and well-being. Poor sleep patterns can lead to increased risk of heart disease. Aim for 7-9 hours of quality sleep each night by establishing a consistent sleep schedule, creating a relaxing bedtime routine, and ensuring your sleep environment is comfortable and free from distractions.

Water plays a crucial role in maintaining cardiovascular health. It helps with nutrient absorption, digestion, and the elimination of waste products from the body. Make sure to drink enough water throughout the day, and consider herbal teas like hibiscus or green tea, which can offer additional heart benefits.

Smoking and excessive alcohol consumption are major risk factors for heart disease. If you smoke, seek support to quit, and aim to limit alcohol intake to moderate levels—generally up to one drink per day for women and two drinks per day for men.

Being overweight or obese can increase your risk of heart disease. Achieving and maintaining a healthy weight through a combination of balanced eating and regular physical activity is key. If you need to lose weight, do so gradually and with the support of a healthcare provider or nutritionist.

Positive social relationships can support heart health by providing emotional support, reducing stress, and encouraging healthy behaviors. Surround yourself with supportive friends and family, and engage in social activities that bring you happiness.

Routine check-ups with your healthcare provider can help you monitor your heart health and catch any potential issues early. Regular screenings for blood pressure, cholesterol levels, and blood sugar can help you stay on top of your cardiovascular health and make necessary adjustments to your lifestyle.

Eating mindfully means paying attention to your food and how it affects your body. Slow down and savor each bite, listen to your hunger and fullness cues, and avoid emotional eating. This approach can help you make healthier food choices and improve digestion.

Conclusion

Congratulations on making it through this comprehensive journey of natural healing! As we reach the end, it's important to reflect on the core message of Barbara O'Neill's philosophy: the power of nature and the body's innate ability to heal. By nourishing ourselves with wholesome food, detoxifying regularly, and using nature's remedies, we can promote lasting health and prevent illness.

Throughout this book, we've explored a wide range of topics, from supporting gut health to managing stress, and from healing chronic conditions to enhancing longevity. Each chapter offers practical advice that can be easily implemented in everyday life. Whether you're looking to improve your skin, balance your hormones, or strengthen your immune system, there's a natural solution waiting for you.

The beauty of natural healing is that it's accessible to everyone. You don't need complicated treatments or expensive medications to improve your well-being. With a bit of knowledge, patience, and commitment, you can start making positive changes that benefit your body and mind. As Barbara O'Neill often emphasizes, small, consistent steps lead to big, transformative results over time.

Remember, true health is a holistic journey. It's about more than just treating symptoms—it's about nurturing your whole self. This includes paying attention to your nutrition, emotional well-being, and spiritual balance, and using nature's wisdom to guide you.

As you move forward, we encourage you to keep exploring and learning. Let this book be your guide, but don't hesitate to adapt its teachings to your unique needs and lifestyle. Healing is a deeply personal journey, and you have the power to shape it in a way that best serves you.

Video Bonus:

Access hours of exclusive videos by Barbara O'Neill

Made in the USA
Columbia, SC
11 October 2024